Nutrition Counseling Skills
for the Nutrition Care Process

FOURTH EDITION

Linda G. Snetselaar, RD, PhD, LD

Departmental Executive Officer in Community and Behavioral Health
Professor, Department of Epidemiology
University of Iowa
Iowa City, Iowa

JONES AND BARTLETT PUBLISHERS
Sudbury, Massachusetts
BOSTON   TORONTO   LONDON   SINGAPORE

World Headquarters

Jones and Bartlett Publishers
40 Tall Pine Drive
Sudbury, MA 01776
978-443-5000
info@jbpub.com
www.jbpub.com

Jones and Bartlett Publishers
Canada
6339 Ormindale Way
Mississauga, Ontario L5V 1J2
Canada

Jones and Bartlett Publishers
International
Barb House, Barb Mews
London W6 7PA
United Kingdom

Jones and Bartlett's books and products are available through most bookstores and online booksellers. To contact Jones and Bartlett Publishers directly, call 800-832-0034, fax 978-443-8000, or visit our website www.jbpub.com.

Substantial discounts on bulk quantities of Jones and Bartlett's publications are available to corporations, professional associations, and other qualified organizations. For details and specific discount information, contact the special sales department at Jones and Bartlett via the above contact information or send an email to specialsales@jbpub.com.

The authors, editor, and publisher have made every effort to provide accurate information. However, they are not responsible for errors, omissions, or for any outcomes related to the use of the contents of this book and take no responsibility for the use of the products and procedures described. Treatments and side effects described in this book may not be applicable to all people; likewise, some people may require a dose or experience a side effect that is not described herein. Drugs and medical devices are discussed that may have limited availability controlled by the Food and Drug Administration (FDA) for use only in a research study or clinical trial. Research, clinical practice, and government regulations often change the accepted standard in this field. When consideration is being given to use of any drug in the clinical setting, the health care provider or reader is responsible for determining FDA status of the drug, reading the package insert, and reviewing prescribing information for the most up-to-date recommendations on dose, precautions, and contraindications, and determining the appropriate usage for the product. This is especially important in the case of drugs that are new or seldom used.

Production Credits
Publisher: Michael Brown
Associate Editor: Katey Birtcher
Production Director: Amy Rose
Associate Production Editor: Mike Boblitt
Marketing Manager: Andrea DeFronzo
Manufacturing Buyer: Amy Bacus

Composition: Pageworks
Proofreader: Donna Marton
Cover Design: Brian Moore
Cover Image: © Trutta55/Shutterstock, Inc.
Printing and Binding: Malloy, Inc.
Cover Printing: Malloy, Inc.

Library of Congress Cataloging-in-Publication Data
Snetselaar, Linda G.
    Nutrition counseling skills for the nutrition care process / Linda G. Snetselaar Jones and
        Bartlett Publishers. -- 4th ed.
        p. ; cm.
    Rev. ed. of: Nutrition counseling skills for medical nutrition therapy / Linda G. Snetselaar.
        Gaithersburg, Md. : Aspen Publishers, 1997.
    Includes bibliographical references and index.
    ISBN-13: 978-0-7637-2960-8
    ISBN-10: 0-7637-2960-4
    1. Nutrition counseling.   I. Snetselaar, Linda G. Nutrition counseling skills for medical nutrition therapy
II. Title.
    [DNLM: 1. Counseling--methods. 2. Nutrition Physiology. 3. Diet Therapy. QU 145 S671na 1997]
    RM218.7.S66 2009
    615.8'54--dc22
                                        2007047746
6048

Printed in the United States of America
12 11 10 09 08   10 9 8 7 6 5 4 3 2 1

DEDICATION

10 05788006

To my husband, Gary, and my children, Tyler, Jordan, and Daniel

NEW TO THIS EDITION

- Reference to the Nutrition Care Process
- Focus on Intervention, Step 3 in the Nutrition Care Process
- New information on theories and strategies for behavior change
- Updated references along with historic classic citations
- Applied examples of stages of change and strategies to achieve dietary modifications

CONTENTS

PART II   Application of Interviewing and Counseling Skills

6 Nutrition Counseling in Treatment of Diabetes

7 Nutrition Counseling in Treatment of Renal Disease

PART III   Ending Counseling Sessions

10 Evaluation and Follow-Up

PREFACE

In its fourth edition, this text focuses on using nutrition counseling and communication skills within the context of the American Dietetic Association Nutrition Care Process. It may be used as a companion to the American Dietetic Association text entitled *Nutrition Diagnosis and Intervention: Standardized Language for the Nutrition Care Process.*[1] The overall goal of this edition is to increase the effectiveness of nutrition counselors as facilitators of behavioral change. The term "nutrition counselor" refers to registered dietitians and will involve other health professionals—medical doctors, nurses, psychologists, or behavioral therapists—who interact with registered dietitians.

Readers of this text will acquire or enhance the following abilities:

1. Demonstrate effective use of tools for nutrition counseling and communication skills in the nutrition care process.
2. Select and apply appropriate strategies when presented with dietary problems.
3. Evaluate and monitor progress, achievements, and failures in both clients and themselves.
4. Adapt counseling strategies based on client and self-evaluations.

This text does not replace discussions on basic nutrition, and the information in the text will be most useful to readers with a sound grasp of the subject as taught in a college curriculum. The intent of the text is to (1) apply communication and counseling skills and strategies to the discipline of nutrition and specifically the nutrition care process and (2) initiate practice in situations that require dietary modifications. Ideally, a course in counseling psychology will expand the nutrition counselor's knowledge and skills as presented in this text.

Each chapter begins with objectives and ends with reference lists for further study. Part I covers basic theories on communication and counseling skills with an emphasis on identifying the client's readiness to change. Part II demonstrates how to use counseling skills in chronic disease states where changes in dietary behavior are required. Part III provides suggestions for evaluating and terminating counseling sessions.

The text frequently uses the term "eating pattern" rather than "diet." The rationale for this substitution of terminology is that "diet" tends to denote the adherence to an eating regimen for a short time with regression to old eating habits as an eventual outcome. In treating or preventing chronic disease, changes in eating behaviors are long-term, and the nutrition counselor's goal is to assist the client/patient/group in maintaining change over time.

Finally, the new title of this text in its fourth edition has replaces the term "medical nutrition therapy" with "nutrition care process." The nutrition care process is an umbrella term used to include medical nutrition therapy. The nutrition counselor who uses the nutrition care process follows steps that define the methods used to provide medical nutrition therapy and other dietary behavioral change strategies that may not fall into the realm of medical nutrition therapy, such as referral to a community program.[1]

Linda G. Snetselaar

1. American Dietetic Association. *Nutrition Diagnosis and Intervention: Standardized Language for the Nutrition Care Process.* Chicago: American Dietetic Association, 2007.

PART I

THE BASICS OF COMMUNICATION AND COUNSELING SKILLS FOR NUTRITION: INTERVENTIONS IN THE NUTRITION CARE PROCESS

Part I, The Basics of Communication and Counseling Skills for Nutrition: Interventions in the Nutrition Care Process, covers theoretical aspects of communication and counseling. The entire nutrition care process involves four steps: nutrition assessment, nutrition diagnosis, nutrition intervention (the step focused on in this book), and nutrition monitoring and evaluation.

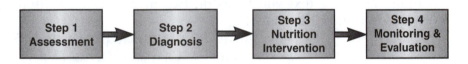

Step 1, nutrition assessment, is the process of interviewing the client to determine whether a dietary problem exists and interpreting this data to identify a nutrition diagnosis. Without appropriate nutrition assessment, the entire nutrition care process breaks down, often headed in a direction that is not tailored to the needs of the client. Step 2, the nutrition diagnosis, describes a problem that the nutrition counselor labels and is responsible for treating. This label is independent of the medical diagnosis that identifies a disease or pathology of organs or body systems. The nutrition diagnosis will change as intervention proceeds. The medical diagnosis does not change and is often a descriptor of a lifelong condition. This nutrition diagnosis step includes a PES statement with three distinct elements: the problem (P), the etiology (E), and the signs and symptoms (S). Information from Step 1, nutrition assessment, is used to determine the PES statement. Step 3, nutrition intervention, follows the first two steps and provides strategies to remedy a nutrition diagnosis or problem. The goal is to change a nutrition-related behavior to improve lifestyle and related health outcomes. Within the intervention, planning and implementation occur. Planning is a tailored process that involves prioritizing the nutrition diagnoses, establishing negotiated goals when appropriate, and defining the nutrition strategies needed to implement the intervention. The client and nutrition counselor are in the action phase when implementing the nutrition intervention. This phase involves carrying out and communicating the plan of care. Using cues from the client the intervention is revised and tailored to lifestyle and associated needs. Finally, Step 4, nutrition monitoring and evaluation, allows for reviewing which nutrition intervention strategies are working and which must be retooled. The nutrition care process is distinct from medical nutrition therapy (MNT). The nutrition care process defines specific steps a practitioner uses when providing MNT. MNT is just one aspect of the nutrition care process.[1]

Within Step 3 of the nutrition intervention process, the terminology is classified into four sets: Food and/or Nutrient Delivery, Nutrition Education, Nutrition Counseling, and Coordination of Nutrition Care. This text will focus on two of the sets: nutrition education and nutrition counseling.

In Part I, the first chapter provides an historical perspective of counseling for the nutrition care process. Chapter 2 discusses basic communication skills that provide strategies to facilitate our interactions with clients. These skills are particularly important for both nutrition assessment and nutrition diagnosis. Learning to listen to the client's perspective will help assure that an appropriate diagnosis is identified. With an appropriate diagnosis, the nutrition intervention that follows forms the basis of the third chapter, which focuses on the client's readiness to change as an essential element in dietary behavior modification. This chapter on motivational interviewing departs from assigning blame to the client for past adherence problems and focuses on constructive ways to provide the client with feedback that can result in positive dietary change.

Reference

1. American Dietetic Association. *Nutrition Diagnosis and Intervention: Standardized Language for the Nutrition Care Process.* Chicago: American Dietetic Association, 2008.

CHAPTER 1

OVERVIEW OF NUTRITION COUNSELING

Chapter Objectives

1. Discuss the influence of counseling on the client.

2. Describe three theories that influence the nutrition counselor.

3. Discuss two ways in which counseling within the nutrition care process is important to the work of the nutrition counselor.[1]

4. Identify the components of counseling skills.

5. Diagram the counseling spectrum.

Definition of Nutrition Counseling

Nutrition is both a science and an art. The nutrition counselor converts theory into practice and science into art. This ability requires both knowledge and skill.[2]

Nutrition counseling is a combination of nutrition expertise and psychological skill delivered by a trained nutrition counselor who understands how to work within the current medical setting. It focuses on both foods and the nutrients contained within them, emphasizing our feelings as we experience eating.

Nutrition counseling has moved from a brief encounter as the patient leaves the hospital with suitcase in hand to an in-depth discovery of tailoring dietary change to individual situations and emotions. Today nutrition counseling sessions include analysis of factors such as nutrition science, psychology and physiology, and an eventual negotiated treatment plan followed by an evaluation. Research has shown that this in-depth approach can produce excellent dietary adherence based on biological markers, even with complicated dietary regimens that are difficult to accommodate in the real world.[3,4] Large long-term randomized controlled trials (RCT) have shown the importance of nutrition counseling in reversing dietary adherence problems.[5-7]

History of Nutrition Counseling

Over the years, nutrition advice has been a part of nearly every culture. Early Greek physicians recognized the role of food in the treatment of disease.[8] In the United States in the early 1800s, Thomas Jefferson described his eating habits in a letter to his doctor in what may be one of the first diet records (Exhibit 1–1).[9] After World War II, advances in chemical knowledge allowed nutrition researchers to define metabolic requirements.[10] This marked the beginning of the study of patterns of nutrients needed by all persons in relation to their age, sex, and activity. These patterns are vital to the assessment phase of counseling.

Exhibit 1–1   A Colonial Era Diet Report

". . . I have lived temperately, eating little animal food, & that . . . as a condiment for the vegetables, which constitute my principal diet. I double however the doctor's glass and a half of wine."

—From Thomas Jefferson to his Doctor

Source: Original in Jefferson Papers, Library of Congress, Washington, DC.

Selling and Ferraro, in discussing the psychology of diet and nutrition in 1945, recommended what at that time must have been an unconventional view:

1. knowing the client's personality
2. knowing the client's psychological surroundings
3. eliminating emotional tension

4. assisting the client in knowing his own limitations
5. arranging the diet so that it has the effect of encouraging the client
6. allowing for occasional cheating [on the diet][11]

In 1945, the flood of scientific knowledge relating nutrition to disease obscured this advice. Nutrition counselors expended only minor efforts to put these critical ideas into practice.

Over the years, the counselor's role has changed. In the past, the role fell more on the authoritarian side of a continuum; today a counselor must be able to function in all roles at appropriate times (Figure 1–1). Ivey et al. describe the role of counseling as knowing which strategy to use for which individual given specific conditions.[12]

Pioneers in the Field

In the early 1900s, Frances Stearn started a nutrition clinic at the New England Medical Center. Her work continues today with dietitians who emphasize the counseling aspects of nutrition.

In the mid-1940s, Selling and Ferraro stated that there was no longer justification for prescribing a diet without also recognizing the psychological factors in a case. They recommended a diagnostic study to determine the right psychodietetic approach.[11] Indeed, they argued that the thrust in counseling should be matching the treatment to each individual case.[12]

In 1973, Margaret Ohlson stressed the importance of creating an interviewing atmosphere in which the client can respond freely. Ohlson warned against a common problem in dietetic counseling sessions: speaking at the expense of missing important factors during the interview.[10]

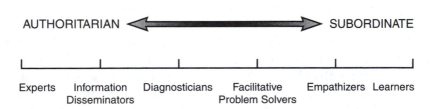

FIGURE 1–1 Roles of the nutrition counselor today.

Theories of Nutrition Counseling

Theories form the basis for developing counseling skills to change eating habits. Both clients and nutrition counselors use theories and beliefs in determining what will take place during an interview.

Theories Influence Clients

In assessing and determining a nutrition diagnosis (steps 1 and 2 in the nutrition care process), nutrition counselors must rely on their ability to identify the client's perspective on counseling and the role of the counselor. Without this knowledge, the nutrition counselor is forced into a position of mandating an intervention without the ability to negotiate strategies that are tailored to the client. The concepts below illustrate types of preconceived ideas that clients may have prior to a counseling session. These ideas shape the direction of the session and determine the success of the eventual necessary dietary behavioral change.

Clients approach nutrition counseling sessions with mindsets about themselves and the world around them. They present "a history of being healed or hurt by others, of being accepted or rejected, or of dominating others."[13] They come with a positive or negative self-image and a record of success or failure in diet modification. From this personal background stems their personal theories of what counseling is and should be.

Most nutrition counselors have faced a client who slouches down in the chair, slams a diet instruction sheet on the desk, and demands: "Well, what are you going to do to get me to follow this diet?" This client sees the counselor as an expert, the person with all the answers—and an adversary. Another client may walk into the office, sit down, and speak only in response to direct questions. Still another client may arrive commenting, "Well, how can we work out this problem I've been having with my diet?"

All three clients see the world through different eyes. The first does not want any responsibility for his diet and nutrition. The second may be afraid of authority figures. The last sees the counselor as an advocate, as someone who can help increase self-directed solutions to dietary problems. Experience has shown that, although written many years ago, Lorr's listing of five descriptors of clients' perceptions of counselors was correct: (1) accepting, (2) understanding, (3) independence encouraging, (4) authoritarian, and (5) critical-hostile.[14] These identifiers have proven to be accurate in work with clients in need of dietary and lifestyle changes. Nutrition assessment, step 1 in the nutrition care process, requires an understanding of the feelings a client has toward the counselor.[1] The client's perceptions may affect the nutrition counselor's ability to determine a nutrition diagnosis that adequately describes the nutrition problem.

Communication skills are imperative when assessing and identifying a nutrition diagnosis. Assessing the client's perception of you as a counselor initiates your understanding of how open the client will be when discussing nutrition problems. Prior to the interview, clients may see the nutrition counselor as rejecting, dominating, or hostile. Consequently, they resort to behavior they have used in the past in dealing with an unapproachable person. Other clients, on the basis of past experience, see counselors as friendly, supportive, respectful, and positive. Both of these perceptions can create self-fulfilling prophecies. Counselors can become trapped into behaving in accordance with the clients' views of the world. Thus, it is important to be open with a client and to discuss interpersonal factors that may influence both client and counselor. Many years ago, Gerber recommended frank, open discussion of any interpersonal factors that may negatively affect counseling for dietary change.[15] This is still noteworthy advice today in using the nutrition counseling process.

Clients also come to a nutrition counseling session with feelings about themselves. Some may want to succeed in changing yet seek to sabotage any efforts toward change so their routines will stay the same.[13] Clients may say, "New eating habits may be healthy, but what changes will they make in my family life?" A familiar image of themselves as overweight can give obese persons a sense of identity and security that they can lose when the pounds come off. A client may say, "Why should I change my feeling of security to a feeling of having to shape up to what people want me to be?" Clients may come to counselors feeling confused, disturbed, and self-defeated by new knowledge that their health is threatened.[15] Identifying and tagging these feelings is a primary method of assessment prior to making the nutrition diagnosis.

In summary, clients come to counseling with:

- attitudes and beliefs about people
- ideas and feelings about counselors and counseling
- self-images
- basic incongruities in desired outcomes:
  1. a desire to continue along a familiar course
  2. a desire to make changes to improve health and well-being[13]

Counseling and communication skills provide the potential to correct or validate clients' preconceived beliefs. They enable counselors to behave as empathic persons in spite of the "provocation to be less or the seduction to be more than they are."[13]

Theories Influence Counselors

Many theories influence the way a nutrition counselor conducts a session. This text will focus on the following specific theories:

1. behavior modification
2. cognitive-behavioral theory and rational-emotive therapy (RET)
3. social learning theory
4. standard behavioral therapy
5. transtheoretical model
6. person-centered therapy
7. theory of planned behavior and theory of reasoned action
8. Gestalt therapy
9. family therapy
10. self-management approach
11. the health belief model
12. developmental skills training.

An analysis of their characteristics as they apply to the nutrition counseling session follows. Many concepts within these theories overlap.

Behavior Modification

Behavioral counseling, as described by Pavlov, Skinner, Wolpe, Krumboltz, and Thoreson, states that people are born in a neutral state. Environment, consisting of significant others and experience, shapes their behavior.[16] Three modes of learning are basic to behavioral counseling:

1. Operant conditioning holds that if spontaneous behavior satisfies a need, it will occur with greater frequency. For example, a person who switches to a high-fiber eating pattern and finds that constipation problems decrease will probably increase fiber in all meals.
2. Imitation does not involve teaching a new behavior; instead, the emphasis is on mimicking. For example, a client with elevated lipids selects a snack low in saturated fat after a spouse or friend has just ordered one in a restaurant.
3. Modeling extends the concept of imitation, which tends to be haphazard, by providing a planned demonstration. Modeling implies direct teaching of a certain behavior.[17] For example, an overweight client watches a videotape of someone who has lost a large amount of weight. The model's description or demonstration of successful weight loss behaviors helps the client begin a weight-loss program.

Behavioral counseling obviously varies from client to client, as each individual is responsible for shaping the environment to accommodate changes in behavior. Problem behaviors result from faulty learning, and the goal is to eliminate faulty learning and substitute more healthful patterns of behavior.[12]

Behavior modification is often described by using the ABCs of behavior: A is the antecedent of a behavior or the environmental cue that triggers an act. B is the behavior itself. C is the consequence of that behavior.[18] A person who eats while watching TV would identify the antecedent of this behavior or the trigger as television watching with a bowl of candy nearby. The behavior then is the act of eating. The consequence is the weight gain associated with eating. The goal in changing a behavior is to stop this chain of events by modifying components within the chain. For example, by eliminating the bowl of candy the chain of events would stop prior to the behavior of eating. The consequence of weight gain would be averted.

Cognitive Behavioral Therapy, Rational-Emotive Therapy, and Disinhibition

Cognitive behavioral therapy (CBT) focuses on the way we think about actions we take. Dobson describes this form of therapy as focusing on thinking and its effect on behavior.[19] When changing behavior, relevant beliefs may be identified and altered. Desired dietary behavioral change may be the result of changing thought processes or cognitions.[20,21] For example, negative thoughts that tell clients that they have failed may trigger unhealthy eating behaviors that require change for a more healthy lifestyle. Cognitive restructuring is a concept that requires the client to change the way he or she thinks about slips in positive dietary habits.[22] For example, the client who says, "I might as well give up—I just ate that forbidden cake. What is the use in even trying?" This client might restructure his/her internal monologue by saying, "If I have one piece at this special event, that is fine. I will just stop with one slice. This can still be a positive experience." This example of cognitive restructuring avoids the all-or-nothing concept of always having to be perfect.

Rational-emotive therapy (RET) was founded by Albert Ellis. As one of many models of CBT, it has definite similarities to Dobson's approach. Ellis determined that irrationality is the most frequent source of individuals' problems. Self-talk—the monologues individuals have with themselves—is the major source of emotion-related difficulties.[23] The major purposes of RET are to demonstrate to clients that negative self-talk, the cause of many of their problems, should be reevaluated and eliminated along with illogical ideas.[23] Clients' major goals in RET are to look to themselves for positive reinforcement of behaviors. In one commentary contrasting CBT and RET, the writer states that while there are strong similarities in the two theories, RET is a more unified theory of rational thinking and living.[24] RET sets therapeutic goals beyond small very specific behavioral changes. It focuses on sustained changes in emotions, life philosophy, and behavioral changes designed to emphasize overall values.[25] For example, in dietary counseling, a client with hyperlipidemia might say: "I know that I need to cut down on saturated fat to maintain a healthy lifestyle overall. But it is hard to think of avoiding all of those foods I love for the rest of my life. Is that really living?" The RET counselor in this case can help change negative self-talk to more positive thoughts by questioning what the changes in eating patterns might do relative to overall lifestyle. The client might respond: "I know that in the long run, eating in a healthful way is best. It will allow me to be more active with my grandchildren, something very dear to me. Yes, my goal will be to focus my thoughts on how changes in eating will affect my entire life, and especially those things I value most."

In working with clients seeking weight reduction, the concept of disinhibition as a part of CBT surfaces as an important indicator for sustained weight loss. In this context, disinhibition is defined as overeating triggered by emotional and external factors. One study supported the use of only moderate caloric restriction in clients with a high risk of disinhibition. Data from this study showed that rigid caloric regimens fostered feelings of hunger and disturbance of healthy eating behaviors. These researchers found that disinhibition can be diminished by enhancing self-control without a focus on restrained eating, and by negotiation of more appropriate ways of dealing with feelings than overeating.[26]

Four theories or models that have developed from the cognitive behavioral theory are the PRECEDE-PROCEED model,[27] social cognitive theory,[28] and two similar theories, the theory of reasoned action[29] and the theory of planned behavior.[30]

The PRECEDE-PROCEED Model

The PRECEDE-PROCEED model included factors that precede a behavior or those that allow it to continue, or proceed. It proposes three factors driving behavior: predisposing factors, enabling factors, and reinforcing factors. The predisposing factors are those that drive a behavior and include knowledge, beliefs, attitudes, and values. Because these factors are considered the motivation for many behaviors, it is important to examine these factors during the assessment phase of the nutrition care process. For example, knowing what a client values in life often can assist in generating the desire to make changes in dietary practices. Enabling factors are basically those aspects of daily living that allow a positive eating behavior to occur. For example, the thought that it would be a good idea to walk more often may need the enabling factor of knowing what type of shoe is best for walking and where it might be purchased. Reinforcing factors are those things that promote maintenance of a dietary behavior. This aspect of the PRECEDE-PROCEED model focuses on family members, peers, and health care providers who help in sustaining a positive lifestyle change.[27]

Social-Cognitive Theory

Social-cognitive theory emphasizes the importance of factors around us that influence our social environment. Each client's interpretation of behavioral outcomes can affect his or her ability initially to achieve that outcome and ultimately to maintain it. The expectations of what an outcome should be influence the client's ability to achieve that outcome. For example, the client who expects to always eat perfect meals may be disappointed at the actual outcome of lifestyle change-related dietary patterns. This disappointment may result in failure to continue trying to make changes.[28]

Theory of Reasoned Action and Theory of Planned Behavior

The theory of reasoned action proposes that behavior is shaped by the beliefs and attitudes of a person.[29] A later version of this theory, the theory of planned behavior, adds the concept of personal control as a predictor of eventual behavioral change.[30] For example, the person who believes that he/she *can* make a dietary behavioral change (self-efficacy) will be more likely to achieve that change.

Standard Behavioral Therapy

A review of most lifestyle change programs reveals that both cognitive and behavioral strategies are used simultaneously to promote diet and exercise change. During the process of tailoring the programs to each client's needs, different components of the program may be emphasized. This process often involves a mixture of both cognitive and behavioral strategies—and with the melding comes the new label, *standard behavioral therapy*. Fabricatore and Foster discuss the collapsing of cognitive and behavioral strategies into this one overall category.[31,32]

Social Learning Theory

Social learning theory builds on the idea of modeling. The concept is that people learn through seeing someone model a positive behavior. In group counseling, one participant who is doing well might describe or model her experiences. By seeing how someone else handles a difficult situation, it becomes more feasible for a client to take on that experience and succeed.

Bandura has written about this theory and focuses on the importance of self-efficacy.[33-35] The client who is able to say, "I can do this," is more likely to achieve success in changing dietary behaviors. Those clients who see the task as too monumental will have difficulty realizing success.

Transtheoretical Model

The transtheoretical model focuses on the concept of behavioral change and occurs in stages of motivation as clients move to a more healthful lifestyle. Clients may begin in initial precontemplation stage with thoughts like: "I really don't need to change my diet. Things are fine as they are." They may then move to contemplation, in which the client looks at the pros and cons of making a behavioral change. A third stage is preparation, in which planning and motivation to commit to a behavioral change occur. A fourth stage is action, in which actual behavior in a positive direction is observed. The fifth and final stage is maintenance, in which the behavioral change has become a habit and is sustained as a long-term part of daily life.[36,37] Motivational interviewing[38] draws from this model and will be discussed in depth in Chapter 3.

Person-Centered Therapy

Carl Rogers is the founder of person-centered therapy, originally client-centered therapy.[39] His work is still apparent in many of the theories related to behavioral change, including motivational interviewing, that emphasize many Rogerian concepts. Three major concepts form the basis of this theory.

1. All individuals are a composite of their physical being, their thoughts, and their behaviors.
2. Individuals function as an organized system, so alterations in one part may produce changes in another part.
3. Individuals react to everything they perceive; this is their reality.

When counselors try to change dietary behaviors, they also must be concerned with clients' thoughts. Behavioral alterations may produce changes in the clients' physical being as well as the cognitive (thoughtful) being. Counselors must also assess client perceptions thoroughly because what clients perceive as reality influences their ability to follow an eating pattern. The skill of listening is very important to this therapy.

The goals of client-centered therapy include the following:

- promoting a more confident and self-directed person
- promoting a more realistic self-perception
- promoting a positive attitude about self[16]

Rogerian, person-centered therapy focuses on each person's worth and dignity. The emphasis is on the ability to direct one's own life and move toward self-actualization, growth, and health.[12]

Ockene has reestablished the concept of person-centered therapy with her emphasis on the client. Her focus is on tailoring interventions to each client's needs.[40] Her ideas revolve around the concept that work toward modifying behavior in lifestyle change areas requires a thorough assessment of where the client's priorities lie. Her ideas on this topic are key to the nutrition assessment step (step 1) in the nutrition care process. Without a tailored assessment of nutrition behaviors in step 1, the client's needs will not be central to the intervention as it proceeds through the other steps in the nutrition care process.

Nutrition counselors can provide the tools to help clients solve their own problems by assessing their current dietary behavior and establishing realistic goals for change. Also, practitioners can assess clients' thoughts about their body image and food behaviors. Changing thoughts from negative to positive is a first step toward the client's mastery of positive self-reinforcement skills.

Gestalt Therapy

Gestalt counseling, a form of therapy made popular in the 1970s, emphasizes confronting problems. Steps toward solving them involve experiencing these problems in the present rather than the past or the future. The major goal in Gestalt therapy is to make clients aware of all the experiences they have disowned and to recognize that individuals are self-regulating. Being aware of the hidden factors related to a problem is the key to finding an eventual solution.[16]

Using Gestalt therapy to help clients with dietary change involves asking them to recognize how many "disowned" factors can contribute to their dietary problems. Showing clients how to be responsible for regulating their behavior is a practical application of the Gestalt approach to counseling. The goal is for clients to take responsibility for making dietary changes.[12] For example, adolescent clients with diabetes who continuously blame poor glucose control on parents who don't help them control foods or teachers who cause them to be under stress are disowning behaviors that they could control. Helping clients set reasonable behavioral goals when they are ready to change can aid in solving the problem of disowning.

Family Therapy

In family therapy, the family is considered a system of relationships that influence a client's behavior, which is examined as a component of the system. The individual client is always seen in the context of relationships, with emphasis on understanding the total system in which the inappropriate behavior exists. The goal is to help individuals and families to change themselves and the systems within which they live.[41]

One of the major techniques used in family therapy is to involve the client's entire family in solving problems through open and closed questioning. Role-playing may be used to illustrate both the negative aspects of "blaming" and the positive aspects, in which praising behavioral change is emphasized.

Self-Management Approach

Researchers have found that behavioral approaches support short-term change[42] but usually fail to maintain change in the long run.[43,44] Leventhal proposed several reasons for this failure: behavioral techniques fail when contact with a health care professional is less frequent or absent, when initial symptoms of illness lessen, and when relapse into a previous behavior pattern does not provoke any symptoms.[45] Leventhal's theory of self-regulation is based on concepts from the behavioral approach and the health belief model,[46] self-efficacy,[35,47] and self-management.[48] The basic premise in self-regulation allows individuals to choose their own goals based on their perceptions of their illness and related challenges. Individuals seek, discover, and select coping behaviors and evaluate the outcome in emotional and cognitive terms. The nutrition counselor is a guiding expert who reinforces, supports, and encourages individuals as they select, evaluate, and adjust goals and strategies for behavioral change. [49-52]

In the contemporary self-management approach, nutrition counselors and clients are partners. Clients problem solve and use resources beyond those of the nutrition counselor. Clients develop skills and confidence (belief in personal efficacy) through guided mastery experiences, social modeling, social persuasion, and the reduction of adverse physiological reactions. Health care professionals and a social network encourage self-management practices.[53,54]

Health Belief Model

The health belief model focuses on the individual's ability to envision success while moving toward better health by changing behavior. This model includes several assumptions:

1. A person will adopt a behavior if failing to do so has consequences that are a critical threat to lifestyle as it exists. Tied to this is the idea of being in a situation where, without change, the client feels defenseless.
2. Changing a behavior depends on a balance between barriers versus benefits to change.[55]

For example, a client decides to follow a diet low in saturated fat after a heart attack. He feels very vulnerable, and the consequences of not changing to healthier eating behaviors are very real. When he looks at the scale of pros and cons to changing dietary habits, the positive aspects of living a longer life outweigh the barriers of socializing with friends and eating food high in saturated fat.

Developmental Skills Training

Mellin has devised a combination of theories while focusing on what she calls the brain-based intervention program designed to promote two skills: self-nurturing (recognizing feelings and needs and providing support) and effective limit-setting (setting reasonable expectations, accepting difficult situations, and experiencing the reward and benefit of such acceptance). Mellin's writings focus on promoting resilience to daily life stressors and decreasing vulnerability to stress. She emphasizes the tie between daily stressors and their negative effects on mind and body which leads to the onset and progression of chronic disease.[56]

The theories described above are only a few of over 200 orientations to helping clients change their behavior. The communication and counseling skills presented in the next two chapters provide a format through which counselors can consider and use ideas based on these theories. All theories are concerned with change—the generation of ways of thinking, being, deciding, and behaving. When a client changes a dietary behavior in a small way, the nutrition counselor has a foundation upon which to support further change. Integrating tenets of many theories into the treatment of a client's dietary problems is the goal. One theory may work best in promoting change at one stage in a client's treatment; another may work well at a different point. Chapter 3 discusses the client's readiness to change and provides ideas on ways to apply the theories described in this chapter.

Importance of Nutrition Counseling in the Nutrition Care Process

Why is counseling important? Within the nutrition care process model, nutrition counseling provides a logical structure using strategies based on a variety of counseling theories. It has a place in each of the four steps in the model: step 1, assessment; step 2, nutrition diagnosis; step 3, intervention; and step 4, monitoring and evaluation. Nutrition counseling sets the stage for optimum dietary adherence within step 3, intervention.

Dietary adherence should be the ultimate goal of all nutrition counseling sessions. Researchers have found that there are many deterrents to dietary adherence:

- the restrictiveness of the dietary pattern
- the required changes in lifestyle and behavior
- the fact that symptom relief may not be noticeable or may be temporary
- the interference of diet with family or personal habits
- other barriers:
  1. cost
  2. access to proper foods
  3. effort necessary for food preparation[57]

Glanz has found that two positive counseling techniques appear to increase dietary adherence: (1) employing strategies that influence client behavior and (2) involving clients more during the session.[58] She further specifies several strategies for maintaining dietary changes: (1) tailoring the dietary regimen and information about the regimen; (2) using social support inside and outside the health care setting; (3) providing skills and training in addition to information, such as assertiveness training skills and weighing and measuring skills; (4) ensuring effective client provider communication; and (5) paying attention to follow-up, monitoring, and reinforcement.[57]

Hosking lists conditions that increase dietary adherence in hypertensive clients on salt-restricted eating patterns:

- diet programs that are individualized, fully explained, and adapted to the client's preferences and lifestyle
- regular revisits to the same nutrition counselor
- involvement of the family
- reinforcement of the eating pattern from every member of the treatment team[59]

Several research studies have reported that adherence is better when the counselor is warm and empathetic and shows interest ("Call me if there is a problem") and demonstrates genuine concern ("I will call in a week").[60–70] Counselor-client relationships are essential to maintaining dietary change. In a large scale RCT, Jackson showed that counseling staff turnover was directly and negatively correlated with study participant adherence.[71] This relationship between counselor and client is immensely important to maintenance of improved dietary behavior.

Counseling skills help eliminate the hit-or-miss philosophy that allows little assurance for success. This hit-or-miss philosophy tends to be inefficient, because the nutrition counselor must backtrack when strategies fail. To provide structure and organization, Figure 1–2 shows the nutrition care process. This text will focus on the nutrition intervention portion of the nutrition care process. Figure 1–3 provides a simplified schematic of nutrition counseling as it occurs with in this process.

Systems Approach to Nutrition Counseling

Models provide a sequenced path for counselors to follow and list essential components in each step of the process. Figure 1–3 shows one model by which nutrition counselors can avoid missing a vital

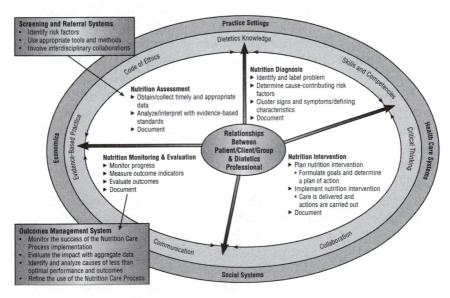

FIGURE 1–2   Nutrition Care Process.[1]

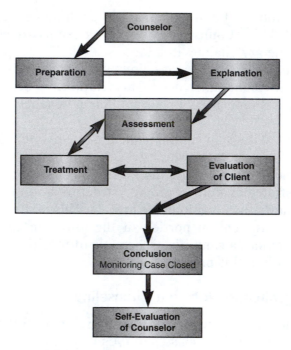

FIGURE 1–3   Model for nutrition counseling.

part of the process. In this model, the counselor wears many hats. The first is that of a diagnostician preparing for the interview by reviewing all available data in the medical record, diet records, diet recalls, diet histories, interviews with family members, and other sources.

The session begins with an explanation of the counseling relationship with enough detail that the client knows precisely what will take place. In this stage, the practitioner is a teacher defining the relationship for the client.

During the assessment and diagnosis phase, once again in the role of diagnostician, the counselor evaluates the client's nutrition status and relates food intake data to behavioral indicators. The practitioner also must establish a safe, trusting, and caring environment, acting as empathizer. In the nutrition intervention portion of the nutrition care process, the counselor's roles are those of expert and mutual problem solver, roles that usually can be combined only through diligent study and practice. Most novices at counseling tend to be either expert or empathizer. When the two roles are used in combination, they can facilitate adherence to diet, but used singly, each can be detrimental to effective client-centered counseling. Steve Berg-Smith has said in reference to counseling for lifestyle change, "The quality of our listening is far greater than the wisdom of our words."[5,72]

Many practitioners are familiar with the all-knowing counselor who approaches clients with an air of authority. Clients are overwhelmed by these experts' self-confidence and taken in by the appearance of wisdom. However, when clients return home, they find it very difficult to follow the diet. They tend to forget much of what was said during the counseling session and are incapable of self-direction in adhering to the new regimen. The clients' solution in such a case is to continue with old eating habits.

On the other hand, counselors who are empathizers can become so involved with the client's problems that they lose sight of their other role of information disseminators. Counselors can run into conflicts when they see a client is in error but feel that revealing the mistake may damage the individual's pride and ability to follow the diet. "Eating cheesecake out a few times won't matter," the counselor says. To the client on a low-saturated-fat diet, this may be a signal to go ahead and continue poor eating habits. Back at home, the client may comment to a family member, "The nutritionist said eating cheesecake in a restaurant just a few times wouldn't hurt. Three nights a week doesn't seem too often."

In evaluating clients, counselors once again become diagnosticians. If no solution to the problem has been reached, counseling reverts to the assessment phase. In some cases the clinicians may decide to refer a client to another practitioner more experienced with the problem.

The intervention phase allows the client to offer ideas with the counselor focused on using those ideas to tailor the strategies for dietary change.

In concluding the counseling session, the counselor should share a few words of wisdom, in which case the counselor becomes the expert again. Ending the program involves more than just closing the case. Monitoring the client's performance in the real world is important to continued dietary adherence. This means calling to check on progress and, with the individual's permission, checking with significant others to determine how they feel the client has progressed.

The last step involves self-evaluation of the counselor's performance. In this case, the counselor becomes the learner, building on past experience to improve present skills.

Counseling Skills

The basic steps just discussed are a part of counseling, but the complexities go beyond what Figure 1–3 indicates. Chapters 2 and 3 review these skills and ways to use them.

Communication Skills

Basic to all counseling is knowledge of communication skills. Without these skills, treatment cannot and will not take place.

Counseling

Once clinicians have acquired this foundation, they then can learn various counseling skills to aid clients in achieving dietary goals. These skills involve nutrition assessment, diagnosis, intervention, and monitoring/evaluation.

Nutrition Assessment

Nutrition counseling involves a process of targeting behaviors involving eating habits. Initially, a careful assessment of current eating behaviors is important. Knowing what food habits exist prior to making a change allows the individual to target specific foods and behaviors.

Assessment involves more than asking clients, "Do you have a problem?" It is a carefully considered plan to determine areas in which problems occur. Assessment in nutrition counseling includes ascertaining what clients are eating and why they make certain food selections.[2] The example that follows illustrates several potential responses to a weight-control client.

A client returns for a visit following the diet instruction and reports a problem: "I just haven't lost any weight on the diet you recommended." There are several counselor responses:

1. "Did you follow all of my advice?"
2. "Well, what have you been eating?"
3. "What is your typical day like?"

These three questions indicate various levels of communication skills. The first question is stated in a way that immediately places the client on the defensive. The client feels compelled to give a glowing picture or a multitude of excuses. The second question focuses only on eating behaviors, disregarding the surrounding circumstances that may have instigated the behavior. Depending on the tone of voice, it also may make the client feel compelled to reply with what the counselor wants to hear. The third question is a sensitive statement that shows caring, characteristic of Rogerian style. It does not imply a reprimand, allows the client time to elaborate on what actually happened, and gives the counselor the information necessary to assess the situation. It sets the stage for client-centered counseling.

For practicing nutrition counselors, the most frequent problem during an interview is a rush to give advice. It is important to stop and take time to assess the situation first. Only after assessment should counselors provide advice, allowing the client to assist by suggesting and describing how he or she expects to apply those recommendations in a true-to-life situation. It is important to remember that the quality of our listening is paramount in achieving successful behavioral change.

Nutrition Diagnosis

The diagnosis of nutrition problems involves identifying and labeling a problem, determining the cause or contributing risk factors, listing signs and symptoms, and documenting the nutrition diagnosis. There are three distinct parts to each nutrition diagnosis:

1. Problem (Diagnostic Label): The diagnostic label defines alterations in the client's nutritional status. The label is an adjective describing the human response: altered, impaired, ineffective, increased/decreased, risk of, acute or chronic.
2. Etiology (Cause/Contributing Risk Factors): Etiology is the term applied to factors that contribute to the existence of the problem. The words "related to" link the etiology to the diagnostic label.
3. Signs and Symptoms (Defining Characteristics): These defining characteristics are identified during the assessment phase. They quantify the problem and describe its severity. The words, "as evidenced by" link these defining characteristics to

the etiology. Signs are objective identifiers of observable changes in health status. Symptoms are subjective changes that the client feels and expresses verbally.

The nutrition diagnosis is written in a PES Statement that states the problem, etiology and signs and symptoms. An example might be: Elevated blood glucose (problem) related to frequent consumption of large portions (etiology) as evidenced by daily intake of calories exceeding recommended amounts by 500 kcal and a 20-pound weight gain in the past 5 months (sign). The client complains of feeling tired and lacks the energy to do daily tasks (symptoms). The client states that her husband is upset because she has no energy to do those things that they previously did together as a couple (symptom, feeling related).

Nutrition Intervention

Beyond understanding initial eating habits, counselors and their clients then make decisions about how to manage change. They determine which foods to modify or substitute to achieve a change in a targeted nutrient. Self-monitoring is crucial.[73,74]

In giving clients strategies to remedy nutrition problems or provide treatment, counselors once again must proceed slowly and focus on the clients in planning and setting attainable goals. Counselors frequently decide before the interview how the problems should be solved and try to force clients into preformed molds. They do not give clients an opportunity to participate. In this phase, mutually decided goals will achieve the most success. Counselors should use the following sequence of steps in setting goals:

1. Identify nutrition goals by listening to the client's ideas.
   - Define desired nutrition behaviors (what to do).
   - Determine conditions or circumstances (where and when to do it).
   - Establish the extent or level (how much or how often to do it).
2. Identify nutrition subgoals (a subgoal for a long-term goal of eliminating snacks would be to eliminate the morning snack and determine a workable substitute behavior).
3. Establish client commitment, which includes identifying obstacles that might prevent goal attainment and listing resources needed for goal achievement.[75]

The strategy chosen to help implement these goals once again requires listening skills to involve the client in reaching solutions. Counselors should ask the following questions to help tailor strategies to each individual's situation:

1. Why is the client here?
2. Is the problem the client describes all or only part of the problem? Many nutrition counselors have thrown their hands up in despair, saying, "He just isn't motivated to follow this diet." In such a case, the real problem may hinge on emotional stress that must be treated before nutrition counseling can take place. The client might be referred to a psychologist or other professional for help before or concurrent with the nutrition counseling session. For those clients who are ready to change the following questions may be helpful:
   • What are the problematic nutrition behaviors and related concerns?
   • Can I describe the conditions contributing to poor nutrition adherence?
   • Am I aware of the present severity and intensity of the nutrition problem?[76]

Chapter 3 discusses motivational interviewing and the importance of identifying readiness to change. Goal setting may be counter productive if the client is not ready to change. The client will fail and the counselor will feel defeated if goals are set when the client is not ready to change. For the client who is not ready, it will be best to send the client home to think about the possibility of change.

For some clients, the problem may be lack of sufficient information to follow the desired regimen. For example, a person with renal disease who follows a low-protein eating pattern routinely has elevated urine urea nitrogen levels inconsistent with diet records that show excellent compliance. After requesting that the cook in her favorite restaurant slice one ounce of chicken off the actual portion of "Chicken Oscar" (her favorite entree), she is surprised: one ounce is much smaller than she guessed. For weeks, her concept of one ounce of meat has been much greater than the actual amount. Providing enough information for the client to follow a new eating pattern is the first step.

The second step may involve solving a problem of a different nature—lack of planning. For example, a guest at a party realizes that he has no idea what ingredients are in the main dish. If before going to the party he has placed a cue on the refrigerator, "Call hostess to check on what is being served for the party tomorrow," the client can avoid a potentially awkward situation. Many clients comment that one of the most important ways to avoid drops in dietary adherence is to plan ahead.

The third step in treating dietary problems is much more difficult. It involves diagnosing a problem involving lack of commitment to a dietary regimen. The term "lack of commitment" is not meant to reflect badly on the client but to diagnose accurately poor dietary adherence. For example, a person with diabetes may decide, "I just want to be free from dietary worries for a while. Life is so complicated. I want to forget my diet and splurge." The counselor cannot say, "Fine, don't worry about it for a week," but the counselor can say, "What can we do to streamline your dietary efforts? Let us begin by identifying when diet is most frequently a problem." Identification may require that the client records in a diary those thoughts related to eating before and after meals. For example, "I ate that chocolate cake even though I knew it would be too high in calories after that huge dinner." If a pattern of negative thoughts seems to occur frequently at dinner time, the client needs strategies to help make that meal a more positive experience.[76–78] By identifying a major problem time, the client may be able to work out menus in advance, elicit help from family in meal preparation on specified nights, rely on precalculated exchanges for each meal, build in time to relax before each meal, and work on more positive self-thoughts. Using the client's suggestions and the counselor's experiences allows for a joint solution to the problem of lack of commitment.

Monitoring and Evaluation

The last phase, monitoring and evaluation, provides a reassessment of progress for both clients and counselors. Much of the questioning used during the assessment phase can be reused here, focusing on the desired objective and whether it was met. The counselor should monitor the client for a time in the client's environment.

Counselor self-evaluation frequently does not take place because of time constraints. It can be very important to review what went on in an interview and then to determine what made it a success and what might have improved its efficacy or quality.

Counseling Spectrum

Nutrition counselors assume a variety of roles. During the sessions some role changes take place automatically; others require a great deal of practice and effort. The role of the counselor falls on a spectrum such as that in Figure 1–4, including some of the positions on both ends. When counseling is totally dominated by client requests and tangential topics, little behavioral change will take place. A session totally dominated by a counselor who only provides information without listening to client concerns can be equally unproductive. The ideal is a mix of client and counselor interaction. Making a trial run of a counseling situation by role-playing with a fellow nutrition counselor can be helpful. When one counselor plays the part of client, he or she will be able to sense where changes in counseling style might be appropriate. For example, after playing the roles, the counselor playing the client might say, "You did a great job, but really asked me too many questions."

In summary, using skills that involve behavioral change may seem unnatural to those who have been mainly involved in providing information to clients. Nutrition counseling strategies elevate the counselor/client interaction to a level that increases self-management and potentially ensures dietary behavioral change success.

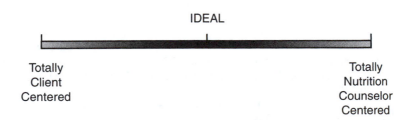

FIGURE 1–4   The nutrition counseling spectrum

References

1. American Dietetic Association. *Nutrition Diagnosis and Intervention: Standardized Language for the Nutrition Care Process.* Chicago: American Dietetic Association, 2008.

2. Mason M. *The Dynamics of Clinical Dietetics,* 2nd ed. New York: John Wiley & Sons, 1982.

3. Reduction of dietary protein and phosphorus in the Modification of Diet in Renal Disease Feasibility Study. The MDRD Study Group. *J Am Diet Assoc* 1994;94(9):986–990; quiz 991–982.

4. Klahr S, Levey AS, Beck GJ, et al. The effects of dietary protein restriction and blood-pressure control on the progression of chronic renal disease. Modification of Diet in Renal Disease Study Group. *N Engl J Med* 1994;330(13):877–884.

5. Berg-Smith SM, Stevens VJ, Brown KM, et al. A brief motivational intervention to improve dietary adherence in adolescents. The Dietary Intervention Study in Children (DISC) Research Group. *Health Educ Res* 1999;14(3):399–410.

6. Bowen D, Ehret C, Pedersen M, et al. Results of an adjunct dietary intervention program in the Women's Health Initiative. *J Am Diet Assoc* 2002;102(11):1631–1637.

7. Gillis BP, Caggiula AW, Chiavacci AT, et al. Nutrition intervention program of the Modification of Diet in Renal Disease Study: a self-management approach. *J Am Diet Assoc* 1995;95(11):1288–1294.

8. Trager J. *Food Book.* New York: Grossman Publishers, 1970.

9. Jefferson T. The Thomas Jefferson Memorial Foundation. In: Utley DV, ed. *Monticello,* Charlottesville, VA, 1819.

10. Ohlson MA. The philosophy of dietary counseling. *J Am Diet Assoc* 1973;63(1):13–14.

11. Selling LS, Ferraro MSS. *The Psychology of Diet and Nutrition.* New York: W.W. Norton & Co., 1945.

12. Ivey AE. *Counseling and Psychotherapy: Integrating Skills and Theory in Practice.* 2nd ed. Englewood Cliffs, NJ: Prentice-Hall, 1986.

13. Stefflre B, Matheny KB. *The Function of Counseling Theory.* Boston: Houghton Mifflin, 1968.

14. Lorr M. Client perceptions of therapists: a study of the therapeutic relation. *J Consult Psychol* 1965;29:146–149.

15. Gerber SK. *A Systematic Approach to Counseling Skills.* New York: Human Science Press, Inc., 1986.

16. Pietrofesa JJ. *Counseling: Theory, Research, and Practice.* Chicago: Rand McNally College Publishing Co., 1978.

17. Spence JT. *Behavioral Approaches to Therapy.* Morristown, NJ: General Learning Press, 1976.

18. Stevens V. Theoretical approaches to counseling for health behavioral change. *J Am Dietetic Assoc* (submitted).

19. Dobson K. *Handbook of Cognitive-Behavioral Therapies.* New York: Guilford Press, 1998.

20. Snetselaar L. *Nutritional Counseling for Lifestyle Change.* New York: CRC Taylor and Francis Group, 2006.
21. Geliebter A, Aversa A. Emotional eating in overweight, normal weight, and underweight individuals. *Eat Behav* 2003;3(4):341–347.
22. Miller PM, Sims KL. Evaluation and component analysis of a comprehensive weight control program. *Int J Obes* 1981;5(1):57–65.
23. Ellis A. *Reason and Emotion in Psychotherapy.* New York: Citadel Press, 1962.
24. Sacks SB. Rational emotive behavior therapy: disputing irrational philosophies. *J Psychosoc Nurs Ment Health Serv* 2004;42(5):22–31.
25. Ellis A, MacLaren C. *Rational Emotive Behavior Therapy: A Therapist's Guide.* Atascadero, CA: Impact Publishers, 1998.
26. Cuntz U, Leibbrand R, Ehrig C, Shaw R, Fichter MM. Predictors of post-treatment weight reduction after in-patient behavioral therapy. *Int J Obes Relat Metab Disord* 2001;25, Suppl 1:S99–S101.
27. Green LW, Kreuter MW. *Health Promotion Planning: An Educational and Environmental Approach.* Mountain View, CA: Mayfield, 1991.
28. Bandura A. *Self-Efficacy in Changing Societies.* New York: Cambridge University Press, 1995.
29. Ajzen I, Fishbein M. *Understanding Attitudes and Predicting Social Behavior.* Englewood Cliffs, NJ: Prentice-Hall, 1980.
30. Ajzen I. From intentions to actions: A theory of planned behavior. In: Kuhl J, Beckman J, eds. *Action-Control: From Cognition to Behavior.* Heidelberg, Germany: Springer, 1985:11–39.
31. Fabricatore AN. Behavior therapy and cognitive-behavioral therapy of obesity: is there a difference? *J Am Diet Assoc* 2007;107(1):92–99.
32. Foster GD. Clinical implications for the treatment of obesity. *Obesity (Silver Spring)* 2006;14, Suppl 4:182S–185S.
33. Bandura A. *Social Learning Theory.* Englewood Cliffs, NJ: Prentice-Hall, 1977.
34. Bandura A. *Self-Efficacy: The Exercise of Control.* New York: W.H. Freeman and Company, 1997.
35. Bandura A. Self-efficacy: toward a unifying theory of behavioral change. *Psychol Rev* 1977;84(2):191–215.
36. DiClemente CC, Prochaska JO. Toward a comprehensive, transtheoretical model of change: Stages of change and addictive behaviors. In: Miller WR, Heather N, eds. *Treating Addictive Behaviors*, 2nd ed. New York: Plenum Press, 1998:3–24.
37. Prochaska JO, Velicer WF, Rossi JS, et al. Stages of change and decisional balance for 12 problem behaviors. *Health Psychol* 1994;13(1):39–46.
38. DiClemente CC, Velasques MM. Motivational interviewing and the stages of change. In: Miller WR, Rollnick S, eds. *Motivational Interviewing, Preparing People for Change*, 2nd ed. New York: Guilford Press, 2002:201–216.
39. Rogers CR. *Client-Centered Therapy.* Boston: Houghton Mifflin, 1951.
40. Ockene JK. Strategies to increase adherence to treatment. In: Burke LE,

Ockene IS, eds. *Compliance in Healthcare and Research.* Armonk, NY: Future Publishing Company, 2001.

41. Bowen M. *Family Therapy in Clinical Practice.* New York: Aronson, 1978.

42. Dunbar JM. Behavioral strategies for improving compliance. In: Haynes RS, ed. *Compliance in Health Care.* Baltimore, MD: The Johns Hopkins University Press, 1979:174–190.

43. Leventhal H, Cameron L. Behavioral theories and the problem of compliance. *Patient Educ Couns* 1987;10:117–138.

44. Wing RR. Behavioral treatment of severe obesity. *Am J Clin Nutr* 1992;55(2 Suppl):545S–551S.

45. Leventhal H. A self-regulation perspective. In: Gentry WD, ed. *Handbook of Behavioral Medicine.* New York: Guilford Press, 1984:369–436.

46. Janz NK, Becker MH. The Health Belief Model: a decade later. *Health Educ Q* 1984;11(1):1–47.

47. Bandura A. Self-efficacy mechanism in physiological activation and health-promoting behavior. In: Madden J, ed. *Neurobiology of Learning, Emotion and Affect.* New York: Raven Press, 1991:229–270.

48. Tobin DL. Self-management and social learning theory. In: Holroyd KA, Greer TL, eds. *Self-Management of Chronic Disease: Handbook of Clinical Interventions and Research.* Orlando, FL: Academic Press, 1986:29–55.

49. Trostle JA. Medical compliance as an ideology. *Soc Sci Med* 1988;27(12):1299–1308.

50. Steele DJ, Blackwell B, Gutmann MC, Jackson TC. The activated patient: dogma, dream, or desideratum? *Patient Educ Couns* 1987;10(1):3–23.

51. Stone GC. Patient compliance and the role of the expert. *J Social Issues* 1979;35:34–59.

52. Szasz TS, Hollender MH. A contribution to the philosophy of medicine: the basic models of the doctor-patient relationship. In: Stockle JD, ed. *Encounters Between Patients and Doctors.* Boston: Massachusetts Institute of Technology Press, 1987:165–177.

53. Holman H, Lorig K. Perceived self-efficacy in self-management of chronic disease. In: Schwarzer R, ed. *Self-Efficacy: Thought Control of Action.* Washington, DC: Hemisphere Publishing Company, 1992:305–323.

54. Lorig K, Seleznick M, Lubeck D, Ung E, Chastain RL, Holman HR. The beneficial outcomes of the arthritis self-management course are not adequately explained by behavioral change. *Arthritis Rheum* 1989;32(1):91–95.

55. Glanz K. *Health Behavior and Health Education: Theory Research and Practice,* 3rd Ed. San Francisco: Pfeiffer, 2002.

56. Mellin L. *The Solution.* New York: Harper Collins, 1997.

57. Glanz K. Nutrition education for risk factor reduction and patient education: a review. *Prev Med* 1985;14(6):721–752.

58. Glanz K. Dietitians' effectiveness and patient compliance with dietary regimens. A pilot study. *J Am Diet Assoc* 1979;75(6):631–636.

59. Hosking M. Salt and hypertension. *Med J Aust* 1979;2(7):351–352.
60. Becker MH, Maiman LA. Strategies for enhancing patient compliance. *J Community Health* 1980;6(2):113–135.
61. Ben-Sira Z. Affective and instrumental components in the physician-patient relationship: an additional dimension of interaction theory. *J Health Soc Behav* 1980;21(2):170–180.
62. Posner RB. Physician-patient communication. *Am J Med* 1984;77(3A):59–64.
63. Dimatteo MR, DiNicola DD. *Achieving Patient Compliance: The Psychology of the Medical Practitioner's Role.* New York: Pergamon Press, 1982.
64. Kayvenhoven MM. Written simulation of patient-doctor encounters. *Family Pract* 1983;1:25–29.
65. Turk DC. *Pain and Behavioral Medicine: A Cognitive-Behavioral Perspective.* New York: Guilford Press, 1983.
66. Stewart M. Patient characteristics which are related to the doctor-patient interaction. *Family Pract* 1983;1:30–36.
67. Peck CL, King NJ. Compliance and the doctor-patient relationship. *Drugs* 1985;30(1):78–84.
68. Glass GV, Kliegl RM. An apology for research integration in the study of psychotherapy. *J Couns Clinical Psychol* 1984;51:28–41.
69. Baker SB. Measured effects of primary prevention strategies. *Personnel Guid J* 1984:459–464.
70. Beck JT, Strong SR. Stimulating therapeutic change with interpretations. *J Couns Psychol* 1982;29:551–559.
71. Jackson M, Berman N, Snetselaar L, Granek I, Boe K, Huber M, Milas C, Spivak J, Chlebowski RJ. Research staff turnover and participant adherence in the Women's Health Initiative. *Journal of Controlled Clinical Trials* 24:422–435, 2003.
72. Berg-Smith S, personal communication, March 20, 2007.
73. Smith DE, Wing RR. Diminished weight loss and behavioral compliance during repeated diets in obese patients with type II diabetes. *Health Psychol* 1991;10(6):378–383.
74. Sperduto WA, Thompson HS, O'Brien RM. The effect of target behavior monitoring on weight loss and completion rate in a behavior modification program for weight reduction. *Addict Behav* 1986;11(3):337–340.
75. Russell ML. *Behavioral Counseling in Medicine.* New York: Oxford University Press, 1986.
76. Cormier WH, Cormier LS. *Interviewing Strategies for Helpers, Fundamental Skills and Cognitive Behavioral Intervention*, 2nd ed. Monterey, CA: Brooks/Cole Publishing, 1985.
77. Mahoney MJ, Mahoney K. *Permanent Weight Control, A Solution to the Dieter's Dilemma.* New York: W.W. Norton & Company, 1976.
78. Mahoney MJ. *Strategies for Solving Personal Problems.* New York: W.W. Norton & Company, 1979.

CHAPTER 2

COMMUNICATION SKILLS

Chapter Objectives

1. List three characteristics necessary to perform optimum nutrition counseling within the nutrition care process.

2. Define the following three forms of nonverbal behavior: (a) kinesics, (b) paralinguistics, and (c) proxemics.

3. Apply appropriate responses to given client nonverbal behaviors.

4. Apply appropriate listening responses to given client statements.

5. Apply appropriate action responses to given client statements.

6. Apply appropriate sharing responses to given client statements.

7. Apply appropriate teaching responses to given client statements.

Effective Counselor-Client Relationships

Communication skills form the foundation for nutrition counseling (Figure 2–1). Every step in the nutrition care process requires an ability to communicate. In step 1, the ability to assess nutrition problems would be impossible without communication skills. It is at this first point in the nutrition care process that the skill of engaging the client in discussion around eating habits is crucial to each of the three steps that follow. The quality of the nutrition counselor's communication skills allows the second step of determining a nutrition diagnosis to occur. No diagnosis will be accurate if communication is not occurring at the highest level during

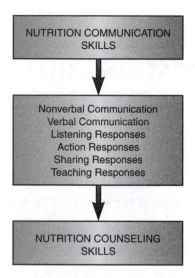

FIGURE 2–1   Communication skills as a foundation for counseling.

step 1, assessment. Step 3 involves negotiating a tailored intervention, and again, communication and counseling skills are crucial to client behavior change success. Finally, in Step 4, accurate information about whether goals were met will only occur if the client feels comfortable communicating with the nutrition counselor, who is the facilitator of client progress.

To learn these skills, practitioners start not by examining their clientele, but by looking at themselves. What characteristics should an effective nutrition counselor possess?

Personal Characteristics of Counselors

Ivey describes counseling as a process of facilitating another person's growth.[1] The way counselors respond to others can greatly influence how clients think and act in the future. The mere act of encouraging clients to talk as opposed to ignoring what they say may influence their lives greatly. Many clients come to a counseling session feeling that no one has really ever listened to them. By finding someone who is focused on them and shows great interest in their past eating problems, they become more willing to discuss those parts of their lives that may be most connected to success and failure in the goal of eating in a healthy manner.

According to Russell, a good rapport between the nutrition counselor and client is essential to behavior change.[2] From the moment of initial contact, the nutrition counselor strives to develop an open, positive relationship in which the client senses the counselor's acceptance and understanding. To change their behavior, clients must feel comfortable freely relating intimate details of lifestyle to the counselor.

Cormier et al. suggest a variety of personal characteristics necessary to be an effective counselor.[3] Practitioners recognize intuitively that being empathetic, conveying respect, and behaving naturally helps to create and maintain a more positively channeled session. The way they view themselves and their priorities, values, and expectations can alter the process positively or negatively.[3]

Nelson-Jones describes some characteristics that helpers bring to a nutrition interview. Nutrition counselors begin an interview with discussion of motives, learning history, thinking skills, capacity to feel, sense of worth, fears and anxieties, sexuality, gender role identity and expectations, values, ethics, culture and cross-cultural skills, race and racial attitudes and skills, and social class.[4]

Researchers have shown an association between the counselor and patient satisfaction resulting from the level of communication skills used by the counselor. Compliance to overall health regimens has also been linked to communication between client and health care provider.[5-7]

Cormier and Cormier focus on three problems with self-image that can result in negative consequences during an interview: competence, power, and intimacy.[8] Counselors' attitudes can involve the concept of competence. Feelings of incompetence can lead to avoidance of controversial issues in counseling sessions. Nutrition counselors may be afraid to say that there are no direct or absolute answers to clients' questions. Counselors or clients may regard a truthful answer, such as, "The evidence is not in at this time," as a sign of incompetence—the very trait that practitioners hope to avoid. Closely tied to feelings of incompetence are those of inadequacy, fear of failure, and fear of success. Counselors with these feelings unconsciously try to keep their negative self-images alive by using several behaviors. They may avoid positive interactions by negating positive feedback and making self-deprecating or apologetic comments. For example, an obese client who has lost weight says, "I really think you're a terrific counselor." A fearful counselor will reply, "Oh, no, I haven't done that much" instead of simply thanking the client for the compliment: "Thank you. Keep in mind you have done all of the work."

The second potential self-image problem, power, can make counselors feel both omnipotent and fearful of losing control or being weak or unresourceful. In the authoritarian role, counselors try to persuade clients to obey suggestions without question; practitioners dominate the content and direction of the interview, thinking, "I am in charge." The nutrition counselor who has the need to always be in control may say, "This is the goal I have for you!" If clients resist or do not respond, the outcome for counselors is resentment and anger. The weak and unresourceful counselor may occupy a subordinate role, complaining, "If you would just do as I say . . ." On the other hand, the powerful practitioner tends to be dictatorial and overly silent, rarely participating in the interview—and, because of this aloof attitude, often loses credibility.

The third potential self-image problem focuses on feelings about intimacy. These can involve two extremes, affection and rejection. Counselors who are fearful of rejection try to elicit only positive feelings from clients, avoiding confrontation at all costs and ignoring negative cues. This type of counselor may even get involved in doing clients favors. Counselors who try to do everything for their clients may be eliminating independent problem-solving. Practitioners at the opposite end of the spectrum try to ignore positive client feelings. They tend to act overly gruff and distant to avoid the closeness they fear. This type of counselor always tries to maintain the authoritarian role of "expert" to maintain distance. (Appendix A presents a counselor self-image checklist.)

Counselors who have tendencies toward self-image problems will find that step 1 in the nutrition care process is difficult, and the steps that follow will often miss targeting the primary cause of the nutrition problem. If competence, power, and intimacy issues prevent communication between client and nutrition counselor, the entire nutrition care process will be flawed and result in lack of success in achieving client goals. If success seems to elude clients, it may be important for the counselor to check on his or her own level of positive self-image.

Counselors as Growth Facilitators

One of the most crucial traits in nutrition counseling is the ability to facilitate growth—the art of helping clients achieve their goals and function on their own. Ivey identifies four potential participants in an interview: the nutrition counselor and his or her cultural and historical background, and the client and his or her cultural and historical background.[1] For example, touching that is appropriate in many South American cultures represents an invasion of privacy among many North Americans. Concreteness is valued highly in North American culture but may be irrelevant to Asians, who communicate ideas more subtly. Facilitative counselors understand that the mode of being in the world differs among cultures. As counselors see the world through their clients' eyes, they facilitate growth and provide concrete and specific strategies for behavior change. (See the segment on strategies in Chapter 3.)

Facilitative Levels

Researchers have delineated growth facilitative levels that counselors assume at various points in acquiring nutrition communication skills.[9] The levels below illustrate a gradual progression in the counselors' ability to respond appropriately to clients' problems.

- Level 1: The response shows no understanding and no direction in relation to the client's position. When the client brings up a crucial personal topic, the counselor starts talking about his or her own personal problems.
- Level 2: The response shows no understanding but some direction. The counselor presents only general advice: when the client expresses difficulty with a weight-loss strategy, the response is, "Well, don't worry about it."
- Level 3: The response shows understanding but no direction. The counselor might say, "You feel afraid because you're not sure how to avoid food offers from friends."
- Level 4: The response shows understanding and some direction. The counselor reacts to the client's deficits and provides details related to the problems, saying, "You feel afraid because you can't say 'no' and you want to avoid eating high-calorie foods."

- Level 5: The response shows understanding and specific direction. It contains the deficit, the goal, and one explicit step for overcoming the problem and reaching the objective: "You feel afraid because you can't say 'no' and want to avoid eating high-calorie foods. How would you feel about exploring positive ways to say 'no'?"

There are no perfect "super counselors" who have all the characteristics to make all sessions successful. Even positive characteristics may not always enhance the interview. Beyond personal characteristics that affect the sessions are the skills that require practice. When these skills are mastered, counseling takes on the characteristics necessary to achieve behavioral change.

Nonverbal Communication

Client Nonverbal Behavior

Clients' nonverbal behavior can affect the direction of the interview. Effective counselors can identify nonverbal cues as signals for unspoken feelings.[10]

Cormier and Cormier describe three forms of client nonverbal behavior: kinesics, paralinguistics, and proxemics. Kinesics includes a variety of physical behaviors (e.g., facial expressions, body language). Paralinguistics refers to how the client's message is delivered (e.g., tone of voice). Proxemics involves environmental and personal space.[8] Evaluation Tool 2–1 at the end of this chapter presents possible meanings associated with behaviors for each region of the body and a general category of autonomic responses. The table is designed to increase awareness of different behaviors; it is not intended to make all nutrition counselors experts on all client feelings. The effect or meaning of each nonverbal behavior varies from person to person and culture to culture.

Ivey contrasts nonverbal attending patterns in European-North American, middle-class culture with patterns of other cultures.[1] European-North American, middle-class cultures consider direct eye contact as a sign of interest. However, even in that culture, people often maintain more eye contact while listening and less while talking. When clients are uncomfortable about a topic, they may avoid eye contact. Some African Americans in the United States may have reverse patterns; they may look more when talking and slightly less when listening. Among some American Indian groups, eye contact by the young is a sign of disrespect. Some cultural groups (American Indian, Inuit, or Aboriginal Australian groups) avoid eye contact when talking about serious subjects.

Passons describes several ways of responding to nonverbal client behaviors "involving congruence, mixed messages, silence, changing cues, and refocusing for direction."[11] Nutrition counselors can use these suggestions to decide on a reply to client statements about dietary adherence.

Congruence. Are the clients' nonverbal messages congruent with the verbal ones? An example might be the individual with diabetes who comes for the first follow-up interview. With furrowed brow, the client sends this confused message to the counselor: "How do I fill in this record? I have forgotten your directions." The counselor can make a mental note of the congruence in behaviors or ask the client to explain the meaning of the nonverbal conduct: "I noticed that you look concerned. What does that mean?" The response could provide specific information on why the record was not completed. Was it too difficult? Did measuring the foods interfere with meal preparation for the family? Was the counselor's description of the information needed on the record unclear?

Mixed messages. Is there a mixed message or discrepancy between the verbal and nonverbal messages? For example, a client comes in after having followed a no-added-salt eating pattern for several weeks and states, "It's going really [pause] well. I've had [pause] very few problems," while looking down and leaning away. The nutrition counselor can deal with these discrepancies in one of three ways: (1) simply take mental note; (2) describe the discrepancy to the client, for example, "You say the diet is really going well and that there are few problems but you were looking down and really spoke with a lot of hesitation"; (3) reply, "I noticed you looked away and paused as you said that. What does that mean?"

Silence. Are there nonverbal behaviors with silence? Silence does not mean that nothing is happening. It can have different meanings from one culture to another. In some cultures silence denotes respect.

Sue points out that for the Chinese and Japanese, silence means a desire to resume speaking after making a point. Once again, the nutrition counselor can mentally note the silence, describe it to the client, or ask the client to explain it.[12]

Changing cues.   Is it necessary to distract or interrupt clients by focusing on nonverbal behavior? If continuation of the topic may be unproductive, interruption may be needed to change the flow of the interview. If clients are pouring out a lot of information or rambling, a change in the direction of the interview may be useful. In such instances, nutrition counselors can distract clients from the verbal content by refocusing on nonverbal behavior. For example, for unproductive content in a client's messages, a counselor might say, "Our conversation so far has been dealing with your inability to cope with your spouse's unsupportive comments about your low-protein eating pattern. Are you aware that you have been gripping the sides of your chair with your hands while you speak?" Nutrition counselors must decide whether such distractions can be destructive or productive to the interview. If the change in flow makes the client feel unable to continue to air feelings, the distraction could be detrimental. Experienced counselors probably will find that their own intuition helps in knowing when to interrupt.

Refocusing for redirection.   Are there pronounced changes in the client's nonverbal behavior? Initially the client may sit with arms crossed, then become more relaxed, with arms unfolded and hands gesturing. Once again, counselors can respond either overtly or covertly. A nutrition counselor might respond to a seemingly more relaxed client by saying, "You seem more relaxed now. Do you feel less tense?"

Counselor Nonverbal Communication

The counselor's nonverbal communication can have a great impact on the relationship. Based on analogue research, Cormier and Cormier report that the nonverbal counselor behaviors that seem to be most important include expressions in the eyes and face, head nodding and smiles, body orientation and posture, some vocal cues, and physical distance between practitioners and clients.[8] Counselors can determine whether they are demonstrating desirable behaviors by asking someone to observe their nonverbal behaviors. Appendix B is a checklist that a third-party observer can mark while evaluating the counselor's nonverbal behavior. One word of caution: counselors should not try to apply these behaviors to themselves in a rigid way. Inflexible conformity to these behaviors can increase the counselor's tension in an interview, and clients will sense their nonverbal expression of that tension.

Verbal Communication

The counselor's knowledge and command of verbal skills can play an important part in directing the interview.

Conversational Style

Beginning counselors tend to fall into a kind of conversational mode that is very comfortable for them. Such a style is typical of a friendly chat with a neighbor. As a part of this conversation, they are under extreme pressure to provide an immediate solution for the client's problem.

Certain aspects of conversational style interfere with the objectives of counseling:[13]

- Informal "small talk": Responding to a client at the beginning of an interview with, "Did you see the diet recipes in today's paper?"
- Expressions of blame, criticism, or judgment: Client: "The diet has gone badly this week." Nutrition Counselor: "I can certainly see that from this weight graph." or "My goal for you is . . ."
- Expressions of advice offered in a preaching or self-righteous tone: "You should really learn to have more self-control with this diet," or "You really ought to lose 20 pounds."
- Expressions of sympathy in a patronizing tone: "I really feel sorry for you. You seem to get absolutely no support from your family in following this diet," or "Now that you've told me your problems with weight loss, I'm sure I can make you feel better."
- Threats or arguing: "You'd better follow the low-protein

eating pattern for your own good," or "I think your constant rejection of my suggestions is uncalled for."

- Rigidity or inflexibility: "There is only one right way to approach a low-cholesterol, fat-controlled eating pattern," or "Your suggestions won't work with a low-sodium diet."
- Overanalyzing, overinterpreting, or intellectualizing: "I think you find being overweight enjoyable, or you would follow the diet."
- Several questions at once: "How do you feel about following a low-cholesterol diet? Does it fit into your family life? If not, why isn't it working out? Could you tell me?"
- Extensive self-disclosure, sharing the counselor's own problems: "I've been thinking a lot about my weight loss attempts as you were talking. I, too, have had several problems. For instance. . . ."

Each of these examples illustrates the importance of using appropriate communication skills during a nutrition counseling session.

Cultural Values

Dietary behavioral change is directly tied to culture. A successful change may depend upon the relationship of the behavior to cultural values. In the text that follows Munoz and Luckmann provide the data to contrast American with several other cultures.[14]

In Asian cultures, group orientation is important in contrast to American ideals of independence, self-reliance, and individualism. The extended family is important in Asian cultures versus the nuclear or blended family found in American homes. The Asian culture places a high value on tradition. In American culture, the concept of innovation is prized. In Asian families, respect for elders and the past is emphasized versus respect for youth and the future in American value systems. The Asian value system focuses on conformity. In American families, the emphasis is often on competition.

In Hispanic culture, again, group orientation and extended family are important. Hispanic culture focuses on person-to-person orientation compared to American culture, in which person-to-object orientation is emphasized. Acceptance and resignation are characteristic of Hispanic values. In American culture these values are replaced with aggression and assertion. American culture also prizes self-determination contrasted with fatalism in Hispanic cultures. Americans live in the future; Hispanic lives revolve around the present.

African American values include family bonding, orientation in the present, matrifocus, and spiritual orientation. In contrast, Anglo American values emphasize individualism, future orientation, patrifocus, and personal mastery.

In Native American culture, the following characteristics are emphasized: bonding to family or group, sharing with others, present orientation, extended family cooperation, and acceptance of nature. In Anglo American culture, the following values are prized: individualism, accumulating for self, future orientation, nuclear family, competition, and mastery over nature.

Culture is very important in each individual's ability to be successful in making healthful behavioral changes. For example, when asking about how ready a person of Hispanic ethnicity is to make a change, the client's orientation may be focused on today. For this reason, the thought of making the change relates to the present not the future. When something happens in the future, that event may alter the ability to make a dietary change; reversion to past unhealthy behaviors is perfectly within the context of acceptable circumstances for this client living in Hispanic culture. This leaves an Anglo American counselor who does not understand Hispanic cultural values wondering why adherence is declining when originally the client was so sure that the change was possible. Our cultural values affect our beliefs, behavior and communication style.

Counselor-Client Focus Identification

Once nutrition counselors have altered their conversational style appropriately, there are several specific ways they can learn to provide direction and focus for an interview. Ivey delineates seven categories of subject focus:[1]

1. Focus on the client: "Laura, you sound upset. Could you tell me more about your feelings as you work to get your blood glucose levels in the 70–100 mg/dL range?"
2. Focus on the main theme or problem: "You had a terrible argument with your husband and then had a hypoglycemic

reaction (encourager for discussion). Could you tell me about your symptoms before having a hypoglycemic reaction (open question)?" Focusing on the person could lead the client to talk more about personal issues, whereas focusing on the main theme or problem encourages discussion of what happened and the facts of the situation. In both cases, listening skills combine with focusing to lead the client in very different directions. Which of the two alternatives is best? Both may be useful in obtaining a complete summary of the situation; at the same time, either could be overused.

3. Focus on others: The "others" might include the husband or other people in the client's life who affect dietary change.
4. Focus on family: Many times, client issues will relate to their families. In Hispanic families including family members in helping the client follow a diet can be very useful in maintaining dietary adherence.
5. Focus on mutual issues or a group: This focus involves the nutrition counselor and client relationship or the entire family.
6. Focus on the nutrition counselor: This focus includes self-disclosure or an "I" statement.
7. Focus on cultural/environmental/contextual issues: These are broader issues often not readily apparent, such as racial or sexual issues, family values, or economic trends. Examples of focus topics include issues of cultural identity, experiences of racism, sexism, or social class. Many clients also represent cultures of cancer survivors, people coping with other illnesses, or those suffering joblessness in a slow economy. People who experience issues such as these may manifest depression or other types of personal distress.[13]

In the North American culture, we are accustomed to making "I" statements and focusing on what an individual can do to help himself or herself. Counselors have to realize that this may clash with the world views of many minority people whose traditions focus on family. It may be hard for them to sever themselves from others in their family and just think of themselves. Their sense of self is often collective in nature, and their self-concept may be defined mainly in terms of others. A balanced focus is needed between individual, family, and cultural expectations.[14]

Listening Responses

Listening responses are the first step in forming a repertoire of communication skills involving clarifying, paraphrasing, reflecting, and summarizing.[15]

Clarifying

Clarification is posing a question, often after an ambiguous client message. Clarification may be used to make the previous message explicit and to confirm the accuracy of the counselor's perceptions of it. An example of incorrect use of clarification is:

Client: "I wish I didn't have to fill in those diet records. They seem so silly to me."
Counselor: "So, are you saying you don't like my diet aids?"
Client: "I like all of them and the record has been useful, but I just don't feel as though it is helping me at this point."

In the next example, a statement of clarification establishes exactly what was said without relying on assumptions and inferences that are not confirmed or explored:

Client: "I wish I didn't have to fill in those diet records. They seem so silly to me."
Counselor: "Are you saying that you don't see any purpose to filling in the diet record?"
Client: "No, I really don't. I just don't think I need them at this point."

Paraphrasing

Paraphrasing is restating or rephrasing the client's message in the counselor's own words. For example, the client says: "I don't mind eating low-protein foods at home, but my job requires that I travel one week of every month. It is impossible to follow the diet when eating in restaurants!" In paraphrasing, counselors can:

- restate the message to themselves;
- identify the content part of the message ("I don't mind eating low-protein foods at home," "My job requires one week of

travel a month," "It is impossible to follow the diet when eating in restaurants");

- translate the message into their own words ("You can follow the diet at home but have problems following it in restaurants.")

Reflecting (Reflective Listening)

Reflection of feelings is used to rephrase the affective part of the message. This form of listening response has three purposes: (1) to encourage expression of more feelings, (2) to help clients experience feelings more intensely so they can become aware of unresolved problems, and (3) to help clients become more aware of feelings that dominate them.

For example, a client comments: "I feel so depressed. Sometimes trying to match the foods I'm eating to insulin dosages seems useless." In reply, counselors can:

- restate the client's message to themselves;
- identify the affective part of the message ("I feel so depressed");
- translate the clients' affective words into their own words ("You sometimes feel frustrated with following the eating pattern for your diabetes.")

One word of caution: a reflection is more than just beginning a statement with the words "You feel . . ." It is a reflecting back of the emotional part of the message with appropriate affect words. (Commonly used affect words are listed in Table 2–1.)

Summarizing

The fourth listening response, summarization, requires extending the paraphrase and reflection responses. It is a rather complex skill that includes paying attention to both content and feelings. It also includes elements of purpose, timing, and effect of the statements (process). Brammer recommends the following guidelines for summarization:[15]

- Attend to major topics and emotions apparent as the client speaks.
- Summarize key ideas into broad statements.

Table 2–1   Commonly Used Affect Words

Happiness	Sadness	Fear	Uncertainty	Anger
Happy	Discouraged	Scared	Puzzled	Upset
Pleased	Disappointed	Anxious	Confused	Frustrated
Satisfied	Hurt	Frightened	Unsure	Bothered
Glad	Despairing	Defensive	Uncertain	Annoyed
Optimistic	Depressed	Threatened	Skeptical	Irritated
Good	Disillusioned	Afraid	Doubtful	Resentful
Relaxed	Dismayed	Tense	Undecided	Mad
Content	Pessimistic	Nervous	Bewildered	Outraged
Cheerful	Miserable	Uptight	Mistrustful	Hassled
Thrilled	Unhappy	Uneasy	Insecure	Offended
Delighted	Hopeless	Worried	Bothered	Angry
Excited	Lonely	Panicked	Disoriented	Furious

Source: From Cormier WH, Cormier LS. *Interviewing Strategies for Helpers: Fundamental Skills and Cognitive Behavioral Interventions.* Copyright © 1991, 1985, and 1975, Brooks/Cole Publishing Company, Pacific Grove, California 93950, a division of International Thomson Publishing Inc. By permission of the publisher.

- Do not add new ideas.
- Decide whether it is wise for you as a counselor to summarize or ask the client to summarize the broad themes, agreements, or plans.

To make this decision, counselors should review the purpose of the summarization:

- Was it to encourage the client at the beginning of the interview?
- Was it to bring scattered thoughts and feelings into focus?
- Was it to close the discussion on the major theme of the interview?
- Was it to check your understanding of the interview's progress?
- Was it to encourage the client to explore the basic theme of the interview more carefully?

- Was it to end the relationship with a progress summary?
- Was it to reassure the client that the interview was progressing well?[15]

Many summarization responses include references to both cognitive and affective messages:

Client: "I want to follow the diet we discussed, but so many things pull me toward food—parties, friends, my family, etc. Above all this, though, I know I want to see my blood cholesterol come down."

Counselor: "You feel torn. You want to reduce your blood cholesterol level, but sometimes you feel reluctant to avoid all of the people and things pulling you toward food" (summarization of emotion) or "You know that you do want to reduce your blood cholesterol level" (summarization of contents).

Action Responses

The previous listening responses deal primarily with the client's message from the client's point of view. For nutrition counseling to progress, the process must move beyond the client's point of view to use of responses based on counselor-generated data and perceptions. These are counselor directed and are labeled active responses. They involve a combination of counselor perceptions and hypotheses, and client messages and behaviors.[8]

The purpose of active responses is to help clients recognize the need for change and positive action in solving nutrition problems. Active replies include probing, attributing, confronting, and interpreting responses.[13]

Probing

In nutrition counseling, an important part of gathering information on clients' eating patterns involves the art of probing. Probing can involve both open and closed questions.[1] Initially, it should be aimed at eliciting the most information possible. The clients should feel free to respond at length on any problem that may limit adherence to the eating pattern. The most direct way to probe is to ask open-ended questions that begin with "what," "when," "how," "where," "could," or "who." Such questions require more than just "yes" or "no" responses. Probing has a variety of purposes, including the following:

- to begin an interview
- to encourage client elaboration or to obtain information
- to elicit specific examples of clients' nutrition-related behaviors, feelings, or thoughts
- to develop client commitment to communicate by inviting the client to talk and by providing guidance toward a focused interaction[8]

The first word of certain open questions can determine client responses. *What* questions most often lead to facts. "What happened?" "What are you going to do?" *How* questions often lead to a discussion about processes or sequences or to feelings. "How could that be explained?" "How do you feel about that?" *Could* questions are considered maximally open and contain some of the advantages of closed questions in that the client is free to say "No, I don't want to talk about . . ." *Could* questions reflect less control and command than others. "Could you tell me more about your situation?" "Could you give me a specific example?" "Could you tell me what you'd like to talk about today?"[1]

Once the clients have provided adequate information for assessment of the nutrition problem, counselors can help focus attention on central issues by using closed questions.[1] When the clients then have a focus on which to concentrate, open invitations to talk may be used again. In becoming skilled interviewers, counselors learn to use a balance of open and closed questions. Various types of interviews use different proportions of open and closed questions.

An example of the use of open-ended probes follows:

Client (a 25-year-old male who is trying to follow a 15 gram saturated fat eating pattern): "I really have problems getting my wife to cook meals low in saturated fat. She says she wants to cook the way her mother taught her. I feel really frustrated about everything."

Counselor: "What else do you think or feel frustrated about?" "How long have you been feeling this way?" "When are some specific times you feel frustrated?" "Who are you with when you feel frustrated?" "What do you do when you feel frustrated?" (It is important to pause for a response from the client after each question. Too many questions may make the counseling session seem like an inquisition.)

Counselors should keep in mind that extensive self-disclosure requests can be damaging to clients. Janis reports that seeking high self-disclosure or asking clients about material they would not usually share with other family members or friends has a detrimental effect on adherence to diet.[16] Asking the client personal questions about current and past sorrows, sex life, guilt feelings, secret longings, and similar private events can result in the client's becoming demoralized despite the counselor's positive comments and acceptance. In contrast, moderate levels of questions about feelings that focus on strengths as well as weaknesses enhance dietary adherence.[17]

After the client has discussed at length several specific frustrating instances, the counselor can focus the interview with closed probes such as:

- "Is your wife aware that you feel frustrated in these situations?"
- "Have you spoken to your wife about these frustrating instances?"
- "Can you speak with your wife about these problem situations?"
- "Do you see any solutions to this particular frustration?"

Attributing or Affirming

Attributing responses point to the client's current potential for being successful in a designated activity. This response has several purposes:

- to encourage the client who lacks initiative or self-confidence to do something
- to expand the client's awareness of personal strength
- to point out a potentially helpful client action[13]

In deciding whether to use this response, counselors focus on inferring how the client will react. Will the attributing response "reinforce the client's action-seeking behavior or the client's feelings of inadequacy?"[13] This response is facilitative only when there is a basis for recognizing the client's ability to pursue a desired action.

It is not simply a pep-talk to smooth over or discount true feelings of discouragement. Feelings should be reflected and clarified first. Finally, the attributing response should be used when the client is ready for action but seems hesitant to initiate a step without some encouragement. An example of an attributing response is as follows:

Client (a 30-year-old woman who has tried repeatedly to lose weight): "I'm really discouraged with trying to lose weight at this point. I feel like I can't do anything right. Not only has it affected me personally, but now it is affecting my family. I just don't feel I can do anything right."

Counselor: "Although you feel discouraged with weight loss right now, you still have those personal qualities you had when you lost weight before. I know that if you can recall what made your behavior change possible then, you will once again be very successful in achieving your healthful living goals."

Confronting

Ivey describes confrontation as a complex of skills resulting in a client's examination of core issues. It may be contained in a *paraphrase* ("You want to see good blood sugars, but you hate watching the amount of foods you eat at parties"), *a reflection of feeling* ("On the one hand, you are angry about having a disease that forces you to watch what you eat, but on the other hand, you are grateful that following an eating pattern can improve your blood sugars"), or any *other skills*. When client discrepancies, mixed messages, and conflicts are confronted skillfully and non-judgmentally, clients are encouraged to talk in more detail and resolve problems.[1]

A confronting response can be a descriptive statement of the client's mixed messages or an identification of an alternate view or perception of something the individual distorts. There are two intended purposes behind a confronting response: *to identify the client's mixed or distorted messages* and *to explore other ways of perceiving the client's self or situation.*[8]

Confronting responses can have very powerful effects. Counselors should keep several basic rules in mind before using them:

- Make the confronting response a description instead of a judgment or evaluation of the client's message or behavior.
- Cite specific examples of the behavior rather than making vague inferences.

- Prior to confronting the client, build rapport and trust.
- Offer the confrontation when the client is most likely to accept it.
- Do not overload the client with confrontations that make heavy demands in a short time.[8]

The timing of a confronting response is important. A confrontation should always take place at a time when clients do not feel threatened, not when it is totally unexpected. Adequate time for talking and listening should be provided in the interview.

Counselors' feelings also are important. Johnson clearly emphasizes confronting clients only if the practitioners are genuinely interested in improving the relationship,[18] never with the idea of punishing or criticizing clients. Before confronting, counselors should try to list their reasons for wanting to challenge discrepancies, distortions, or unproductive behaviors. Exhibit 2–1 describes eight components of effective confrontation by counselors.[18]

Clients' reactions to a confrontation vary. Ivey describes five types of reactions.

Denial. The client may deny that an incongruity or mixed message exists or fail to hear that it is there. ("I'm not angry about having to change my saturated fat intake. I do feel deprived, but definitely not angry.")

Partial examination. The individual may work on a part of the discrepancy but fail to consider the other dimensions of the mixed message. ("Yes, I feel deprived. Perhaps I should be angry, but I can't really feel it.")

Acceptance and recognition, but no change. The client may engage the confrontation fairly completely, but make no resolution. Much of counseling operates at this level or at level 2. Until the client can examine incongruity, immobility, and mixed messages accurately, developmental change will be difficult. ("I guess I do have mixed feelings about it. I certainly miss eating spontaneously. It makes me angry and I ask why I have to deal with this at a time when I want to do whatever I feel like doing.")

Generation of a new solution. The client moves beyond recognition of the incongruity and puts things together in a new and produc-

Exhibit 2–1 Components of Effective Confrontation

1. Personal statements: These opening statements usually begin with the pronoun "I." Included in this statement are expressions of feelings, attitudes, or opinions. Examples are:
   "There is something I've been hearing over and over in our conversation that I would like to speak to you about."
   "I have been confused during this session by something you've been saying."
2. Relationship statements: Define your relationship with the other person. An example is: "Lately we've been trying to work together to come up with some possible solutions to your binge eating."
3. Description of behavior: A description of a specific behavior would include specific time and place of occurrence. An example is: "From your description, binge eating occurs on weekends during parties."
4. Descriptions of your feelings and interpretations of the client's situation: An example: "I am confused when you say that you want to stop eating at parties, but you feel compelled to continue because of social pressure. There seem to be two messages here."
5. Understanding response: This ensures that what you have said is what the client has understood.
   Counselor: "Do you see what I mean?" "Is this the way you see things?"
   Client: "Yes."
6. Perception check: This is stated as a question to the client to double-check thoughts and feelings at this point.
   Counselor: "How do you feel about what I am saying?"
   Client: "I can see that I seem to be giving a mixed message. I want to lose weight, but there are always obstacles when I go to parties. Friends always ask me to eat; I feel compelled to say 'Yes'."
7. Interpretive response: This is a paraphrase of what the client said in 5 and 6. An example is: "From what you have said, you seem to feel this same confusion. You want to lose weight, but there is always someone pushing you to eat to be sociable."
8. Constructive feedback: This component of confrontation calls for working together for a solution. Alternatives are presented and weighed. The counselor, at this point, should allow the client to make suggestions on how to solve the problem. Examples are:
   "Can you think of a solution?"
   "This might be one solution. What else can we come up with?"
   "I'd like to talk about it again after we've thought about it for a while."

Source: From Johnson DW. Reaching Out: Interpersonal Effectiveness and Self-Actualization. Copyright © 1972 by Allyn and Bacon. Adapted with permission.

tive way. ("Yes, you've got it. I've been avoiding my deep feelings of anger, and I think it's getting in my way. If I'm going to move on, I'll have to allow myself to admit that I am angry.")

Transcendence. The client develops new, larger, and more inclusive constructs, patterns, or behaviors—moving beyond the original problem. A confrontation is most successful when the client recognizes the discrepancy, works on it, and generates new thought patterns or behaviors to cope with and perhaps resolve the incongruity. ("I like the plan we've worked out. You've helped me see that mixed feelings and thoughts are part of every change situation.")[1]

If clients seem confused about the meaning of the confrontation, the counselors may not have been specific or concise enough; or confessed lack of understanding may be a way of avoiding the impact of the confrontation.

Sometimes clients may seem to accept the confrontation. If they show a sincere desire to change behavior, their acceptance probably is genuine. However, they may agree verbally with the counselor but, instead of pursuing the confrontation, may do so only to entice the practitioner not to discuss the topic in the future.

There is no defined way to deal with negative reactions to a confrontation, but the components of effective confrontation (Exhibit 2–1) can be used to repeat the relationship statement or describe the counselor's own feelings and perceptions. The sequence might go like this:

Counselor: "Both of our goals are to help eliminate binge eating at parties." (relationship statement)
Client: "Actually, I'm not sure I can ever achieve that, even though I do want to lose weight." (mixed message)
Counselor: "You say you want to lose weight but one of the major causes is too difficult to overcome." (description of counselor feelings and perceptions)
Client: "No, I guess you just don't understand. You've never been in my shoes." (discredit the counselor)
Counselor: "Because I've never been in your shoes doesn't mean we can't work on a solution together. I have had experience with many cases like yours. You seem to exhibit many qualities that show me that you can handle this problem." (attributing statement) "You are open about the difficulties you face and can describe specific instances where problems occur."

(attributing statement) "Let's look at those specifics and try to come up with some solutions." (constructive feedback)

Ivey indicates that an overly confronting, charismatic counselor can prevent client growth.[1] In a confrontation, the counselor tries to point out discrepancies in attitudes, thoughts, or behaviors. Clients who come to nutrition counselors for help invariably give double messages: "I want to follow this diet, but I don't want to change my life to do it." Because almost all clients either overtly or covertly make this statement, confrontation becomes an important skill for nutrition counselors in facilitating behavior change.

Confrontation must be used with great sensitivity to individual and cultural differences. Within the United States and Canada, there are a variety of cultures and peoples who may object to strong confrontations. In regard to Native American, Canadian Inuit, and traditional Latina/Latino people, confrontational statements may not be helpful, particularly in the early stages of the helping process. Moreover, any individual who is particularly sensitive may prefer softer, more indirect confrontations.

Keeping caution in mind, any time the counselor can encourage clients to confront themselves and think about situations in new ways, the counselor can greatly facilitate growth. Some clients respond best to direct, assertive confrontations. Again, flexibility and the counselor's ability to respond to the unique person are essential. Also, motivational interviewing skills can be a value when clients are unsure of readiness to change (as discussed in Chapter 3).

Interpreting

An interpreting response is an active reply that gives a possible explanation of or association among various client behaviors. It has three intended purposes:

1. to identify the relationship between the client's behavior and nonverbal messages;
2. to examine the client's behavior using a variety of views or different explanations;
3. to help the client gain self-understanding as a basis for behavior change or action.

There are several specific ground rules for interpreting responses.[8]

Counselors must be careful about timing, and clients should demonstrate some degree of readiness for self-exploration or self-examination before an interpreting response is used. This response is best given at the beginning or middle phase of an interview so both the counselor and client have sufficient time to work through the client's reaction. It is important for the counselor's interpretation to be based on the client's actual message. Practitioners must eliminate their own biases and values and offer the interpretive response tentatively, using such words as, "I wonder if," "It's possible that," "Perhaps," or "Maybe." Finally, counselors ask clients whether the message is accurate.

Brammer offers these guidelines for counselors in interpreting responses:

- Look for the client's basic message.
- Paraphrase the message to the client.
- Add your own understanding of what the message means (motive, defense, needs, style, etc.).
- Keep the language simple and the level close to the client's message.
- Indicate that you are offering tentative ideas.
- Elicit the client's reactions to your interpretations.[15]

Ivey describes the interpreting response as a part of the essence of what the clients have said (emotionally and intellectually) and as a summary that adds other relevant data.[1] An interpreting response provides the client with a new way to view the situation. Such a change in view may result in changes in thoughts and behaviors.

The following is an interpreting response:

Client (an overweight middle-aged man): "I'm really discouraged with this dieting. I am at the point where I feel like I can't win. I've been to doctors and weight-loss groups. I've taken diet pills. It's at the point where I can't think straight at work because my thoughts are always on dieting. I feel very frustrated."

Counselor: "I wonder if you're allowing your preoccupation with weight loss to interfere with your ability to cope?" (This interpreting response makes an association between the client's desire to lose weight and resulting feelings and behavior.)

Or: "Is it possible that you're trying to find an easy, magic way to lose weight when that solution may not exist?" (This interpreting response offers a possible explanation of the client's weight-loss behaviors.)

The interpreting response can be a powerful influencer for clients who are locked into feelings of failure. It is a core skill that is vital to encouraging behavior change.

Sharing Responses

The sharing responses involve counselor self-expression and content that refers to the practitioner, the client, or the emotions of either one. Counselors can use two sharing responses: self-disclosure and immediacy.

Self-Disclosure

Self-disclosure is a response in which counselors verbally share information about themselves. Cormier and Cormier describe four purposes:

1. to provide an open, facilitative counseling atmosphere
2. to increase the client's perceived similarity between self and the counselor to reduce the distance resulting from role differences
3. to provide a model to assist in increasing the client's disclosure level
4. to influence the client's perceived or actual behavioral changes[8]

There are several basic ideas to keep in mind before using self-disclosure. First, self-disclosure is a controversial communication skill. Cormier, Cormier, and Weisser caution that if the counselor's beliefs differ significantly from the client's on a given issue, it is probably better for the counselor to remain silent.[3]

Ivey states that extensive self-disclosures take the focus away from the client and should be avoided, but that moderate levels of self-disclosure help show clients how they come across to others. For example, "Oh, I really have trouble resisting desserts, too. It's tough isn't it? But I figure it's worth it to resist them and work toward a normal weight."[1]

Moderate levels of self-disclosure help establish a basis for similarity and enhance interpersonal influence. Counselors who rarely self-disclose may add to the distance between themselves and their clients. Self-disclosing statements should be similar in content and mood to the clients' message. Self-disclosure can be demographic, personal, positive, or negative.

In demographic disclosures, counselors talk about non-intimate events. For example:

"I have had some failures in low-cholesterol meal preparation, also."
"I have not always used good self-control skills in following a balanced diet."

In personal disclosures, counselors reveal private personal events. For example:

"Well, I don't always feel loving toward my husband (wife), especially when he (she) is unsupportive of my efforts in meal preparation."
"I think it is very natural to want to please close friends. There are times when I've accepted food at parties when I really didn't want it, but I cared so much about the person offering it that I couldn't say 'no'. "

In positive self-disclosure, counselors reveal positive strengths, coping skills, or positive successful experiences. For example:

"I'm really a task-oriented person. When I decide what must be done, I work until the task is completed."
"It's important to be as open with my husband (wife) as possible. When he (she) upsets me, I try to tell him (her) honestly exactly how I feel."

In negative self-disclosure, counselors provide information about personal limitations or difficult experiences. For example:

"I also have trouble expressing opinions, I guess I am wishy-washy some of the time."
"Sometimes I'm also afraid to tell my husband (wife) how I really feel. Then my frustration builds to a climax and I just explode."

1. Personal pronouns. A counselor self-disclosure inevitably involves "I" statements or self-reference using the pronouns I, me, and my.

2. Verb for content or feeling or both. "I think . . . ," "I feel . . . ," and "I have experienced . . . " all indicate some action on the part of the counselor.
3. Object coupled with adverb and adjective descriptors. "I feel happy about your being able to assert yourself more directly in restaurants. My experience with asserting myself in restaurants was similar to yours."[1]

Two examples of self-disclosure can apply to the same situation: the client is feeling like a failure because no one supports weight loss. The counselor responds: "I, too, have felt down about myself at times," or "I can remember feeling frustrated when everyone seemed to take lightly something that was important to me, like eating a favorite dish at my favorite restaurant."

Immediacy

The second sharing response, immediacy, involves the counselor's reflections on a present aspect of a thought or feeling about self, clients, or a significant relationship issue. The verbal expression of immediacy may include the listening responses of reflection and summation, the active responses of confrontation and interpretation, or the sharing response of self-disclosure. Examples of the three categories of immediacy are:

1. Counselor immediacy: The counselor reveals personal thoughts of immediacy at the moment they occur: "It's good to see you again," or, "I'm sorry, I didn't follow that. I seem to have trouble focusing today. Let's go over that again."
2. Client immediacy: The counselor states something about the client's behavior or feeling as it occurs in the interview: "You seem uncomfortable now," or "You're really smiling now. You must be very pleased."
3. Relationship immediacy: The counselor reveals personal feelings or thoughts about experiencing the relationship: "I'm glad that you are able to share those feelings you have about following the diet with me," or, "It makes me feel good that we've been able to resolve some of the problems with your diet."

Immediacy has two purposes: first, it can bring expressed feelings or unresolved relationship issues into the open for discussion, and second, it can provide immediate feedback about the counselor's and client's feelings and aspects of the relationship as they occur in the session. When making an immediacy response, counselors should (1) describe what they see as it happens, (2) reflect the present the experience, and (3) reserve this response for initiating exploration of the most significant or most influential feelings or issues.

Teaching Repsonses

Much of nutrition counselors' work involves teaching clients how to change eating behaviors. Change means clients learn new ways to deal with themselves, others, or environmental situations. Counselors may teach new eating behaviors, new awareness or new perceptions of past and present behaviors, or methods by which clients can teach themselves. Three verbal responses associated with teaching and learning can give structure to what ordinarily might be haphazard teaching: instructions, verbal setting operations, and information giving.[13] Usually this response is used when clients are in the "action" stage of change as discussed in Chapter 3.

Instructions

Instructions involve one or more statements in which the counselors tell clients what changes in current intake are necessary to achieve new eating behaviors, how new eating behaviors might occur, and what the allowable limits are. When using instruction responses, counselors instruct, direct, or cue the clients to do something. Instructions may deal with what should happen within or outside the interview and can be both informing and influential. Instructions have two main purposes: (1) to influence or give cues to help clients respond in a certain way, and (2) to provide information necessary to acquire, strengthen, or eliminate a response.

After giving instructions, counselors should ascertain whether the clients really understand the directions. Clients are asked to repeat what was said to help the counselors know whether they communicated the message accurately. The counselors then ask clients to use the instructions.

Instructions can be worded in many ways. "You should do something" is likely to put a client on the defensive. It is too demanding. More useful words are "I'd like you to . . . ," "I'd appreciate it if . . . ," or "I think it would help if . . . ." Clients are more likely to follow instructions that are linked to positive or rewarding consequences.

Verbal Setting Operation

The second teaching response, the verbal setting operation, attempts to predispose someone to view a situation or an event in a certain way before it takes place. This response includes a statement describing a treatment and the potential value of counseling and/or treatment for clients. The purposes of verbal setting operations are to motivate clients to understand the purpose of and to use counseling and/or treatment.

Goldstein suggests that some initial counseling structure may prevent negative feelings in clients that result from lack of information about what to expect.[19] Initial structuring should focus upon and clarify counselor and client role expectations. This type of structuring should be detailed, deliberate, and repeated.

The following are examples of verbal setting operations:

- To provide an overview of nutrition counseling, the counselor says: "I believe it would be helpful if I first talked about what nutrition counseling involves. We will spend some time talking together to find out first the kinds of nutrition concerns you have and what you want to do about them. Then we will work as a team to identify solutions for each concern. Sometimes I may ask you to do some things on your own outside the session."
- To discuss the purpose of nutrition counseling, the counselor says: "These sessions may help you change eating behaviors to achieve weight loss. The action plans you'll carry out, with my assistance, can help you learn to eat wisely in situations that may be of concern to you."
- To check the client's understanding of nutrition counseling, the counselor asks: "How does this fit with your expectations?"

Information Giving

Much of the nutrition counselor's responsibility involves the third teaching response, information giving. Information giving should be done only when clients are in the "action" stage described in Chapter 3. Below are specific guidelines to follow when giving information:

- Identify information presently available to client.
- Evaluate client's present information. Is it valid? Are databases sufficient? Insufficient?

The following guidelines can be used in determining what information to give:

- Identify the kind of information useful to the client.
- Identify possible reliable sources of information.
- Identify any preferred sequencing of information (i.e., option A before option B).

The following guidelines indicate how to deliver information:

- Limit the amount of information given at one time.
- Ask for and discuss client's feelings and biases about information.
- Know when to stop giving information so action is not avoided.
- Wait for the client's cue of readiness for additional information after providing a group of facts.
- Present all relevant facts; don't protect client from negative information.
- Be specific, clear, detailed, concrete, concise, and simple in communicating and giving instructions.
- Organize the material. Information given in the first third of communication is remembered longer. The first instruction given is usually remembered the longest.
- Provide advanced organizers. (For example, "First, we will look at your current eating habits. Second, you will describe the changes you might make in the types of foods you currently eat.").
- Repeat important information.
- Use concrete illustrations, anecdotes, and self-disclosure to heighten the personal relevance of the material.

- Use oral and written material together. Supplement with slides, audiotapes, videotapes, films, anatomical models, diagrams, charts, and other aids.
- Check the client's comprehension, asking for a restatement of key features of a message.
- Involve significant others.[20–27]

Table 2-2 presents examples of information giving both inside and outside a nutrition counseling session.

Choosing the Appropriate Response

One of the most important processes in counseling involves deciding when to use the responses just described. Steps toward determining appropriate responses include: (1) identification of the purposes of the interview and of the counselor responses and (2) assessment of the potential effects of the selected replies and strategies on client answers and outcomes. When one response or strategy does not achieve its intended purpose, the counselor can use

Table 2–2   Aspects of Information Giving

Counselor's Instructions	In the Interview	Outside the Interview
What to do	"Please repeat what I have asked you to do in responding to your husband's (wife's) nonsupportiveness toward your diet. I want to be sure I am communicating the request accurately."	"Please keep a record of your thoughts before your conversations with your husband (wife)."
How to do	"When you say this, pretend that I am your husband (wife). Look at me and maintain eye contact while you say it."	"Write your thoughts down on a note card and bring them in next week."
Allowable limits	"Say it in a strong, firm voice. Don't speak in a soft, weak voice. Look at me while you say it."	"Remember to record these thoughts before, not after, you speak."

discrimination to identify and select another that is more likely to achieve the desired results or focus.

Cormier and Cormier describe three parts of an interview that can be used in determining which responses or strategies to select:

1. Counselor identifies purposes of the interview and responses.
2. Counselor selects and implements the response.
3. Counselor determines if resulting client verbal and nonverbal responses achieve the purpose or distract from the purpose.[13]

These authors also describe a step-by-step process for counselors in conducting an effective interview:

1. Define the purpose of the interview.
2. Define the purpose of your initial response.
3. Make your initial response.
4. Identify client verbal and nonverbal responses.
5. Label those client responses as goal related or distracting.
6. Set a plan for the next response.[13]

The nutrition counselor's first step is to listen carefully to each of the client's statements. The counselor must think about whether each statement is related to or distracts from the purpose of the interview. Having made this determination, the counselor can select and use responses he or she believes will achieve the objective. If client responses are goal-related, practitioners may decide that their own replies and comments are on target; however, if they note several statements that are distracting, it may be necessary to analyze what they have been saying.

For example, one of the major goals of a counseling session may be to identify steps to help change eating behaviors in an overweight adult male. The counselor has suggested cutting down on midmorning snacking by switching from high-calorie snack foods that are low in nutrients to low-calorie, high-nutrient foods. The client indicates that this change will not work for him. After determining that this is a distracting client response, the practitioner will need to formulate and use an alternate response, perhaps a new action step. Regardless of what that next response is, the important point is that the counselor can identify a purpose or direction, assess whether the client's answers are related to that goal, and select alternative replies with a rationale in mind. Counselors should make these assessments cognitively. This step-by-step procedure should be used in thinking through an interview.

What follows is an example of how those steps might apply in a nutrition counseling session in which the purpose of the interview is to listen to the client (a 26-year-old woman) describe factors contributing to her inability to lose weight over the past two years.

Counselor: "According to your chart, Dr. B. sent you to see me again today. He writes here that you've been trying to lose weight and need some help in determining what factors have contributed to the lack of weight loss. Is that correct?" (The purpose of the initial response is to double-check the client's rationale for attending the interview.)

Client (fidgeting): "Well, that's true. Sometimes I think that all I have to do is to look at food and I gain weight."

(Counselor thinks: The client admits that she has a weight problem (indirectly). She seems to be discounting the contributing factors (distracting response). In frustration, she tries to absolve herself from blame by attributing her problem to some unknown phenomenon that makes her gain weight at the very sight of food. For my next response I will check her thoughts as to her control over the weight gain.)

Counselor: "From what you have said you seem to think that your weight gain is out of your control. How well does that describe what you are thinking?"

Client: "Well, sometimes I feel that way, but I suppose I do have some control."

(Counselor thinks: Okay, the client is now admitting to having some control. I will focus next on areas where she may feel she has some control.)

Counselor: "What are some areas related to your weight gain that you do feel you can control?"

Client: "Well, I guess I could just stop buying groceries."

(Counselor thinks: She either did not understand my question or she is feeling defensive about having to discuss situations where she might have control but doesn't exercise the option. My next response will focus on the idea of shopping and I will give her some examples using a self-disclosing response.)

Counselor: "Well, sometimes when I go shopping and I'm very hungry, I tend to buy more food and high-calorie snacks."

Client (voice pitch goes up, tone gets louder): "How would you know what it's like to go shopping and want foods you shouldn't have? You're not overweight."

(Counselor thinks: My example seemed to make the client avoid the issue of contributing factors even more. She seems to have built up a great deal of frustration. Perhaps exploring her feelings about grocery buying might give me some clues. I will respond to her question and then direct the focus to her concern about buying groceries.)

Counselor: "I really can't know what it's like to be in your shoes. I can only express a situation similar to yours that I have been in. I guess buying groceries is a very important concern for you because it is tied so closely to your desire to lose weight. What feelings do you have while you're shopping?"

Client (loud voice): "I feel like a child in a candy store. Here is everything I love, everything that gives me pleasure, but I am forbidden to touch any of it. Then my kids and my husband are saying, 'Oh, go on honey (or mom) buy it; we love it. We shouldn't have to suffer just because you don't have any willpower.'"

(Counselor thinks: That's the most verbal she has been. It's the first indication that she is willing to explore the situation. It seems that one of the factors contributing to her lack of ability to lose weight is her non-supportive husband and children. I might check this theory out further.)

Counselor: "Are you saying that your family really doesn't give you a lot of support in losing weight?"

Client: "Yes. Being overweight is bad enough but, when your own family gives you no support, losing weight is almost impossible."

(Counselor thinks: The client seems to feel very strongly about this lack of family support. I will try to get at how this affects the way she feels in specific situations where nonsupport is apparent.)

Counselor: "Having your family respond negatively when you try to buy low-calorie foods and avoid high-calorie snacks seems to make you feel very frustrated. You would like them to praise your efforts. I guess having your family reject your efforts at weight loss may affect the way you see yourself, too."

Client (avoids eye contact): "What do you mean?"

(Counselor thinks: From the lack of eye contact and the client's verbal message, I believe either my response was unclear or she isn't ready to look at her self-image yet. I will approach this indirectly by asking her to describe some situations in which she has felt frustrated by lack of support from her family.)

Counselor: "Well, I'm not sure. Maybe you could tell me exactly what happens in a situation where your family is non-supportive."

At this point the interview enters the area where additional counseling skills are necessary. Chapter 3 discusses those skills and how they can help nutrition counselors in formulating plans and applying strategies during interviews.

References

1. Ivey AE. *Intentional Interviewing and Counseling: Facilitating Client Development in a Multicultural Society*, 3rd ed. Pacific Grove, CA: Brooks/Cole Publishing, 1994.
2. Russell ML. *Behavioral Counseling in Medicine: Strategies for Modifying At-Risk Behavior*. New York: Oxford University Press, 1986.
3. Cormier LS, Cormier WH, Weisser RJ. *Interviewing and Helping Skills for Health Professionals*. Belmont, CA: Wadsworth Health Sciences Division, 1984.
4. Nelson-Jones R. *Lifeskills Helping: Helping Others Through a Systematic People Centered Approach*. Pacific Grove, CA: Brooks/Cole Publishing, 1993.
5. Lask B. Patient-clinician conflict: causes and compromises. *J Cyst Fibros* 2003;2(1):42–45.
6. Jung HP, Wensing M, Olesen F, Grol R. Comparison of patients' and general practitioners' evaluations of general practice care. *Qual Saf Health Care* 2002;11(4):315–319.
7. Cooper-Patrick L, Gallo JJ, Gonzales JJ, et al. Race, gender, and partnership in the patient-physician relationship. *JAMA* 1999;282(6):583–589.
8. Cormier WH, Cormier LS. *Interviewing Strategies for Helpers, Fundamental Skills and Cognitive Behavioral Intervention*, 2nd ed. Monterey, CA: Brooks/Cole Publishing, 1985.
9. Carkhuff RR, Pierce RM. *The Art of Helping: Trainer's Guide*. Amherst, MA: Human Resources Development Press, 1975.
10. Egan G. *The Skilled Helper: A Problem Management Approach to Helping*. Pacific Grove, CA: Brooks/Cole Publishing, 1994.

11. Passons WR. *Gestalt Approaches in Counseling.* New York: Rinehart and Winston, 1975.
12. Sue DW. Culture specific strategies in counseling: a conceptual framework. *Prof Psychol Res Pract* 1990;21(6):426.
13. Cormier WH, Cormier LS. *Interviewing Strategies for Helpers: A Guide to Assessment, Treatment and Evaluation.* Monterey, CA: Brooks/Cole Publishing, 1979.
14. Munoz C, Luckmann J. *Transcultural Communication in Nursing,* 2nd ed. Clifton Park, NY: Delmar Learning, 2005.
15. Brammer LM. *Helping Relationship Process and Skills.* Englewood Cliffs, NJ: Prentice-Hall, 1985.
16. Janis IL. Improving adherence to medical recommendations: prescriptive hypotheses derived from recent research in social psychology. In: Baum A, ed. *Handbook of Psychology and Health,* Vol. 4. Hillsdale, NJ: Erlbaum, 1984:113–148.
17. Dimatteo MR, DiNicola DD. *Achieving Patient Compliance: The Psychology of the Medical Practitioner's Role.* New York: Pergamon Press, 1982.
18. Johnson DW. *Reaching Out: Interpersonal Effectiveness and Self-Actualization.* Englewood Cliffs, NJ: Prentice-Hall, 1972.
19. Goldstein AP. Relationship-enhancement methods. In: Kanfer FH, ed. *Helping People Change.* New York: Pergamon Press, 1975:18.
20. Warpeha A, Harris J. Combining traditional and nontraditional approaches to nutrition counseling. *J Am Diet Assoc* 1993;93(7):797–800.
21. Baldwin TT, Falciglia GA. Application of cognitive behavioral theories to dietary change in clients. *J Am Diet Assoc* 1995;95(11):1315–1317.
22. Johnston JM, Jansen GR, Anderson J, Kendall P. Comparison of group diet instruction to a self-directed education program for cholesterol reduction. *J Nutr Edu* 1994;26:140–145.
23. Dunbar J. Adhering to medical advice: a review. *Int J Mental Health* 1980;9:70–87.
24. Eraker SA, Kirscht JP, Becker MH. Understanding and improving patient compliance. *Ann Intern Med* 1984;100(2):258–268.
25. Leventhal H, Zimmerman R, Gutmann M. Compliance: A self-regulation perspective. In: Gentry WD, ed. *Handbook of Behavioral Medicine.* New York: Guilford Press, 1984:369–435.
26. Ley P. Giving information to patients. *Social Psychology and Behavioral Medicine.* New York: Wiley, 1982:339–373.
27. Turk DC, Holzman AD, Kerns RD. Chronic pain. In: Holroyd KA, Creer TL, eds. *Self-Management of Chronic Disease: Handbook of Clinical Interventions and Research.* Orlando, FL: Academic Press, 1986:446.

Evaluation Tool 2–1   Client Nonverbal Behavior Checklist

Behaviors	Description of Counselor–Client Interaction	Possible Effect or Meanings
KINESICS		
Eyes		
Direct eye contact	Client has just shared concern with counselor. Counselor responds; client maintains eye contact.	Readiness or willingness for interpersonal communication or exchange; attentiveness
Lack of sustained eye contact	Each time counselor brings up the topic of client's family, client looks away. Client demonstrates intermittent breaks in eye contact while conversing with counselor.	Withdrawal or avoidance of interpersonal exchange; or respect or deference. Respect or deference
	Client mentions sexual concerns, then abruptly looks away. When counselor initiates this topic, client looks away again.	Withdrawal from topic of conversation; discomfort or embarrassment; or preoccupation
Lowering eyes—looking down or away	Client talks at some length about alternatives to present job situation. Pauses briefly and looks down. Then resumes speaking and eye contact with counselor.	Preoccupation
Staring or fixating on person or object	Counselor has just asked client to consider consequences of a certain decision. Client is silent and gazes at a picture on the wall.	Preoccupation; possibly rigidness or uptightness; pondering; difficulty in finding an answer
Darting eyes or blinking rapidly—rapid eye movements; twitching brow	Client indicates desire to discuss a topic yet is hesitant. As counselor probes, client's eyes move around the room rapidly.	Excitation or anxiety; or wearing contact lenses
Squinting or furrow on brow	Client has just asked counselor for advice. Counselor explains role and client squints, and furrows appear in client's brow.	Thought or perplexity; or avoidance of person or topic

continued

Evaluation Tool 2–1   *continued*

Behaviors	Description of Counselor– Client Interaction	Possible Effect or Meanings
Eyes		
	Counselor suggests possible things for client to explore in difficulties with parents. Client doesn't respond verbally; furrow in brow appears.	Avoidance of person or topics
Moisture or tears	Client has just reported recent death of father; tears well up in client's eyes.	Sadness; frustration; sensitive area of concern
	Client reports real progress during past week in marital communication; eyes get moist.	Happiness
Eye shifts	Counselor has just asked client to remember significant events in week; client pauses and looks away; then responds and looks back.	Processing or recalling material; or keen interest; satisfaction
Pupil dilation	Client discusses spouse's sudden disinterest and pupils dilate.	Alarm; or keen interest
	Client leans forward while counselor talks and pupils dilate.	Keen interest; satisfaction
Mouth Smiles	Counselor has just asked client to report positive events of the week. Client smiles, then recounts some of these instances.	Positive thought, feeling, or action in content of conversation; or greeting
	Client responds with a smile to counselor's verbal greeting at beginning of interview.	Greeting
Tight lips (pursed together)	Client has just described efforts at sticking to a difficult living arrangement. Pauses and purses lips together.	Stress or determination; anger or hostility

Evaluation Tool 2-1 *continued*

Behaviors	Description of Counselor– Client Interaction	Possible Effect or Meanings
Mouth		
	Client has just expressed irritation at counselor's lateness. Client sits with lips pursed together while counselor explains the reasons.	Anger or hostility
Lower lip quivers or biting of lip	Client starts to describe her recent experience of being laughed at by colleagues at work because she is trying hard to follow her new eating pattern. As client continues to talk, her lower lip quivers; occasionally she bites her lip.	Anxiety, sadness, or fear
	Client discusses loss of parental support after a recent divorce. The problems associated with this home situation make following a new eating pattern difficult. Client bites her lip after discussing this.	Sadness
Open mouth without speaking	Counselor has just expressed feelings about a block in the relationship. Client's mouth drops open; client says was not aware of it.	Surprise; or suppression of yawn–fatigue
	It has been a long session. As counselor talks, client's mouth parts slightly.	Suppression of yawn– fatigue
Facial Expressions		
Eye contact with smiles	Client talks very easily and smoothly, occasionally smiling; maintains eye contact for most of session.	Happiness or comfortable- ness
Eyes strained; furrow on brow; mouth tight	Client has just reported strained situation with a spouse who dislikes her efforts to cut down on fat intake. Client then sits with lips pursed together and frowns.	Anger; or concern; sadness

continued

Evaluation Tool 2–1   *continued*

Behaviors	Description of Counselor–Client Interaction	Possible Effect or Meanings
Facial Expressions		
Eyes rigid, mouth rigid (unanimated)	Client states: "I have nothing to say"; there is no evident expression or alertness on client's face.	Preoccupation; anxiety; fear
Head		
Nodding head up and down	Client has just expressed concern over own health status and what the new eating pattern will do to improve health; counselor reflects client's feelings. Client nods head and says "That's right."	Confirmation; agreement; or listening, attending
	Client nods head during counselor explanation.	Listening; attending
Shaking head from left to right	Counselor has just suggested that client's continual lateness to sessions may be an issue that needs to be discussed. Client responds with "No," and shakes head from left to right.	Disagreement; or disapproval
Hanging head down, jaw down toward chest	Counselor initiates topic of termination. Client lowers head toward chest, then says, "I am not ready to stop the counseling sessions."	Sadness; concern
Shoulders		
Shrugging	Client reports that spouse just walked out with no explanation. Client shrugs shoulders while describing this.	Uncertainty; or ambivalence
Leaning forward	Client has been sitting back in the chair. Counselor discloses something personal; client leans forward and asks counselor a question about the experience.	Eagerness; attentiveness; openness to communication

Evaluation Tool 2–1 *continued*

Behaviors	Description of Counselor–Client Interaction	Possible Effect or Meanings
Shoulders		
Slouched, stooped, rounded, or turned away from person	Client reports feeling inadequate and defeated because of snacking; slouches in chair after saying this.	Sadness or ambivalence; or lack of receptivity to interpersonal exchange
	Client reports difficulty in talking. As counselor pursues this, client slouches in chair and turns shoulders away from counselor.	Lack of receptivity to interpersonal exchange
Arms and Hands		
Arms folded across chest	Counselor has just initiated conversation. Client doesn't respond verbally; sits back in chair with arms crossed against chest.	Avoidance of interpersonal exchange; or dislike
Trembling and fidgety hands	Client expresses fear of weight gain; hands tremble while talking about this.	Anxiety or anger
	In a loud voice, client expresses resentment; client's hands shake while talking.	Anger
Fist clenching of objects or holding hands tightly	Client has just come in for initial interview. Says that he or she feels uncomfortable; hands are closed together tightly.	Anxiety or anger
	Client expresses hostility toward husband; clenches fists while talking.	Anger
Arms unfolded—arms and hands gesturing in conversation	Counselor has just asked a question; client replies and gestures during reply.	Accenting or emphasizing point in conversation; or openness to interpersonal exchange
	Counselor initiates new topic. Client readily responds; arms are unfolded at this time.	Openness to interpersonal exchange
Rarely gesturing, hands and arms stiff	Client arrives for initial session. Responds to counselor's questions with short answers. Arms are kept down at side.	Tension or anger

continued

Evaluation Tool 2–1   *continued*

Behaviors	Description of Counselor–Client Interaction	Possible Effect or Meanings
Arms and Hands		
	Client has been referred; sits with arms down at sides while explaining reasons for referral and irritation at being here.	Anger
Legs and Feet		
Legs and feet appear comfortable and relaxed	Client's legs and feet are relaxed without excessive movement while client freely discusses personal concerns.	Openness to interpersonal exchange; relaxation
Crossing and uncrossing legs repeatedly	Client is talking rapidly in bursts about problems; continually crosses and uncrosses legs while doing so.	Anxiety; depression
Foot-tapping	Client is tapping feet during a lengthy counselor summary; client interrupts counselor to make a point.	Anxiety; impatience—wanting to make a point
Legs and feet appear stiff and controlled	Client is open and relaxed while talking about job. When counselor introduces topic of marriage, client's legs become more rigid.	Uptightness or anxiety; closed to extensive interpersonal exchange
Total Body		
Facing other person squarely or leaning forward	Client shares a concern and faces counselor directly while talking; continues to face counselor while counselor responds.	Openness to interpersonal communication and exchange
Turning of body orientation at an angle, not directly facing person, or slouching in seat	Client indicates some difficulty in "getting in to" interview. Counselor probes for reasons; client turns body away.	Less openness to interpersonal exchange
Rocking back and forth in chair or squirming in seat	Client indicates a lot of nervousness about an approaching conflict situation. Client rocks as this is discussed.	Concern; worry; anxiety

Evaluation Tool 2–1 *continued*

Behaviors	Description of Counselor– Client Interaction	Possible Effect or Meanings
Total Body		
Stiff—sitting erect and rigidly on edge of chair	Client indicates some uncertainty about direction of interview; sits very stiff and erect.	Tension; anxiety; concern

PARALINGUISTICS

Behaviors	Description of Counselor– Client Interaction	Possible Effect or Meanings
Voice Level and Pitch		
Whispering or inaudibility	Client has been silent for a long time. Counselor probes; client responds, but in a barely audible voice.	Difficulty in disclosing
Pitch changes	Client is speaking at a moderate voice level while discussing job. Then client begins to talk about unsupportive friends at work and voice pitch rises considerably.	Topics of conversation have different emotional meanings
Fluency in Speech		
Stuttering, hesitations, speech errors	Client is talking rapidly about feeling uptight in certain social situations; client stutters and makes some speech errors while doing so.	Sensitivity about topic in conversation; or anxiety and discomfort
Whining or lisp	Client is complaining about having a hard time losing weight; voice goes up like a whine.	Dependency or emotional emphasis
Rate of speech slow, rapid, or jerky	Client begins interview talking slowly about a bad weekend. As topic shifts to client's feelings about self, client talks more rapidly.	Sensitivity to topics of conversation; or topics have different emotional meanings
Silence	Client comes in and counselor invites client to talk; client remains silent.	Reluctance to talk; or preoccupation
	Counselor has just asked client a question. Client pauses and thinks over a response.	Preoccupation; or desire to continue speaking after making a point; thinking about how to respond

continued

Evaluation Tool 2–1 *continued*

Behaviors	Description of Counselor–Client Interaction	Possible Effect or Meanings
Fluency in Speech		
	A Chinese client talks about own family. Pauses; then resumes conversation to talk more about the same subject	Desire to continue speaking after making a point
Autonomic Responses		
Clammy hands, shallow breathing, sweating, pupil dilation, paleness, blushing, rashes on neck	Client discusses the exciting prospect of having two desirable job offers. Breathing becomes faster and client's pupils dilate.	Arousal—positive (excitement, interest) or negative (anxiety, embarrassment)
	Client starts to discuss binge eating; breathing becomes shallow and red splotches appear on neck.	Anxiety, embarrassment
PROXEMICS		
Distance		
Moves away	Counselor has just confronted client; client moves back before responding verbally.	Signal that space has been invaded; increased arousal, discomfort
Moves closer	Midway through session, client moves chair toward helper.	Seeking closer interaction, more intimacy
Position in Room		
Sits behind or next to an object in the room, such as table or desk	A new client comes in and sits in a chair that is distant from counselor.	Seeking protection or more space
Sits near counselor without any intervening objects	A client who has been in to see counselor before sits in chair closest to counselor.	Expression of adequate comfort level

Source: From Cormier WH, Cormier LS. *Interviewing Strategies for Helpers: Fundamental Skills and Cognitive Behavioral Interventions.* Copyright © 1991, 1985, and 1975, Brooks/Cole Publishing Company, Pacific Grove, California 93950, a division of International Thomson Publishing Inc. By permission of the publisher.

CHAPTER 3

COUNSELING SKILLS TO FACILITATE SELF-MANAGEMENT

Chapter Objectivs

1. List the stages through which clients pass in the course of changing a behavior within step 3, intervention, in the nutrition care process.

2. Describe each stage.

3. Apply the skills described in assessing the readiness-to-change stages.

4. Apply scaling by using the adherence thermometer to evaluate motivation, confidence, and readiness-to-change in a variety of nutrition situations where adherence may be a problem.

5. Apply eight motivational strategies to nutrition-related adherence problems.

6. Apply the stages of change to goal setting by asking appropriate questions.

This chapter describes ways in which nutrition counselors motivate people to change. The secret to change lies in self-management. Emphasis is on client responsibility for behavior and for planning the future. This type of counseling is highly individualized and evolves over time. It is not a short-term intervention emphasizing only education. At the core of the counseling situation is the counselor/client relationship.[1,2]

The nutrition counselor sets up an environment that is a transient support system that prepares the client to handle social and personal demands more effectively. The nutrition counselor's role is to provide the most favorable conditions for change.[3]

Within the nutrition care process, counseling skills in the assessment step and then eventual diagnosis step, items in the Behavioral/ Environmental category (Exhibit 3–1) often will be important as the client has difficulties in adhering to a dietary regimen. Then, beyond the assessment and diagnosis steps, the intervention will require an understanding of the staging process. Success in navigating through the nutrition care process is based on the level of counseling skills possessed by the nutrition counselor. Without appropriate skills the nutrition counselor is merely an information provider not a behavioral change facilitator.

The Stages of Change

Communication skills discussed in Chapter 2 provide a basis for facilitating a state of readiness or eagerness to change. DiClemente and Prochaska describe a model of how change occurs.[4] They describe a series of six stages through which people pass in the course of changing a behavior:

Exhibit 3–1   Step 1, Diagnosis, Behavioral, and Environmental Category

Behavioral–Environmental   **NB**
Defined as "nutritional findings/problems identified that relate to knowledge, attitudes/beliefs, physical environment, access to food, or food safety"[1]

• Food and nutrition-related deficit	NB-1.1
• Harmful beliefs/attitudes about food or nutrition-	NB-1.2
related topics (use with caution)	NB-1.3
• Not ready for diet/lifestyle change	NB-1.4
• Self-monitoring deficit	NB-1.5
• Disordered eating pattern	NB-1.6
• Limited adherence to nutrition-related	NB-1.7
recommendations	
• Undesirable food choices	NB-1.7

[1]**Knowledge and Beliefs:** Defined as "actual knowledge and beliefs as related, observed, or documented"

1. precontemplation
2. contemplation
3. preparation
4. action
5. maintenance

Miller and Rollnick illustrate the Prochaska–DiClemente model with the concept that a client may move in and out of stages with a kind of spiral affect as shown in Figure 3–1.[5]

The spiral indicates that it is normal for everyone involved in changing eating habits to go around the process several times before achieving stable changes. In research with smokers, Prochaska and DiClemente found that smokers ordinarily went around the spiral between three and seven times (with an average of four) before finally quitting completely. This wheel recognizes relapses in changing behaviors as a normal stage in change. Knowing this, the self-managing client avoids feeling disheartened when relapse occurs. By distinguishing different stages of readiness for change, the nutrition counselor approaches clients differently, depending

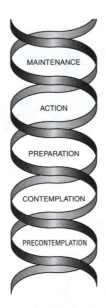

FIGURE 3–1 A Spiral Model of the Stages of Change. From Miller WR, Rollnick S. *Motivational Interviewing: Preparing People for Change*, 2nd ed. New York: Guilford Press, 2002.

on where they are in the process of change.[6] Each stage requires a different skill. Problems of clients being unmotivated or resistant occur when a nutrition counselor uses inappropriate strategies for a client's current stage of change. Figure 3–1 illustrates these stages and how they relate to and occur in an actual nutrition-counseling situation. Figure 3–2 shows tasks that are important in each stage as the nutrition counseling process occurs.

Precontemplation

As illustrated in Figure 3–1, the entry point to the process of change is the precontemplation stage. This is the point at which the client has not even contemplated having a problem or needing to make a change. Statements like, "I'm not interested in what I eat," may be common. A person in the precontemplative stage needs information and feedback to raise his or her awareness of the problem and possibility of change. Nutrition advice for eating changes is counterproductive at this point.[7] Tasks within this stage of change are aimed at consciousness-raising.[8]

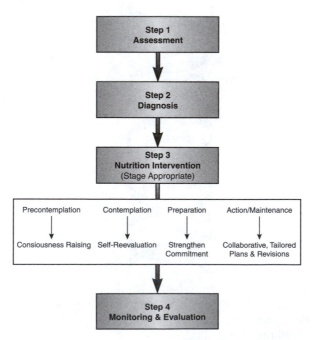

FIGURE 3–2   Nutrition Care Process with Stages of Change and Key Tasks.

To raise consciousness, the nutrition counselor uses concepts and skills discussed in Chapter 2 to involve the client in discovering what is important in his/her life and how that relates to the nature of the dietary problem. Self-reevaluation is one aspect of consciousness-raising that asks the client to envision how he/she might be different once the dietary problem behavior is overcome. The client is asked to determine when and how the problem behavior conflicts with personal values. Often the process of self-reevaluation may strike an emotional chord that arouses very deep feelings of the importance of making a lifestyle change. When the client recalls an emotional experience related to a dietary problem, this act of remembering allows for a greater awareness of defenses against change. Through this process, the client moves from precontemplation to contemplation.

Contemplation

Once some awareness of the problem arises, the person enters a period of ambivalence: the contemplation stage. The contemplator considers change and rejects it. As nutrition counselors listen to the contemplator, they hear reasons for concern and justification for excitement if change were to happen. This is a normal and characteristic stage of change, although sometimes it is erroneously attributed to pathological personality traits or defense mechanisms. The contemplator seesaws between reasons to change and reasons to stay the same. A person who falls into this stage may say the following: "I really do eat low-fat foods most of the time. Probably I do eat out too often, but my friends and my husband always talk me into going to high-fat restaurants. But at home I do a really good job. It is just that lately we seem to eat out all of the time."

The nutrition counselor's task at this stage is to help tip the balance in favor of change. This is the most common stage for clients to come to the nutrition counselor for assistance in changing eating behaviors. A nutrition counselor who launches into strategies appropriate for the action stage at this point is likely to engender resistance. However, working on advantages and disadvantages to continuing or discontinuing a nutrition therapy may help the client see change differently.

An example of how a counselor might facilitate change in a client moving from precontemplation to contemplation is presented below.

Counselor: Hi, Ellen, it's nice to see you again. The last time you were here, you were considering smaller, more frequent meals to help you get your blood sugars under better control. Today, if it's OK with you, I thought we might continue this discussion.

Ellen: That's OK, but I've been too busy to really make any changes.

Counselor: So your busy schedule might make this kind of change difficult?

Ellen: Yes, I thought about what we discussed last time, but so many things got in the way.

Counselor: If you are willing, might we make a list of the disadvantages and advantages of eating smaller, more frequent meals?

Ellen: Sure.

Counselor: Let's start with the negatives. You mentioned your busy schedule. What are some of the other downsides to changing the way you eat?

Ellen: If I start eating earlier in the day, it seems to make me hungrier, and then I eat too much.

Counselor: So eating more frequently makes you hungrier and more likely to overeat.

Ellen: Right; it's like once I start, I can't stop.

Counselor: OK, what else?

Ellen: I've eaten whenever I want all my life, and to tell you the truth I'm not ready to let diabetes rule my life.

Counselor: You resent being asked to change your eating schedule because of diabetes.

Ellen: Yes, it doesn't really seem fair, and it constantly reminds me that I have something wrong.

Counselor: OK, Ellen, let me see if I understand the negative side of changing. It's difficult to adjust your frequency of eating because of time constraints, you are concerned about a tendency to overeat, and it's a constant reminder that you have diabetes.

Ellen: (nods head)

Counselor: Now let's take a few minutes to explore the positives. What do you see as some benefits to eating more frequently?

Ellen: Well, maybe I'd have more energy. Mornings are especially hard—I just can't seem to get going.

Counselor: So eating more frequently might increase your energy—what else?

Ellen: The structure of eating more frequently would probably help me remember to take my pills better too. I usually get them in, but sometimes I forget.

Counselor: So eating more frequently could make it easier to remember to take your medications. Other benefits? (Pause)

Ellen: Well, as you know, my doctor mentioned it would help improve my blood sugar levels. I know good blood sugar control is important to prevent diabetic complications.

Counselor: So diabetic complications concern you.

Ellen: Yes, my father had diabetes, and towards the end his eyesight got so bad he wasn't able to drive. That was really devastating to him, and things went downhill from there.

Counselor: So you don't want to end up like your father.

Ellen: Yes, I have my grandchildren to think of; I want to stay well enough so that I can go to all their ball games and dance recitals. I want to be a fun grandma who can do things with them, not someone who sits on the sidelines.

Counselor: Taking care of your health is important so you can maintain your quality of life.

Ellen: Yes, I want to be able to do the things I want to do.

Counselor: OK, let me see if I got this right, Ellen. On the one hand making changes in the way you eat is difficult because of your busy schedule. You're concerned that eating more frequently may increase your hunger encouraging you to overeat, and you resent the demands your diabetes is making on your life. On the other hand, eating more frequently might give you more energy and help you take your medications more regularly. It would also promote better blood sugar control which would help prevent diabetic complications like loss of vision so you could continue to do the things you enjoy doing for a long time to come.

Ellen: That pretty much sums it up.

Counselor: Looking at the negatives versus the positives for changing the frequency of your eating, what seems to be the strongest right now?

Ellen: I think it's pretty obvious that the positives outweigh the negatives. All things considered making the effort to eat a little more frequently is something I certainly could try especially if I remind myself that I'm doing it for my grand-kids.

The questions below provide additional ways of helping the client make a list of the disadvantages of making a dietary behavioral change.

- What makes you worry about your current eating habits?
- What makes you think about a possible change in your eating habits?
- What are some of the negatives about your current physical symptoms when, as you have said, you may eat "too much food"?
- How has this dietary problem stopped you from doing things in your life that are important to or fun for you?
- What do you think will happen if you do not change anything in your daily eating pattern?

It is equally important to look at the advantages of change. Some of the questions and requests below will facilitate the client's ability to analyze uncertainty about making dietary changes.

- In what ways would you like for your eating habits to be different?
- What would be good things about making dietary changes?
- How important is making changes in your diet to you? And further, how much do you really want to start eating in a different manner?
- If you could imagine, what would you like for your life to be like in 5 years?
- If by magic, you could make a change in the way you eat, how might things be better for you?
- Just the fact that you came to this appointment shows me that you want to do something differently. Describe for me some of the main reasons you want to make changes in your diet.

Beyond these questions related to the disadvantages and advantages of change are some questions and requests that emphasize the positive nature of making a change.

- Tell me, what makes you feel encouraged that you can make a change if you decide to make it happen?

- If you decided to change, what would make dietary changes a realistic option for you?
- Are there other things in your life that you have changed in the past? What did you do to make those changes possible?
- Think about actually making these dietary changes. How confident are you that these changes are possible?
- You have talked about other times that you have had successes in behavioral changes. What about your personal abilities made that work for you?
- If you were to need support, where might that help come from in your daily relationships?
- In a perfect world, what would you like to see happen if dietary change were possible?

In summary, to work through ambivalence begin with the disadvantages and end with the advantages. This order means that the client has a positive focus as the counseling session ends.

Preparation

When the balance tips and the advantages outweigh the disadvantages, the client is in the preparation stage. At this stage, the client may say the following: "I've got to start eating more low-fat dairy products! This is serious! Something has to change. What can I do? How can I change?"

The preparation stage is like a window of opportunity that opens for a brief period of time. If the person enters into action during this time, the change process continues. If not, the person slips back into contemplation. The nutrition counselor's task when a client is in the preparation stage is not one of motivating, but rather, matching. At this point, the client needs help in finding a change strategy or a goal that is acceptable, accessible, appropriate, and effective.

Action

The action stage is what is most often termed *counseling*. The client engages in actions that bring about change. The goal during this stage is to produce a change in the problem area. This stage is characterized by client commitment to making change. This is the time at which the helping relationship between nutrition counselor and client is focused on fine-tuning those strategies that allow the client to change behavior.

Maintenance

Making a change does not guarantee maintenance of that change. Obviously, human experience includes good intentions and initial changes, followed by minor ("slips") or major ("relapses") steps backward. During the maintenance stage, the challenge is to sustain the change accomplished by previous action and to prevent relapse.[9] Maintaining a change may require a different set of skills and strategies from those needed to accomplish the change in the first place. Reducing dietary fat may be an initial step, followed by the challenge of maintaining reduced fat intake. If relapse occurs, the individual's task is to start around the spiral again rather than becoming stuck in this stage. Slips and relapses are normal, expected occurrences as a person seeks to change any long-standing pattern of behavior. The nutrition counselor's task here is to help the client avoid discouragement and demoralization, continue contemplating change, renew preparation, and resume action and maintenance efforts.

Assessment of the Client's Readiness for Change

Assessing which stage a person is in is a very important part of the process of counseling. The adherence thermometer in Figure 3–3 identifies adherence to dietary patterns. Figure 3–4 provides a way of helping clients work through the process of identifying which stage they are currently in or whether relapse is occurring. Using the thermometer is a process called *scaling*.

When the nutrition counselor is assessing where the clients fit into the model, it is important to ask, "How ready are they?" Giving advice is not appropriate at this point. Avoid lists of dos and don'ts. It is important to use the listening skills discussed in Chapter 2 to hear where clients feel they are in the process of change. This is when open-ended questions can help to explore current eating behavior and progress. "Tell me more about _____."
"Tell me more about 'sometimes.' At what times do you follow your low-saturated fat eating pattern, and at what times don't you?"

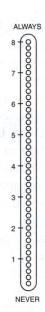

FIGURE 3–3 Adherence Thermometer. Courtesy of Kaiser Permanente, Portland, OR.

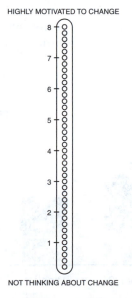

FIGURE 3–4 Motivation, Confidence, and Readiness-to-Change Thermometer. Courtesy of Kaiser Permanente, Portland, OR.

"How are you feeling about limiting the saturated fat in foods you choose?" "The last time we met, you were working on _____. How is that going?" As clients speak, use positive responses to affirm, compliment, and reinforce.

At this point, it is appropriate to provide objective feedback about dietary intake. Show clients feedback forms indicating changes in lipids or saturated fat or blood glucose levels. Compare client results with normative data or other interpretative information. After giving feedback by showing data, ask about the client's overall response, "What do you make of all this information?" (Figure 3–5 shows differences in carbohydrate intake for a specific time.)

Determine the client's readiness to change by showing the readiness-to-change thermometer (Figure 3–4). Ask the question, "How interested are you in making changes to eat foods lower in saturated fat and cholesterol?" This thermometer provides the clues to where a client is in readiness to change. Points on the thermometer include different stages of change. "Not interested in changing what I eat" falls into the precontemplative stage. "Thinking about changing some dietary habits in the next month" is suggestive of the contemplation phase. "Thinking about changing dietary behaviors in the next week" implies preparation. "Already starting to act on change in my eating behaviors" shows the action stage. The final stage of maintenance involves implementing the

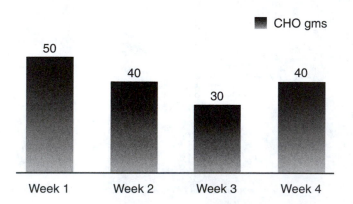

FIGURE 3–5   Carbohydrate Eaten on Tuesdays for Breakfast in 4 Weeks (Goal = 40 gms).

new behavior and feeling that "not doing the behavior would require effort."

Motivational Strategies

Keeping in mind the stages of change, the nutrition counselor might ask this question, "What strategies can a counselor use to enhance motivation for change?" Researchers have found that there are identifiable factors that motivate people to change. Miller provides a detailed review of this extensive literature.[10] From that research, eight general motivational strategies can be identified:

1. giving advice
2. identifying and removing barriers
3. providing choices
4. decreasing desirability of a present behavior
5. practicing empathy
6. providing feedback
7. clarifying goals
8. active helping

Giving Advice

Advice alone is not likely to be sufficient to induce change in a majority of individuals, but the motivating influence of clear and compassionate advice is valuable. Brief and systematic advice from a physician can increase the likelihood that medical patients will stop smoking or change their alcohol use.[11-15] Miller and Rollnick propose elements of effective advice.[5] Advice should clearly identify the problem or risk area, explain why change is important, and advocate specific change.

Identifying and Removing Barriers

A second effective motivation approach involves identifying and removing significant barriers to change. A contemplator may be willing to consider entering treatment, but also may be inhibited or discouraged from doing so by specific practical barriers, such as cost, transportation, child care, shyness, waiting time, or safety concerns. These barriers may interfere not only with beginning a dietary intervention, but with change efforts more generally. Once the nutrition counselor identifies barriers, the task is to assist the client in practical problem-solving.

Sisson and Mallams provide a good example of the power of simple strategies for overcoming barriers.[16] Their goal was to increase attendance at initial Alcoholics Anonymous (AA) meetings. The counselor gave one group the usual encouragement: an explanation of the importance of attendance, a schedule of available meeting times and places, and exhortation to attend. A second group, chosen at random, received systematic help in overcoming barriers to attendance. While the client was in the office, the counselor placed a prearranged telephone call to an AA member. Acting as a buddy, the AA member then spoke to the client, offering to provide transportation and to accompany the client to the first meeting. They agreed on a meeting time, and the member attained the client's telephone number in order to place a reminder call on the evening before the agreed-upon meeting. Marked results occurred. Every client in the latter group attended AA; in the former (encouragement) group, not a single client made it to the first AA meeting.

Some barriers are very tangible, such as cost or transportation. Other factors are less tangible but also significant: delays, comfort, a sense of belonging, cultural appropriateness. Long delays in a waiting room or assignment to a waiting list can discourage participation. It may be better to offer clients an effective, brief intervention than place them on a waiting list for treatment.[17-19] Child care during intervention is an issue for many women. Transportation and safety may be special concerns for the elderly. Language and cultural sensitivity are issues in counseling people from different racial and cultural backgrounds.

Some barriers to change are more attitudinal than overt. A person may fear that changing will result in adverse consequences[20] or cut off important sources of positive reinforcement. An individual's circle of friends or cultural context may encourage the perception that the "problem" behaviors are really quite normal and acceptable, and that no change is needed. Removal of these barriers to change may require more cognitive and informational strategies that require the client to think about alternatives. For example, in Hispanic culture where family is important, involving a family member in assisting the client to stay on course for a dietary change may be a strategy for barrier elimination.

Providing Choices

The effective nutrition counselor provides choices. Offering clients choices among alternative approaches may decrease resistance a nd dropout rates and may improve goal attainment and out-comes.[18,21–23] Similarly, acknowledging freedom of choice with regard to treatment goals may enhance client motivation.

Decreasing Desirability of a Present Behavior

Decreasing the desirability of a present behavior is important in the contemplation stage. At this point, the client is weighing the bene-fits and costs of change against the merits of continuing as before. Motivation strategies for the contemplation stage involve removing weights from the status quo side of the balance, and increasing weights on the change side of the scales. An important task for the nutrition counselor is to identify the client's positive incentives for continuing his or her present behavior. How and why is this behavior desirable to the client? Clear positive client incentives allow the nutrition counselor to seek effective approaches for decreasing or counterbalancing the behavior. Change in affective or value dimensions of desirability alter behavior.[24,25] Relation-ships and environment, along with individual desire, work to change behavior as well.

Practicing Empathy

Practicing empathy toward all clients favors motivation for change. Experimental and correlational studies show that an empathic counseling style results in low levels of client resistance and greater long-term behavioral change.[26,27]

As discussed in Chapter 2, empathy is not an ability to identify with a person's experiences. It is a learnable skill to understand another's meaning through the use of reflective listening, whether or not the listener has actually had similar experiences. Although a nutrition counselor skilled in empathic listening can make it look easy and natural, this is a demanding counseling style. It requires sharp attention to each new client statement, and a continual gen-eration of hypotheses as to the underlying meaning. Nutrition counselors reflect back to the client their best guesses as to mean-ing, often adding to the client's content. The client responds, and the whole process starts over again. Reflective listening is easy to copy or do poorly, but quite challenging to do well. It is a key element to behavioral change.

Providing Feedback

Providing clients with feedback on changes in dietary intake is valuable to future change. If the clients do not know where they are, it is difficult to plan how to get somewhere else. People sometimes fail to change because they do not receive sufficient feedback about their current situation. Clear knowledge of the present situation is a crucial element of motivation for change. Checkups that provide information about how a behavior is harmful yield long-term changes.[13,27] Self-monitoring dietary behaviors can be very helpful to clients on a daily basis as they change behaviors.[28-31]

In the world of nutrition, feedback from the nutrition counselor is often overemphasized. It is important, but feedback alone cannot achieve change. It is this process of self-evaluation—comparing perceived status with personal standards—that influences whether change will occur.[32]

This process is most effective in achieving change if the client identifies where change might occur. The graph on page 88 shows the normal ups and downs of dietary change. As the client reviews this graph, he or she remembers what triggered positive change and relapses. Knowing this information can help the client move forward. Asking open questions will provide even more information: "What was happening in your life when you were meeting your goal?" and "What were barriers when you were not meeting your goal?"

Clarifying Goals

Helping clients set clear goals facilitates change.[33] Clients must see goals as realistic and attainable, or they will expend little effort to reach the goal, even if they acknowledge it as important.[34] Goals are of little use if clients lack feedback about the present situation. Motivation for change occurs when goals and feedback work together.

Goal setting involves asking the right questions to elicit the stage in which the client falls. An initial stage of goal setting (which corresponds with the precontemplation or contemplation stage of change) may involve unreadiness or ambivalence. The goal for the nutrition counselor is to build motivation and help tip the client's decisional balance in favor of change. Important questions to ask include the following:

- What do you think about eating food high in saturated fat and cholesterol? Any dislikes?
- What are some of the good reasons for not making changes in your eating habits?
- Are there any reasons why you might want to make a change in your eating habits?
- Ideally, how would you like to be eating?
- What do you think might happen if you keep eating like this the rest of your life?

In this stage, it is important to address the client's ambivalence. Explore reasons for ambivalence without controlling or passing value judgments on responses to the above questions. Use of confrontation skills described in Chapter 2 may be important now if clients are in precontemplative stages. In the contemplation stage, assessing thoughts and feelings about self and the problem is important.

The second stage of goal setting (which corresponds with the preparation stage of change) involves a serious consideration of making changes in eating habits. The nutrition counselor's goal is to strengthen commitment to change by eliciting from the client reasonable goals and strategies for change. The following questions would be helpful in this stage:

- What are your reasons for wanting to eat foods lower in saturated fat and cholesterol?
- What has helped you eat foods low in saturated fat and cholesterol in the past?
- What do you think needs to change?
- What are your ideas for making a change in your eating?

In this stage, the window is open for action. The questions above provide ways to let the client know that there are ways to approach the action stage.

The third stage of goal setting corresponds with the action/

maintenance stage of change. In this stage, the goal of the nutrition counselor is to help the client take additional steps to change and deal with backward slips. At this point, the following questions are helpful:

- What do you like about low-fat eating?
- What are you doing that is working?
- How would you change what you are now doing?
- Is there anything else you see as a challenge?

In this action/maintenance stage, client and nutrition counselor negotiate a plan. The questions above provide ideas that tell the nutrition counselor what the client wants to do. The goal is to balance the differences between what the nutrition counselor wants and what the client wants to do.

It is important to follow up on whether goals are being met. The time of contact should be shortly after the client tries the goal. If the client is not able to meet the goal, the goal is faulty. Recycling (revising goals) is a positive step and not a sign of failure. Help the client set contingency plans. If plan X does not work, use plan Y.

Active Helping

At the end of a session, keep directions clear. Always be sure to leave clients with a sense of hope, not shame. Exhibit 3–2 provides the client with a few clear positive steps toward dealing with backward slips.

Conclusion

Each of the chapters that follow on eating pattern change related to chronic disease states provides information on how to move clients to appropriate stages on the spiral of change (Figure 3–1). To make these moves, knowledge about risk factors (the behaviors or conditions that place one at risk) and the ways in which risk factors can be reduced is necessary.[35]

Chapters 4 through 9 give ideas for tools that provide knowledge. Beyond knowledge, clients need skills that can first be modeled by the nutrition counselor and then practiced by the client.[36]

Exhibit 3–2   Dealing with Backward Slips

1. Stay calm and listen to any negative thoughts and turn them into positive thoughts.
   a. Listen to your thoughts.
   b. Decide if your thoughts help or hurt your progress.
      i.   What messages are you giving yourself?
      ii. Are they positive and helpful, or negative and limiting?
   c. Stop your negative thoughts.
   d. Reword your negative thoughts to make them into positive messages.
      i.   Think about the successful changes you've already made.
      ii. Be specific.
      iii. Use the present tense.
      iv. Forget what should be.
   e. Replace the negative thought with the positive message.
   f. Repeat your positive message to yourself, as often as possible.
2. Learn from your slip.
   a. What type of high-risk situation triggered your slip?
   b. What went wrong in your high-risk situation?
   c. What strategies have you successfully used before to prevent a slip in this type of situation?
3. Make a plan to get back on track.
   a. What two steps can you take today to get yourself back on track?
   b. How can you reward yourself when you get back on track?

Finally, clients must be confident that they are capable of changing their behavior.[37]

To move within the spiral of change, a variety of behavioral skills are necessary. The interventions needed to move a client toward the desired behavior vary by stage.[38–40] To move from precontemplation to contemplation, a knowledge of past performance is necessary. A graph of dietary intake is suggested in many of the following chapters. Encouragement and reevaluation of the positive new information can then begin to have the desired effect.

Moving from contemplation to preparation requires practicing new behaviors. Writing a menu is suggested in the chapters that follow. Once again, giving feedback on change in diet over time is very important. To move from the preparation stage to the action stage requires several different behavioral techniques. Cueing devices are described in the following chapters (e.g., a reminder on the refrigerator). This is the point at which social support is very important. Setting specific goals or designing contracts are important behavioral devices in this change step. Learning how to cope with problems and acquiring social and self-reinforcement is important in this move.

To move from action to maintenance is a process of refining. Seeing a set-back as an example of how to cope is important in this stage of change. The nutrition counselor bolsters the ability to handle change by referring to times when change was achieved. At this point the nutrition counselor encourages people to feel encouraged as they progress toward a goal and have positive thoughts.

In summary, the behavioral change spiral (Figure 3–1) includes numerous behavioral strategies. As change occurs, the strategies used may change also. Figure 3–2 on page 80 is a description of the nutrition care process with the stages of change and their key task. This process has the potential for assuring behavioral change when stages of change are used in the intervention step.

References

1. Jackson M, Berman N, Huber M, et al. Research staff turnover and participant adherence in the Women's Health Initiative. *Control Clin Trials* 2003;24(4):422–435.
2. Kratina K, King NL, Hayes D. *Moving Away from Diets: Healing Eating Problems and Exercise Resistance*, 2nd ed. Lake Dallas, TX: Helm Publishing, 2003.
3. Kanfer H, Gaelic-Buys L. Self-management methods. In: Kanfer H, Goldstein PJ, eds. *Helping People Change: A Textbook of Methods*, New York: Pergamon Press, 1991:306.
4. DiClemente CC, Prochaska JO. Toward a comprehensive, transtheoretical model of change: Stages of change and addictive behaviors. In: Miller WR, Heather N, eds. *Treating Addictive Behaviors*. Vol 3–24, 2nd ed. New York: Plenum Press, 1998:276–288.
5. Miller WR, Rollnick S. *Motivational Interviewing: Preparing People for Change*, 2nd ed. New York: Guilford Press, 2002.

6. Davidson R. *Counseling Problem Drinkers.* London: Tavistock/Routledge Publishers, Inc., 1991.
7. Rollnick S, MacEwan I. Alcohol counselling in context. In: Davidson R, Rollnick S, MacEwan I, eds. *Counseling Problem Drinkers.* London: Tavistock/Routledge Publishers, Inc., 1991:97–114.
8. Prochaska JO, Norcross JC, DiClemente CC. *Changing for Good.* New York: William Morrow & Co; 1994.
9. Marlatt GA, Cognitive assessment and intervention procedures for relapse prevention. In: Marlatt GA, Gordan JR, eds. *Relapse Prevention: Maintenance Strategies in the Treatment of Addictive Behaviors.* New York: Guilford Press, 1985.
10. Miller WR. Motivation for treatment: a review with special emphasis on alcoholism. *Psychol Bull* 1985;98(1):84–107.
11. Chick J, Lloyd G, Crombie E. Counselling problem drinkers in medical wards: a controlled study. *Br Med J (Clin Res Ed)* 30 1985;290(6473):965–967.
12. Elvy GA, Wells JE, Baird KA. Attempted referral as intervention for problem drinking in the general hospital. *Br J Addict* Jan 1988;83(1):83–89.
13. Kristenson H, Ohlin H, Hulten-Nosslin MB, Trell E, Hood B. Identification and intervention of heavy drinking in middle-aged men: results and follow-up of 24–60 months of long-term study with randomized controls. *Alcohol Clin Exp Res* 1983;7(2):203–209.
14. Russell MAH. Effect of general practitioner's advice against smoking. *Br Med J* 1988;297:663–668.
15. Wallace P, Cutler S, Haines A. Randomised controlled trial of general practitioner intervention in patients with excessive alcohol consumption. *Br Med J* 1988;297(6649):663–668.
16. Sisson RW, Mallams JH. The use of systematic encouragement and community access procedures to increase attendance at Alcoholic Anonymous and Al-Anon meetings. *Am J Drug Alcohol Abuse* 1981;8(3):371–376.
17. Harris KB, Miller WR. Behavioral self-control training for problem drinkers: mechanisms of efficacy. *Psychol Addictive Behav* 1990;4:82–90.
18. Sanchez-Craig M. Brief didactic treatment for alcohol and drug-related problems: an approach based on client choice. *Br J Addict* 1990;85(2):169–177.
19. Schmidt MM, Miller WR. Amount of therapist contact and outcome in a multidimensional depression treatment program. *Acta Psychiatr Scand* 1983;67(5):319–332.
20. Hall SM. The abstinence phobia. In: Krasnegor NA, ed. *Behavioral Analysis and Treatment of Substance Abuse.* Rockville, MD: National Institute on Drug Abuse, 1979:55–67.
21. Costello RM. Alcoholism treatment and evaluation: in search of methods. II. Collation of two-year follow-up studies. *Int J Addict* 1975;10(5):857–867.

22. Kissin B, Platz A, Su WH. Selective factors in treatment choices and outcomes in alcoholics. In: Mello NK, Mendelson JH, eds. *Recent Advances in Studies of Alcoholism.* Washington, DC: U.S. Government Printing Office; 1971:781–802.
23. Parker MW, Winstead DK, Willi FJ. Patient autonomy in alcohol rehabilitation. I. Literature review. *Int J Addict* Oct 1979;14(7):1015–1022.
24. Leventhal H. Fear appeals and persuasion: the differentiation of a motivational construct. *Am J Public Health* 1971;61(6):1208–1224.
25. Premack D. Mechanisms of self-control. In: Hunt WA, ed. *Learning Mechanisms in Smoking.* Chicago: Aldine, 1970:107–123.
26. Patterson GR, Forgatch MS. Therapist behavior as a determinant for client noncompliance: a paradox for the behavior modifier. *J Consult Clin Psychol* 1985;53(6):846–851.
27. Miller WR, Sovereign RG. The check-up: a model for early intervention in addictive behaviors. In: Loberg T, Miller WR, Nathan PE, Marlatt GA, eds. *Addictive Behaviors: Prevention and Early Intervention.* Amsterdam: Swets and Zeitlinger, 1989:219–231.
28. Wing RR. Behavioral treatment of severe obesity. *Am J Clin Nutr* 1992;55(2 Suppl):545S–551S.
29. Smith DE, Wing RR. Diminished weight loss and behavioral compliance during repeated diets in obese patients with type II diabetes. *Health Psychol* 1991;10(6):378–383.
30. Sperduto WA, Thompson HS, O'Brien RM. The effect of target behavior monitoring on weight loss and completion rate in a behavior modification program for weight reduction. *Addict Behav* 1986;11(3):337–340.
31. Baker RC, Kirschenbaum DS. Self-monitoring may be necessary for successful weight control. *Behav Therap* 1993;24:395–408.
32. Kanfer H, Gaelick L. Self-Management Methods. In: Kanfer H, Goldstein AP, eds. *Helping People Change*, 3rd ed. Elmsford, NY: Pergamon Press, 1986:283–345.
33. Locke EA, Shaw KN, Saari LM, Latham GP. Goal setting and task performance: 1969–1980. *Psychol Bull* 1981(90):125–152.
34. Bandura A. Self-efficacy mechanism in human agency. *Am Psychol* 1982;37:122–147.
35. Maibach EW, Cotton D. Moving people to behavior change. In: Maibach EW, Parrott L, eds. *Designing Health Messages.* Thousand Oaks, CA: Sage Publications, Inc., 1995:44.
36. Bandura A. Self-efficacy mechanism in physiological activation and health-promoting behavior. In: Madden J, ed. *Neurobiology of Learning, Emotion and Affect.* New York: Raven Press, 1991:46.
37. Wood R, Bandura A. Social cognitive theory of organizational management. *Acad Mgt Rev* 1989;14:361–384.
38. Weinstein ND. The precaution adoption process. *Health Psychol* 1988;7(4):355–386.
39. Prochaska JO, DiClemente CC, Norcross JC. In search of how people change. Applications to addictive behaviors. *Am Psychol* 1992;47(9):1102–1114.
40. Baranowski T. Beliefs as motivational influences at stages in behavior change. *Int J Commun Health Educ* 1992;13:3–29.

PART II

APPLICATION OF INTERVIEWING AND COUNSELING SKILLS

Exhibit 1: Nutrition Diagnostic Terminology[1] shows the summary of the American Dietetic Association's Nutrition Diagnosis labeling sheet. In Part II of the text, the majority of dietary behavioral problems initially would be classified under Behavioral-Environmental (NB) with the subcategory of Knowledge and Beliefs (1) and Not Ready for Diet/Lifestyle Change (NB-1.4) and/or Undesirable Food Choices (NB-1.7).

Exhibit 2: Nutrition Intervention Terminology[1] provides the summary of the American Dietetic Association's Nutrition Intervention labeling sheet. It uses the concepts of nutrition counseling, including the theoretical basis/approach and strategies to use when obstacles to dietary adherence are unrelated to knowledge and planning but reflect instead a lack of commitment by the client.

Exhibit 3: Monitoring and Evaluation Terminology[1] is designed to show follow-up assessment. Its purpose is to monitor and evaluate progress. Goals and expected outcomes are recorded. This type of follow-up on the effectiveness of the intervention is crucial to allowing the client to see progress and readdress goals if progress is not occurring. It includes nutrition-related behavioral-environmental outcomes, knowledge/beliefs, behavior—including ability to plan meals/snacks, ability to select healthful food/meals, ability to prepare food/meals, adherence, goal setting, portion control, self-care management, self-monitoring, social support, and stimulus control—access to food, and physical activity and function.

Exhibit 4 provides the four steps in the **Nutrition Care Process** (NCP). Each step will be a focus in this book with emphasis on the theories and strategies to use when counseling clients.

For the majority of clients' dietary adherence problems, understanding what is needed relative to knowledge and planning has occurred; the major focus is on lack of commitment. This is not meant to be a negative label, but rather a way of characterizing a client who just has not reached a place in his/her life where making a change is realistic.

Part II, Exhibit 1   Nutrition Diagnostic Terminology

INTAKE   **NI**

Defined as "actual problems related to intake of energy, nutrients, fluids, bioactive substances through oral diet or nutrition support"

Energy Balance (1)

Defined as "actual or estimated changes in energy (kcal) balance"

- Unused   NI-1.1
- Increased energy expenditure   NI-1.2
- Unused   NI-1.3
- Inadequate energy intake   NI-1.4
- Excessive energy intake   NI-1.5

Oral or Nutrition Support Intake (2)

Defined as "actual or estimated food and beverage intake from oral diet or nutrition support compared with patient goal"

- Inadequate oral food/beverage intake   NI-2.1
- Excessive oral food/beverage intake   NI-2.2
- Inadequate intake from enteral/parenteral nutrition   NI-2.3
- Excessive intake from enteral/parenteral nutrition   NI-2.4
- Inappropriate infusion of enteral/parenteral nutrition *(use with caution)*   NI-2.5

Fluid Intake (3)

Defined as "actual or estimated fluid intake compared with patient goal"

Fat and Cholesterol (5.6)

- Inadequate fat intake   NI-5.6.1
- Excessive fat intake   NI-5.6.2
- Inappropriate intake of food fats   NI-5.6.3
  (specify)

Protein (5.7)

- Inadequate protein intake   NI-5.7.1
- Excessive protein intake   NI-5.7.2
- Inappropriate intake of amino acids   NI-5.7.3
  (specify)

Carbohydrate and Fiber (5.8)

- Inadequate carbohydrate intake   NI-5.8.1
- Excessive carbohydrate intake   NI-5.8.2
- Inappropriate intake of types of carbohydrates   NI-5.8.3
  (specify)
- Inconsistent carbohydrate intake   NI-5.8.4
- Inadequate fiber intake   NI-5.8.5
- Excessive fiber intake   NI-5.8.6

Vitamin (5.9)

- Inadequate vitamin intake   NI-5.9.1
  (specify)
- Excessive vitamin intake   NI-5.9.2
  (specify)
- A
- C
- D
- E
- K
- Riboflavin
- Niacin
- Folate
- B6
- B12

Biochemical (2)

Defined as "change in capacity to metabolize nutrients as a result of medications, surgery, or as indicated by altered lab values"

- Impaired nutrient utilization   NC-2.1
- Altered nutrition-related laboratory values *(specify)*   NC-2.2
- Food-medication interaction   NC-2.3

Weight (3)

Defined as "chronic weight or changed weight status when compared with usual or desired body weight"

- Underweight   NC-3.1
- Involuntary weight loss   NC-3.2
- Overweight/obesity   NC-3.3
- Involuntary weight gain   NC-3.4

BEHAVIORAL-ENVIRONMENTAL   NB

Defined as "nutritional findings/problems identified that relate to knowledge, attitudes/beliefs, physical environment, access to food, or food safety"

Knowledge and Beliefs (1)

Defined as "actual knowledge and beliefs as related, observed, or documented"

- Food- and nutrition-related knowledge deficit   NB-1.1
- Harmful beliefs/attitudes about food- and nutrition-related topics *(use with caution)*   NB-1.2
- Not ready for diet/lifestyle change   NB-1.3

Part II, Exhibit 1 *continued*

☐ Inadequate fluid intake   NI-3.1
☐ Excessive fluid intake   NI-3.2

Bioactive Substances (4)

Defined as "actual or observed intake of bioactive substances, including single or multiple functional food components, ingredients, dietary supplements, alcohol"

☐ Inadequate bioactive substance intake   NI-4.1
☐ Excessive bioactive substance intake   NI-4.2
☐ Excessive alcohol intake   NI-4.3

Nutrient (5)

Defined as "actual or estimated intake of specific nutrient groups or single nutrients as compared with desired levels"

☐ Increased nutrient needs (specify)   NI-5.1
☐ Evident protein-energy malnutrition   NI-5.2
☐ Inadequate protein-energy intake   NI-5.3
☐ Decreased nutrient needs (specify)   NI-5.4
☐ Imbalance of nutrients   NI-5.5

#1 Problem _____

Etiology _____

Signs/Symptoms _____

☐ Thiamin
☐ Other (specify) _____

Mineral (5.10)

☐ Inadequate mineral intake (specify)   NI-5.10.1
☐ Excessive mineral intake (specify)   NI-5.10.2

☐ Calcium ☐ Phosphorus
☐ Iron ☐ Potassium
☐ Magnesium ☐ Zinc
☐ Other (specify) _____

CLINICAL   NC

Defined as "nutritional findings/problems identified that relate to medical or physical conditions"

Functional (1)

Defined as "change in physical or mechanical functioning that interferes with or prevents desired nutritional consequences"

☐ Swallowing difficulty   NC-1.1
☐ Biting/Chewing (masticatory) difficulty   NC-1.2
☐ Breastfeeding difficulty   NC-1.3
☐ Altered GI function   NC-1.4

#2 Problem _____

Etiology _____

Signs/Symptoms _____

☐ Self-monitoring deficit   NB-1.4
☐ Disordered eating pattern   NB-1.5
☐ Limited adherence to nutrition-related recommendations   NB-1.6
☐ Undesirable food choices   NB-1.7

Physical Activity and Function (2)

Defined as "actual physical activity, self-care, and quality-of-life problems as reported, observed, or documented"

☐ Physical inactivity   NB-2.1
☐ Excessive exercise   NB-2.2
☐ Inability or lack of desire to manage self-care   NB-2.3
☐ Impaired ability to prepare foods/meals   NB-2.4
☐ Poor nutrition quality of life   NB-2.5
☐ Self-feeding difficulty   NB-2.6

Food Safety and Access (3)

Defined as "actual problems with food access or food safety"

☐ Intake of unsafe food   NB-3.1
☐ Limited access to food   NB-3.2

Date Identified	Date Resolved

#3 Problem _____

Etiology _____

Signs/Symptoms _____

Part II, Exhibit 2   Nutrition Intervention Terminology

Problem _____
Etiology _____
Signs/Symptoms _____

Nutrition Prescription
The patient's/client's individualized recommended dietary intake of energy and/or selected foods or nutrients based on current reference standards and dietary guidelines and the patient's/client's health condition and nutrition diagnosis. (specify) _____

Intervention #1 _____
Goal(s) _____

Intervention #2 _____
Goal(s) _____

Intervention #3 _____
Goal(s) _____

FOOD AND/OR NUTRIENT DELIVERY   ND

Meal and Snacks (1)
Regular eating event (meal); food served between regular meals (snack).

☐ General/healthful diet	ND-1.1
☐ Modify distribution, type, or amount of food and nutrients within meals or at specified time	ND-1.2
☐ Specific foods/beverages or groups	ND-1.3
☐ Other	ND-1.4
(specify)	

Enteral and Parenteral Nutrition (2)
Nutrition provided through the GI tract via tube, catheter, or stoma (enteral) or intravenously (centrally or peripherally) (parenteral).

☐ Initiate EN or PN	ND-2.1
☐ Modify rate, concentration, composition, or schedule	ND-2.2

Bioactive Substance Supplement (3.3)
Supplemental bioactive substances.

☐ Initiate	ND-3.3.1
☐ Dose change	ND-3.3.2
☐ Form change	ND-3.3.3
☐ Route change	ND-3.3.4
☐ Administration schedule	ND-3.3.5
☐ Discontinue	ND-3.3.6
(specify)	

Feeding Assistance (4)
Accommodation or assistance in eating.

☐ Adaptive equipment	ND-4.1
☐ Feeding position	ND-4.2
☐ Meal set-up	ND-4.3
☐ Mouth care	ND-4.4
☐ Other	ND-4.5
(specify)	

Feeding Environment (5)
Adjustment of the factors where food is served that impact food consumption.

Comprehensive Nutrition Education (2) *cont'd*

☐ Result interpretation	E-2.4
☐ Skill development	E-2.5
☐ Other	E-2.6
(specify)	

NUTRITION COUNSELING   C

Theoretical Basis/Approach (1)
The theories or models used to design and implement an intervention.

☐ Cognitive-Behavioral Theory	C-1.1
☐ Health Belief Model	C-1.2
☐ Social Learning Theory	C-1.3
☐ Transtheoretical Model/ Stages of Change	C-1.4
☐ Other	C-1.5
(specify)	

Strategies (2)
Selectively applied evidence-based methods or plans of action designed to achieve a particular goal.

☐ Motivational interviewing	C-2.1

Part II, Exhibit 2 *continued*

- ☐ Discontinue EN or PN — ND-2.3
- ☐ Insert enteral feeding tube — ND-2.4
- ☐ Site care — ND-2.5
- ☐ Other — ND-2.6

(specify) _____

Supplements (3)

Medical Food Supplements (3.1)

Commercial or prepared foods or beverages that supplement energy, protein, carbohydrate, fiber, fat intake.

Type
- ☐ Commercial beverage — ND-3.1.1
- ☐ Commercial food — ND-3.1.2
- ☐ Modified beverage — ND-3.1.3
- ☐ Modified food — ND-3.1.4
- ☐ Purpose — ND-3.1.5

(specify) _____

Vitamin and Mineral Supplements (3.2)

Supplemental vitamins or minerals.

- ☐ Multivitamin/mineral — ND-3.2.1
- ☐ Multi-trace elements — ND-3.2.2
- ☐ Vitamin — ND-3.2.3
  - ☐ A
  - ☐ C
  - ☐ D
  - ☐ E
  - ☐ K
  - ☐ Thiamin
  - ☐ Riboflavin
  - ☐ Niacin
  - ☐ Folate
  - ☐ B6
  - ☐ B12
  - ☐ Other (specify)
- ☐ Mineral — ND-3.2.4
  - ☐ Calcium
  - ☐ Iron
  - ☐ Magnesium
  - ☐ Phosphorus
  - ☐ Potassium
  - ☐ Zinc
  - ☐ Other (specify)

- ☐ Lighting
- ☐ Odors
- ☐ Distractions
- ☐ Table height
- ☐ Table service/set up
- ☐ Room temperature
- ☐ Other

(specify) _____

Nutrition-Related Medication Management (6)

Modification of a drug or herbal to optimize patient/client nutritional or health status.

- ☐ Initiate — ND-6.1
- ☐ Dose change — ND-6.2
- ☐ Form change — ND-6.3
- ☐ Route change — ND-6.4
- ☐ Administration schedule — ND-6.5
- ☐ Discontinue — ND-6.6

(specify) _____

NUTRITION EDUCATION   E

Initial/Brief Nutrition Education (1)

Build or reinforce basic or essential nutrition-related knowledge.

- ☐ Purpose of the nutrition education — E-1.1
- ☐ Priority modifications — E-1.2
- ☐ Survival information — E-1.3
- ☐ Other — E-1.4

(specify) _____

Comprehensive Nutrition Education (2)

Instruction or training leading to in-depth nutrition-related knowledge or skills.

- ☐ Purpose of the nutrition education — E-2.1
- ☐ Recommended modifications — E-2.2
- ☐ Advanced or related topics — E-2.3

- ☐ Goal setting — C-2.2
- ☐ Self-monitoring — C-2.3
- ☐ Problem solving — C-2.4
- ☐ Social support — C-2.5
- ☐ Stress management — C-2.6
- ☐ Stimulus control — C-2.7
- ☐ Cognitive restructuring — C-2.8
- ☐ Relapse prevention — C-2.9
- ☐ Rewards/contingency management — C-2.10
- ☐ Other — C-2.11

(specify) _____

COORDINATION OF NUTRITION CARE   RC

Coordination of Other Care During Nutrition Care (1)

Facilitating services with other professionals, institutions, or agencies during nutrition care.

- ☐ Team meeting — RC-1.1
- ☐ Referral to RD with different expertise — RC-1.2
- ☐ Collaboration/referral to other providers — RC-1.3
- ☐ Referral to community agencies/ programs *(specify)* — RC-1.4

_____

Discharge and Transfer of Nutrition Care to New Setting or Provider (2)

Discharge planning and transfer of nutrition care from one level or location of care to another.

- ☐ Collaboration/referral to other providers — RC-2.1
- ☐ Referral to community agencies/ programs *(specify)* — RC-2.2

_____

Part II, Exhibit 3   Nutrition Monitoring and Evaluation Terminology

During nutrition monitoring and evaluation, practitioners list the signs and symptoms from the PES statement that are the targets of the nutrition intervention. Then, practitioners list the nutrition interventions and goals/expected outcome along with the indicators and criteria to provide evidence for the nutrition monitoring and evaluation. There may be more than one indicator per goal, and one indicator may be used for multiple goals.

Nutrition Intervention(s) and Goal/expected outcome(s)	Indicator(s)	Signs/Symptoms from PES statement(s)	Criteria
Intervention ____			
#1 Goal ____			
#2 Goal ____			
Intervention ____			
#1 Goal ____			
#2 Goal ____			
Intervention ____			
#1 Goal ____			
#2 Goal ____			

NUTRITION-RELATED BEHAVIORAL-ENVIRONMENTAL OUTCOMES   **BE**

Knowledge/Beliefs (1)
Improved understanding of nutrition concepts and change in beliefs and attitudes that increase the probability that the patient/client will successfully implement nutrition prescription/goal.

Beliefs and attitudes (1.1)
□ Readiness to change   BE-1.1.1
□ Perceived consequence   BE-1.1.2
   of change

Portion control (2.6)
□ Portion size eaten   BE-2.6.1
Self-care management (2.7)
□ Self-care management ability   BE-2.7.1
Self-monitoring (2.8)
□ Self-monitoring ability   BE-2.8.1
Social support (2.9)
□ Ability to build and utilize   BE-2.9.1
   social support
Stimulus control (2.10)
□ Ability to manage behavior in   BE-2.10.1
   response to stimuli

FOOD AND NUTRIENT INTAKE OUTCOMES   **FI**

Energy Intake (1)
Total energy intake from all sources, e.g., food, beverages, supplements, and via enteral and parenteral routes.
Energy intake (1.1)
□ Total energy intake   FI-1.1.1
Food and Beverage (2)
Foods and food groups and fluids from all sources, e.g., food, beverages, supplements.
Fluid/beverage intake (2.1)

Part II, Exhibit 3   *continued*

- ☐ Perceived costs versus benefits of change — BE-1.1.3
- ☐ Perceived risk — BE-1.1.4
- ☐ Outcome expectancy — BE-1.1.5
- ☐ Conflict with personal/family value system — BE-1.1.6
- ☐ Self-efficacy — BE-1.1.7
  (breastfeeding, eating, weight loss)

Food and nutrition knowledge (1.2)
- ☐ Level of knowledge — BE-1.2.1
  (e.g., none, limited, minimal, substantial, and extensive)
- ☐ Areas of knowledge — BE-1.2.2
  (food/nutrient requirements, physiological functions, disease/condition, nutrition recommendations, food products, consequences of food behavior, food label understanding, self-management parameters)

Behavior (2)
Patient/client activities and actions necessary to achieve nutrition-related goals.

Ability to plan meals/snacks (2.1)
- ☐ Meal/snack planning ability — BE-2.1.1

Ability to select healthful food/meals (2.2)
- ☐ Food/meal selection — BE-2.2.1

Ability to prepare food/meals (2.3)
- ☐ Food/meal preparation ability — BE-2.3.1

Adherence (2.4)
- ☐ Self-reported adherence — BE-2.4.1

Goal setting (2.5)
- ☐ Goal setting ability — BE-2.5.1

Access (3)
Availability of a sufficient quantity of safe, healthful food.

Access to food (3.1)
- ☐ Access to a sufficient quantity of healthful food — BE-3.1.1
- ☐ Access to safe food — BE-3.1.2

Physical Activity and Function (4)
Improved physical activity and ability to engage in specific tasks (e.g., breastfeeding).

Breastfeeding success (4.1)
- ☐ Initiation of breastfeeding — BE-4.1.1
- ☐ Duration of breastfeeding — BE-4.1.2
- ☐ Exclusive breastfeeding — BE-4.1.3
- ☐ Breastfeeding problems — BE-4.1.4

Nutrition-related ADLs and IADLs (4.2)
- ☐ Acceptance of assistance with eating — BE-4.2.1
- ☐ Ability to use adaptive eating devices — BE-4.2.2
- ☐ Time taken to eat and consume meals — BE-4.2.3
- ☐ Ability to shop for food — BE-4.2.4
- ☐ Nutrition-related ADL — BE-4.2.5
- ☐ Nutrition-related IADL — BE-4.2.6

Physical activity (4.3)
- ☐ Consistency/frequency — BE-4.3.1
- ☐ Duration — BE-4.3.2
- ☐ Intensity — BE-4.3.3
- ☐ Strength — BE-4.3.4

- ☐ Oral fluids amounts — FI-2.1.1
  (water, coffee/tea, juice, milk, soda)
- ☐ Food derived fluids — FI-2.1.2
- ☐ IV fluids — FI-2.1.3
- ☐ Liquid meal replacement — FI-2.1.4

Food intake (2.2)
- ☐ Food variety — FI-2.2.1
- ☐ Number of food group servings — FI-2.2.2
  (grains, fruits, vegetables, milk/dairy, meat/protein substitutes)
- ☐ Healthy Eating Index — FI-2.2.3
- ☐ Children's Diet Quality Index — FI-2.2.4
- ☐ Revised Children's Diet Quality Index — FI-2.2.5

Enteral and Parenteral (3)
Specialized nutrition support intake from all sources, e.g., enteral and parenteral routes.

Enteral/parenteral nutrition intake (3.1)
- ☐ Access — FI-3.1.1
- ☐ Formula/solution — FI-3.1.2
- ☐ Discontinuation — FI-3.1.3
- ☐ Initiation — FI-3.1.4
- ☐ Rate/schedule — FI-3.1.5

Bioactive Substances (4)
Alcohol, plant stanol and sterol esters, soy protein, psyllium and β-glucan, and caffeine intake from all sources, e.g., food, beverages, supplements, and via enteral and parenteral routes.

Alcohol intake (4.1)
- ☐ Drink size/volume — FI-4.1.1
- ☐ Frequency — FI-4.1.2

Part II, Exhibit 3 *continued*

Bioactive substance intake (4.2)
☐ Plant sterol and stanol esters   FI-4.2.1
☐ Soy protein   FI-4.2.2
☐ Psyllium and β-glucan   FI-4.2.3

Caffeine intake (4.3)
☐ Total caffeine   FI-4.3.1

Macronutrients (5)
Carbohydrate, fiber, protein, and fat and cholesterol intake from all sources, e.g., food, beverages, supplements, and via enteral and parenteral routes.

Fat and cholesterol intake (5.1)
☐ Total fat   FI-5.1.1
☐ Saturated fat   FI-5.1.2
☐ Trans fatty acids   FI-5.1.3
☐ Polyunsaturated fat   FI-5.1.4
☐ Monounsaturated fat   FI-5.1.5
☐ Omega-3 fatty acids   FI-5.1.6
(marine/plant derived, alphalinolenic acid)
☐ Dietary cholesterol   FI-5.1.7

Protein intake (5.2)
☐ Total protein   FI-5.2.1
☐ High biological value protein   FI-5.2.2
☐ Casein   FI-5.2.3
☐ Whey   FI-5.2.4
☐ Soy protein   FI-5.2.5
☐ Amino acids   FI-5.2.6
☐ Essential amino acids   FI-5.2.7

Carbohydrate intake (5.3)
☐ Total carbohydrate   FI-5.3.1
☐ Sugar   FI-5.3.2
☐ Starch   FI-5.3.3
☐ Glycemic index   FI-5.3.4
☐ Glycemic load   FI-5.3.5

Fiber intake (5.4)
☐ Total fiber   FI-5.4.1
☐ Soluble fiber   FI-5.4.2

☐ Body fat percentage
☐ Triceps skin fold
☐ Waist circumference
☐ Waist-hip ratio
☐ Bone age
☐ Bone mineral density

Biochemical and Medical Tests (2)
Lab values or medical tests such as glucose, lipids, electrolytes, and fecal fat test.

Acid-base balance (2.1)
☐ pH, serum   S-2.1.1
☐ Bicarbonate   S-2.1.2
☐ Partial pressure of carbon dioxide in arterial blood   S-2.1.3

Electrolyte and renal profile (2.2)
☐ BUN   S-2.2.1
☐ Creatinine   S-2.2.2
☐ BUN-creatinine ratio   S-2.2.3
☐ Glomerular filtration rate   S-2.2.4
☐ Sodium   S-2.2.5
☐ Chloride   S-2.2.6
☐ Potassium   S-2.2.7
☐ Magnesium   S-2.2.8
☐ Calcium   S-2.2.9
☐ Calcium, ionized   S-2.2.10
☐ Phosphorus   S-2.2.11
☐ Serum osmolality   S-2.2.12
☐ Parathyroid hormone   S-2.2.13

Essential fatty acid profile (2.3)
☐ Triene:Tetraene ratio   S-2.3.1

Gastrointestinal profile (2.4)
☐ Amylase   S-2.4.1
☐ Alkaline phosphatase   S-2.4.2
☐ Alanine aminotransferase   S-2.4.3
☐ Aspartate aminotransferase   S-2.4.4
☐ Gamma glutamyl transferase   S-2.4.5

☐ Total iron-binding capacity   S-2.8.12
☐ Transferrin saturation   S-2.8.13

Protein profile (2.9)
☐ Albumin   S-2.9.1
☐ Prealbumin   S-2.9.2
☐ Transferrin   S-2.9.3
☐ Phenylalanine, plasma   S-2.9.4
☐ Tyrosine, plasma   S-2.9.5

Respiratory quotient (2.10)
☐ RQ   S-2.10.1

Urine profile (2.11)
☐ Urine color   S-2.11.1
☐ Urine osmolality   S-2.11.2
☐ Urine specific gravity   S-2.11.3
☐ Urine tests   S-2.11.4
(e.g., ketones, sugar, protein)
☐ Urine volume   S-2.11.5

Vitamin profile (2.12)
☐ Vitamin A   S-2.12.1
(serum or plasma retinol)
☐ Vitamin C   S-2.12.2
(plasma or serum)
☐ Vitamin D   S-2.12.3
(25-hydroxy)
☐ Vitamin E   S-2.12.4
(plasma alpha-tocopherol)
☐ Thiamin   S-2.12.5
(activity coefficient for erythrocyte transketolase activity)
☐ Riboflavin   S-2.12.6
(activity coefficient for erythrocyte glutathione reductase activity)
☐ Niacin   S-2.12.7
(urinary N'methyl-nicotinamide concentration)
☐ Vitamin B6   S-2.12.8

Part II, Exhibit 3   *continued*

□ Insoluble fiber   FI-5.4.3
(fructo-oligosaccharides)

Micronutrients (6)
Vitamins and minerals intake from all sources, e.g., food, beverages, supplements, and via enteral and parenteral routes.

Vitamin intake (6.1)
□ A   □ Riboflavin
□ C   □ Niacin
□ D   □ Folate
□ E   □ B6
□ K   □ B12
□ Thiamin
□ Other (specify)

Mineral/element intake (6.2)
□ Calcium   □ Potassium
□ Iron   □ Sodium
□ Magnesium   □ Zinc
□ Phosphorus
□ Other (specify)

NUTRITION-RELATED PHYSICAL SIGN/SYMPTOM OUTCOMES   S

Anthropometric (1)
Measure such as weight, body mass index (BMI) percentile/age, waist circumference, and length.

Body composition/growth (1.1)
□ Body mass index (kg/m2)   S-1.1.1
□ IBW or UBW percentage   S-1.1.2
□ Growth pattern   S-1.1.3
(head circumference, length/height, weight for length/stature, BMI percentile/age, also see Weight change)
□ Weight/weight change   S-1.1.4
(e.g., % change, weight gain/day)
□ Lean body mass, fat free mass   S-1.1.5
□ Mid-arm muscle circumference   S-1.1.6

□ Bilirubin, total   S-2.4.6
□ Ammonia, serum   S-2.4.7
□ Prothrombin time   S-2.4.8
□ Partial thromboplastin time   S-2.4.9
□ INR *(ratio)*   S-2.4.10
□ Fecal fat   S-2.4.11

Glucose profile (2.5)
□ Glucose, fasting   S-2.5.1
□ Glucose, casual   S-2.5.2
□ HgbA1c   S-2.5.3
□ Pre-prandial capillary plasma glucose   S-2.5.4
□ Peak postprandial capillary plasma glucose   S-2.5.5

Lipid profile (2.6)
□ Cholesterol, serum   S-2.6.1
□ Cholesterol, HDL   S-2.6.2
□ Cholesterol, LDL   S-2.6.3
□ Triglycerides, serum   S-2.6.4

Mineral profile (2.7)
□ Copper, serum   S-2.7.1
□ Iodine, urinary excretion   S-2.7.2
□ Thyroid stimulating hormone   S-2.7.3
□ Zinc, plasma   S-2.7.4

Nutritional anemia profile (2.8)
□ Hemoglobin   S-2.8.1
□ Hematocrit   S-2.8.2
□ Mean corpuscular volume   S-2.8.3
□ Red blood cell folate   S-2.8.4
□ Red cell distribution width   S-2.8.5
□ Serum B12   S-2.8.6
□ Serum methylmalonic acid   S-2.8.7
□ Serum folate   S-2.8.8
□ Serum homocysteine   S-2.8.9
□ Serum ferritin   S-2.8.10
□ Serum iron   S-2.8.11

(plasma or serum pyridoxal 5'phosphate concentration)

Physical Examination (3)
Physical exam parameters such as edema, nausea, vomiting, bowel function, skin integrity, and blood pressure.

Nutrition physical exam findings (3.1)
□ Cardiovascular-pulmonary   3.1.1
(pulmonary edema)
□ Extremities, musculo-skeletal   3.1.2
(e.g., nails, subcutaneous fat, muscle)
□ Gastrointestinal   3.1.3
(e.g., nausea, vomiting, bowel function)
□ Head and neck   3.1.4
(e.g., tongue, mouth, and hair changes)
□ Neurological   3.1.5
(e.g., confusion, fine/gross motor)
□ Skin   3.1.6
(e.g., appearance, turgor, integrity)
□ Vital signs   3.1.7
(blood pressure, respiratory rate)

NUTRITION-RELATED PATIENT/ CLIENT-CENTERED OUTCOMES   PC

Nutrition Quality of Life (1)
Patient/client's perception of his/her nutrition intervention and its impact on life.

Nutrition quality of life (1.1)
□ Food impact   PC-1.1.1
□ Physical state   PC-1.1.2
□ Psychological factors   PC-1.1.3
□ Self-image   PC-1.1.4
□ Self-efficacy   PC-1.1.5
□ Social/interpersonal factors   PC-1.1.6
□ Nutrition quality of life score   PC-1.1.7

Satisfaction (2)   To be added

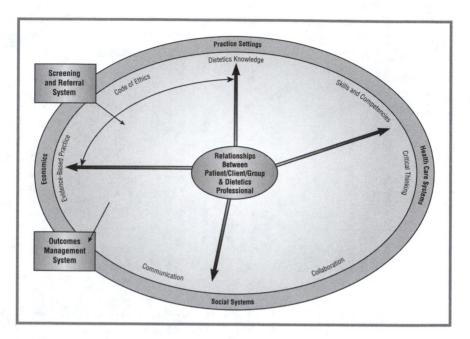

Part II, Exhibit 4   Nutrition Care Process

Exhibit V: Stages of Change with Corresponding Processes[1] shows the tasks that are a part of stages of change. Note that the time where a helping relationship occurs is when the client is ready to make a change (action or ready to change stage). The other stages involve concepts that do not include the counselor giving information or offering help.

Under precontemplation (not ready to change) it is important to counsel with a focus on consciousness-raising. An example is given below.

Client: "I just don't see how changing my diet will make a difference. I am retired now and just want to be spontaneous."

Counselor: "You just want to be free of worry about watching what you eat." (Reflection)

Client: "Yes!"

Counselor: "What do you see as a positive to making dietary changes?" (Open Question)

Client: "The doctor says that I will have more energy."

Counselor: "More energy . . . How might that change things that are going on in your life now?" (Open Question)

Client: "Life might be more fun."

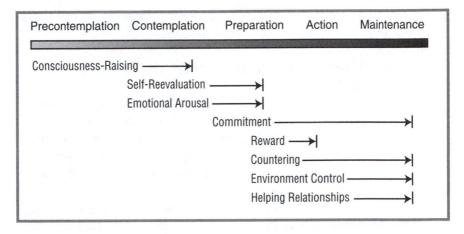

Part II, Exhibit 5   Stages of Change with Corresponding Processes
Adapted from *Changing for Good,* Prochaska et al., 2002, pg. 54.

In this case, we have just opened the door to thinking about making a change. This is not the time to set a goal specifically focused on changing foods that are eaten on a daily basis. It is the point at which the client thinks about the possibility of change. Goal setting at this time will result in feelings of failure on the part of the client and counselor. In reality, this may mean sending the client home to think about changing eating behaviors, or, going in a different direction, it may mean that the client is ready to explore (contemplation or unsure about change) the pros and cons of making a change before leaving the counseling session.

Contemplation (unsure about change) warrants counseling to try to determine those things that are positive and negative, pros and cons, or costs and benefits of making a change. In this task the counselor tries to uncover those aspects of change that allow for ambiguous thoughts about making a dietary change. It is important to start with the negatives and end with the positives when counseling in this fashion.

Client: "I know that I should change my dietary habits, but I just don't seem to be able to achieve those changes I know are important to my health."
Counselor: "You are frustrated because you know you should change your eating habits, but this seems to be out of your reach to achieve." (Reflection)
Client: "Yes!"

Counselor: "Would it be OK with you to explore some of the costs and benefits of making dietary changes?"

Client: "Sure."

Counselor: "To begin, what are some of the costs of changing your eating habits?"

Client: "One is that I just won't be able to do anything in a spontaneous fashion. I always thought that retirement would mean having fun and doing whatever at the moment seemed like fun. It was one of those blessings of your golden years. Now I have to constantly worry about what I eat. That just doesn't make life enjoyable."

Counselor: "You have looked forward to fun in retirement and these dietary changes just force you to be worried about something that you feel should be spontaneous and fun." (Reflection)

Client: "Yes!"

Counselor: "What are other things that make change difficult?" (Open Question)

Client: "I sometimes ask myself whether a difficult diet is really worth it. This happens when I am discouraged and wish for a way out."

Counselor: "You sometimes wonder if the diet is really of value." (Reflection)

Client: "Yes, when I am discouraged. I know that from all of the information that I have been given, the research shows that it will make me healthier."

Counselor: "Is it OK if we move to the benefits of changing your eating habits?"

Client: "Yes. I am told that I will have more energy and will feel better if I eat in a healthier way."

Counselor: "What might another benefit be?" (Open Question)

Client: "My doctor says that I will have more energy. I love to play with my grandchildren and would have more energy to do things with them."

Counselor: "To summarize, on the negative side you really want to be spontaneous in your retirement and are unsure about the health benefits of making dietary changes. On the positive side you have been told that you will have more energy if you follow a healthy dietary pattern and that energy might mean more fun with your grandchildren. (Summary) What are your thoughts now about changing your eating habits?" (Open Question)

Client: "It really isn't a contest. I love my grandchildren. They come first and are really the joy and fun in my life. I should try harder to follow a healthy eating pattern."

This client has moved from contemplation or being unsure about change to really feeling positive about beginning to make dietary changes. Note that this change happened because the counselor facilitated thoughts on the part of the client. The counselor is not providing a goal or a solution. The counselor listened in an active way and helped to provide an open mind to hear what the client felt.

Because the client was not in the action stage or ready to change, advice on diet was not given, solutions were not offered, goals that involved diet change were not set, lists of dos and don'ts on what to eat were not given. When the client reaches the action stage or is ready to change, goal setting and advice giving are appropriate tasks.

Counselor: "On a scale of 1 to 10, how ready are you to begin to make very small changes in your diet?"

Client: "I think that I am at a 9."

Counselor: "Why are you not a 10?"

Client: "I am very ready but want to proceed slowly. I really want to succeed."

Counselor: "That is great. Please know that I also only want your success. The goal you decide upon must be yours, not mine. I want to be sure that the dietary changes are tailored to your needs and life's activities."

The chapters that follow are designed to focus on tailoring the diet to the client. The chapters are organized around theories and facts about nutrition as it relates to specific disease states, dietary adherence to diet patterns that are connected to diseases states, inappropriate eating behaviors, assessing eating behaviors, and dietary treatment.

Reference

1. American Dietetic Association. *International Dietetics and Nutrition Terminology (IDNT) Reference Manual Standardized Language for the Nutrition Care Process.* Chicago: ADA, 2008: pp. 8, 32, 39, 171, 182, 230, 244–245.

CHAPTER 4

NUTRITION COUNSELING IN TREATMENT OF OBESITY

Chapter Objectives

1. Identify common, inappropriate behaviors associated with weight gain or overeating.

2. Identify individual eating behaviors using strategies that are a part of step 1, assessment.

3. Identify theories and strategies to treat inappropriate eating behaviors contributing to weight gain as a part of step 3, intervention.

4. As a part of step 3, generate appropriate strategies to counsel overweight clients in facilitating control of eating patterns.

5. As a part of step 3, recommend dietary adherence tools for weight-loss clients.

Theories and Facts About Nutrition Obesity

The Obesity Education Initiative (OEI) classifies overweight and obesity by BMI and waist circumference (Table 4–1).

Obesity is one of the most common medical disorders in the United States. From statistics collected in 2003–2004, 34% of adults were overweight and 32% were obese,[1] and the prevalence of obesity reached 30% of non-Hispanic white adults, 45% of non-Hispanic black adults, and 36.8% of Mexican Americans.[1,2]

Epidemiology studies show a positive association between mortality and obesity and increased risk for diabetes, heart disease, stroke, hypertension, gallstones, and certain types of cancer.[3-6] Assessment of the obese client requires both clinical and laboratory techniques. Epidemiologists predict that the current generation of

Table 4–1   Classification of Overweight and Obesity by BMI, Waist Circumference, and Associated Disease Risk*

	BMI (kg/m2)	Obesity Class	Disease risk* (Relative to Normal Weight and Waist Circumference)†	
			Men ≤ 40 in (≤ 102 cm) Women ≤ 35 in (≤ 88 cm)	> 40 in (> 102 cm) > 35 in (> 88 cm)
Underweight	< 18.5		–	–
Normal	18.5–24.9		–	–
Overweight	25.0–29.9		Increased	High
Obesity	30.0–34.9	I	High	Very High
	35.0–39.9	II	Very High	Very High
Extreme obesity	≥ 40	III	Extremely High	Extremely High

*Disease risk for type 2 diabetes, hypertension, and CVD.
†Increased waist circumference can also be a marker for increased risk even in persons of normal weight.

Adapted from Preventing and Managing the Global Epidemic of Obesity. Report of the World Health Organization Consultation of Obesity. WHO, Geneva, June 1997, by National Institutes of Health, National Heart, Lung, and Blood Institute, Obesity Education, Initiative PEI, North American Association for the Study of Obesity. The practical guide: Identification, evaluation, and treatment of overweight and obesity in adults, 2000. NIH Publication Number 00-4084.

children will live nearly one decade less than their parents due to the obesity pandemic.[7] The major diseases associated with obesity (coronary heart disease, diabetes, and high blood pressure) and their nutritional associations are discussed in Chapters 5, 6, and 8.

Identification, Measurement, and Classification of Obesity

Obesity is an excessive amount of weight in relation to height. It is also defined as an excessive amount of total body fat (adipose tissue) compared to lean body tissue. Regional adiposity targets specific areas of the body (abdominal area, hips, and thighs) in which there is an excess amount of adipose tissue. Additionally, researchers use statistical definitions of overweight or obesity, based on body dimensions and connect these with risk for adverse health outcomes.[8]

Several laboratory-based methods often used in research studies provide estimates of body fat. Body density determined using underwater weighing allows for a conversion equation to estimate a proportion of body fat. This methodology is considered the gold standard procedure for estimating body fat. It assumes that a two-compartment model of body composition will be adequate to obtain a valid measure of body fat content. This is reasonable, if one also assumes that the density of fat-free tissue is constant with little variation. Unfortunately, density does fluctuate with disease (e.g., osteoporosis), growth, aging, exercise, and malnutrition. While errors in estimating body fat content occur in many circumstances, the magnitude of these errors in terms of percentage of body fat is relatively small.

Nutrition counselors use other methods to estimate body fat content that do not require the density of lean tissue to be constant from person to person. Most notable is the dual emission x-ray absorptiometry (DEXA). It exposes the body to a very small dose of radiation and is thought to provide an accurate measure of total body fat content. Several other techniques of estimating total body fat are used in laboratories. They include isotopic dilution to assess body water, body potassium content to assess skeletal muscle mass, computed tomography (CT) scanning and magnetic resonance imaging (MRI) to assess body fat at a large number of sites or over the whole body. All these methods are expensive; require elaborate instrumentations using routine calibration; and, in some instances,

provide data that are difficult to analyze. These methods are con-
fined to the laboratory and are used almost exclusively for research
purposes.

Simple approaches to estimate body fat content include body
mass index (BMI)—the prediction of body fat from simple anthropometric measurements (see Appendix C) such as skinfolds and cir-
cumferences, and bioelectric impedance analysis (BIA).[9,10]

The BMI (kg/m^2), typically used in large-scale population studies, is a valid marker of body mass for height but is only a moderately valid surrogate for measuring body fat content. Fatness can
be measured by a number of techniques, but in epidemiologic studies it is usually measured by the skinfold thickness. When the BMI
is above 30 kg/m^2, skinfold measurements and BMI are positively
associated for the top 5 to 10% of the population. BIA may have
the potential to be a useful measure, but more research is needed
on its limitations and on the conditions under which it is best used.
In general, these methods provide estimates of mean total body fat
for a group of patients, but are not accurate for an individual.

Criteria for Defining Overweight in the United States

Statistical reports from the U.S. government as well as from academic researchers reporting in scientific and medical journals use a
survey-based BMI definition of overweight. Height and weight dis-
tributions of adult participants in the Second National Health and
Nutrition Examination Survey (NHANES II) of the National Center
for Health Statistics provide data for this definition. The overweight
category includes adults ages 20 years or older who have a BMI
greater than 27.8 for males and greater than 27.3 for females. This
is a statistical definition that corresponds to the 85th percentile of
BMI for persons ages 20 to 29 years in the NHANES II.[11]

Fat Distribution

Excessive amounts of weight involve excess body fat content but
may also be associated with a large skeletal and muscle mass. The
OEI monograph indicates that BMI may be misleading in very muscular individuals.[12] Very muscular persons may have a higher BMI
but little body fat. Excess fat occurs in variable patterns of distribution in the upper body and lower body. In addition, some individuals have more fat than others in the abdominal visceral

(intra-abdominal) compartment. Normal weight and obese men have more visceral fat on the average than normal weight and obese women. In both genders, the amount of visceral fat is thought to increase naturally with age.

Various types of obesity carry different levels of risk for heart disease, diabetes, and other common diseases. Researchers have found that upper body obesity and visceral obesity are the high-risk types of obesity.[12-16]

Calculating Body Mass Index and Waist-to-Hip Ratio

A body mass nomogram[17] or table in Table 4–2 provides a quick and simple way to determine BMI. BMI is calculated by dividing weight in kilograms by height in meters squared (kg/m^2), and waist-to-hip ratio (W:H) is calculated by dividing the waist measure by the hip measure. The OEI determined that the waist measurement alone was more highly associated with obesity and related disease. Due to the difficulties with measuring hip circumference it is often not a reliable measure. The OEI recommendations use only waist circumference in connecting obesity and disease.[12]

Recommended Energy and Nutrient Levels

Government authorities such as the U.S. Food and Nutrition Board's Committee on Recommended Dietary Allowances and the Canadian Ministry of Health and Welfare have published estimated energy requirements for various groups by age and sex.[17,18] An energy deficit of 3,500 calories is necessary for the loss of a pound of body fat. This means that with a deficit of 500 calories per day, an individual will lose a pound of weight each week. Whitney and Hamilton found that the loss of more than two pounds of body fat a week rarely can be maintained; they cautioned that a diet supplying less than 1,200 calories per day can be made adequate in vitamins and minerals only with great difficulty.[19]

Nutrient levels are important in promoting adequate nutrition. When weight loss is the goal, often the nutrient content of the eating pattern is a secondary concern but should be a major priority. To ensure adequate nutrient levels while reducing calories, attention must be given to Recommended Dietary Allowances (RDAs). For adults, the RDAs are 0.8 grams of protein per kilogram of body weight per day.[18] For a 70-kilogram man, that would be 56

Table 4–2   Body Mass Index (BMI) Table

BMI Height	19	20	21	22	23	24	25	26	27	28	29	30	31	32	33	34	35
								Weight (in pounds)									
4'10" (58")	91	96	100	105	110	115	119	124	129	134	138	143	148	153	158	162	167
4'11" (59")	94	99	104	109	114	119	124	128	133	138	143	148	153	158	163	168	173
5' (60")	97	102	107	112	118	123	128	133	138	143	148	153	158	163	168	174	179
5'1" (61")	100	106	111	116	122	127	132	137	143	148	153	158	164	169	174	180	185
5'2" (62")	104	109	115	120	126	131	136	142	147	153	158	164	169	175	180	186	191
5'3" (63")	107	113	118	124	130	135	141	146	152	158	163	169	175	180	186	191	197
5'4" (64")	110	116	122	128	134	140	145	151	157	163	169	174	180	186	192	197	204
5'5" (65")	114	120	126	132	138	144	150	156	162	168	174	180	186	192	198	204	210
5'6" (66")	118	124	130	136	142	148	155	161	167	173	179	186	192	198	204	210	216
5'7" (67")	121	127	134	140	146	153	159	166	172	178	185	191	198	204	211	217	223
5'8" (68")	125	131	138	144	151	158	164	171	177	184	190	197	203	210	216	223	230
5'9" (69")	128	135	142	149	155	162	169	176	182	189	196	203	209	216	223	230	236
5'10" (70")	132	139	146	153	160	167	174	181	188	195	202	209	216	222	229	236	243
5'11" (71")	136	143	150	157	165	172	179	186	193	200	208	215	222	229	236	243	250
6' (72")	140	147	154	162	169	177	184	191	199	206	213	221	228	235	242	250	258
6'1" (73")	144	151	159	166	174	182	189	197	204	212	219	227	235	242	250	257	265
6'2" (74")	148	155	163	171	179	186	194	202	210	218	225	233	241	249	256	264	272
6'3" (75")	152	160	168	176	184	192	200	208	216	224	232	240	248	256	264	272	279

Evidence Report of Clinical Guidelines on the Identification, Evaluation, and Treatment of Overweight and Obesity in Adults, 1998. NIH/National Heart, Lung, and Blood Institute (NHLBI).

Evidence Report of Clinical Guidelines on the Identification, Evaluation, and Treatment of Overweight and Obesity in Adults, 1998. NIH/National Heart, Lung, and Blood Institute (NHLBI).

grams of protein per day, and for a 55-kilogram woman, 44 grams. Patients who have renal insufficiency may have other prescribed protein levels (see Chapter 7).

There is a considerable difference of opinion as to whether carbohydrates or fats should be reduced in an energy-restricted diet. Table 4–3 illustrates macronutrients in relation to different types of diets. If restriction of carbohydrates is a focus, Table 4–3 shows that certain food groups that are very beneficial in terms of nutrient content may also be eliminated. In this case, the diet may provide decreased levels of Vitamin A and folate. Any dietary pattern that eliminates a macronutrient, such as carbohydrates, and in so doing eliminates food groups, will eliminate important micronutrients.

Significant weight reductions on very low carbohydrate diets probably result from loss of water bound to glycogen. With reduced carbohydrates in the diet, the body uses stored glycogen to maintain normal blood glucose levels. The water with its electrolytes that are bound to the glycogen is excreted by the kidneys.

The Women's Health Initiative (WHI) looked at caloric intake in elderly women who followed a low-fat, high-carbohydrate diet. The results of this randomized controlled trial showed that women lost weight in the first year and maintained that loss for an average of 7.5 years of follow-up. When stratified by age, ethnicity, or body mass index there was no tendency toward weight regain. Those women who ate lower fat diets tended to have greater weight loss.[20]

Table 4–3   Eliminating Some High Carbohydrate Foods Reduces Nutrient Quality

	Kcal	CHO	PRO	FAT	Vitamin A	Folate
Melon (1 cup)	57	13.7	1.5	.4	3069 IU (decreased cancer risk)	45 mog (prevents birth defects)
Whole Grain/ 7-Grain Healthy Choice Bread (1 slice)	80	18	4	1	——	60 mog (prevents birth defects)

An energy-restricted diet should provide vitamins and minerals at least equivalent to the RDAs. If calorie intake is very restricted, vitamin and mineral supplements may be needed.

The alcohol content of the diet should be assessed carefully at baseline, because clients tend to underestimate consumption. One gram of alcohol provides 7 calories. Beer and wine contain carbohydrates that also contribute calories. The calories from alcoholic beverages may be the difference between losing and gaining weight.

Water and other nonnutritive fluids are not restricted in a reduced calorie diet unless there are heart or kidney complications.

Adherence with Weight-Loss Progams

Behavioral programs are among the most widely used approaches for weight loss. Researchers have indicated that a weight loss of 5–10% is associated with clinically significant improvements in cardiovascular risk profiles and incidence of type 2 diabetes.[21,22]

The National Heart, Lung, and Blood Institute provides key components of weight loss strategies that include diet modification with a reduction of kilocalories per day from 500 to 1000 and increase in physical activity of 30 minutes or more of moderate-intensity 5 or more days per week. The Institute's report includes a focus on behavioral therapy that includes self-monitoring, stress management, stimulus control, problem-solving, contingency management, cognitive restructuring, and social support.[12]

Weight loss during active treatment is of obvious importance, but the more crucial concern is whether obese persons can be helped to achieve long-term weight loss.[23] There is a body of data on follow-ups of one year and longer.[24-29] The results for the first year of follow-up for behavioral treatment of obesity are encouraging. Wilson and Brownell found that weight losses at one year typically are similar to those following treatment and, sometimes, slightly better.[30] These findings for one year lend credence to the value of behavioral interventions. Consistent with one-year follow-up, weight maintenance at one and even two years post-treatment is promising.[23,31]

The OEI panel reviewed evidence from clinical trials and determined that the combined intervention of a low-calorie diet, increased physical activity, and behavioral therapy when compared to other single forms of weight loss intervention resulted in the greatest weight loss and overall weight maintenance.[32] Table 4–4 is a guide to selecting treatment.

Wing describes the success of behavior therapy in producing initial weight loss. She presents the outcome of a behavioral program as achieving a 20-pound weight loss within the first six months. This compares to a 10% loss from an initial body weight. The problem of weight loss maintenance still remains.[33]

Wing and Hill have established a registry of individuals who have lost at least 30 pounds and maintained this weight loss for 1 year. Within this registry there are 2500 persons who have lost 60 pounds and have maintained this loss for 6 years. The reports from these maintainers shows that they are following a low-fat (less than

Table 4–4   A Guide to Selecting Treatment

Treatment	BMI Category				
	25–26.9	27–29.9	30–34.9	35–39.9	≥ 40
Diet, physical activity, and behavior therapy	With co-morbidities	With co-morbidities	+*	+	+
Pharmacotherapy		With co-morbidities	+	+	+
Surgery				With co-morbidities	

- Prevention of weight gain with lifestyle therapy is indicated in any patient with a BMI ≥ 25 kg/m², even without co-morbidities, while weight loss is not necessarily recommended for those with a BMI of 25–29.9 kg/m² or a high waist circumference, unless they have two or more co-morbidities.
- Combined therapy with a low-calorie diet (LCD), increased physical activity, and behavior therapy provide the most successful intervention for weight loss and weight maintenance.
- Consider pharmacotherapy only if a patient has not lost 1 pound per week after 6 months of combined lifestyle therapy.

*The (+) represents the use of indicated treatment regardless of co-morbidities.

National Institutes of Health, National Heart, Lung, and Blood Institute, Obesity Education, Initiative PEI, North American Association for the Study of Obesity. The practical guide: Identification, evaluation, and treatment of overweight and obesity in adults, 2000. NIH Publication Number 00-4084.

24% of calories from fat), low-calorie eating pattern with an activity level that expends 2800 kcal per week. When the strategies to maintain this loss are requested, the maintainers state that they follow a very strict diet, exercise routinely, and weigh themselves daily. Almost half of them lost weight on their own with no help from a professional trainer.[34]

Another researcher who speaks on the topic of the obesity pandemic is Dr. William Dietz. He has made statements about the role of genetics in this problem. In his discussions he indicates that a person may be more susceptible to being overweight or obese because of genetics. Nevertheless, he points out that the gene pool of the United States had not changed dramatically in the past decade, yet weight has. It is clear that the environment and lifestyle, including exercise and diet, contribute significantly to the increasing rate of overweight and obesity.[35]

The medical team has many options available for weight-loss management. Before selecting a strategy, practitioners should analyze numerous methods. In weight-loss programs, unlike other areas of dietary change, practitioners have a great deal of research from which to draw conclusions. In the 1970s, much was written on treatments based on behavioral modification and their effectiveness as compared with traditional dietary methods based on short-term evaluation.[36-38] Although weight losses resulting from behavioral modification treatment strategies are statistically different from control group losses, these changes are small and not clinically significant, especially for grossly overweight persons.

Few long-term follow-up evaluations are available for dietary, medical, or behavioral modification programs. However, 12-month and longer evaluations of behavioral modification programs began to appear in the literature in the late 1970s. In a self-controlled behavioral program, Hall et al. found short-term weight losses that were not maintained over time.[39] Other studies have shown similar results.[40-42] Data from Stuart provide a single exception to these studies.[43] Using two key elements, individual behavioral modification sessions coupled with booster sessions throughout the follow-up, Stuart found an average weight loss of 32 pounds for eight patients at 12 months.

Miller and Sims evaluated components of a weight-loss program to compare the successful client with the unsuccessful one.[44]

Initially, stimulus control and contingency management (contracts) were found useful, but they were not significantly related to long-term success. This finding was corroborated in reports by Brownell and Stunkard[45] and by Wing,[41] suggesting that techniques necessary for weight maintenance may be quite different from those needed for short-term weight loss.[46-49]

The majority of successful clients over a 12-month period used (1) cognitive restructuring techniques (positive self-thoughts), (2) exercise, (3) social skills (assertiveness skills), and (4) eating style changes.[44] Mahoney and Teixeira report that changes in perfectionistic standards, negative beliefs, and self-defeating private monologues are important to success in a 12-month weight-control program.[50,51]

Researchers have found that exercise alone is an ineffective method in losing significant weight.[52-58] In light of this finding, most recent weight-loss programs incorporate a multidisciplinary approach to weight control. The most successful programs utilize a combination of behavior change (exercise and nutrition behavior) and moderate to severe caloric restriction.[59-63]

Many studies have stressed the importance of social support in weight-loss maintenance. Mahoney reported a high correlation between weight loss and family support in a two-year follow-up study.[50] In a more controlled study, Brownell and coworkers evaluated the involvement of spouses in the weight loss program.[64] Subjects whose spouses were trained to be supportive showed three times the weight loss of clients whose spouses were not trained. Clients were also taught the interpersonal skills, such as assertiveness, that are necessary for requesting appropriate support from others.[33,65]

Researchers' findings on eating style are contradictory.[66-70] Researchers have compared duration of eating, size of mouthfuls, time between bites, and chewing time of obese and non-obese individuals, but it is unclear whether these groups differ in these dimensions. Some researchers suggest that the "non-obese" eating style may be important in controlling food intake because it increases awareness of satiety cues and enhances feelings of self-efficacy and self-control.[40,68-70]

More research is needed in the form of controlled clinical trials (the Miller and Sims research was not in this category). Even though social skills training, exercise, and cognitive restructuring appear to influence long-term success, other forms of behavioral therapy should not be discounted. Indeed, combinations of behavioral techniques are provided below as examples of ways to deal with lack of commitment.

There are a variety of general techniques to facilitate weight loss. Honig reviews various psychological and nonpsychological strategies for treating overweight persons:[71]

- calorie counting
- behavioral modification
- self-help groups, such as Jenny Craig and Weight Watchers

Weight Watchers includes group support with a balanced, reduced-calorie diet, exercise and behavioral modification. While there are three randomized, controlled trials to look at results of this commercial weight loss program,[72-74] the largest showed that a comparison of Weight Watchers to a self-help guide, including visits with a registered dietitian and a self-help intervention, indicated a positive effect of the Weight Watchers intervention. Participants in the Weight Watchers program lost 5.3% of their baseline weight at year one (–4.3 kg) and maintained a loss of 3.2% at year two (–2.9 kg). The self-help group lost 1.5% of their baseline weight (–1.3 kg) at year one and did not maintain the loss, with 0% (–0.2 kg) at year two.[72-74]

Other methods used in weight loss are as follows:

- exercise programs
- gastric bypass surgery
- drugs to increase metabolic rate and suppress appetite
- popular "lose-pounds-quickly" diets

The OEI did not recommend use of the latter three treatments without major reasons to justify their use. Van Itallie,[75] Shikora et al.,[76] and Staten[77] carefully review the problems associated with the last three methods listed. Both surgical and pharmacologic treatments of obesity are expensive and carry serious side effects. There are a variety of complications associated with these non-lifestyle change methods for weight reduction: increased blood pressure, tachycardia, inhibition of absorption of fat-soluble vitamins and nutrients, mood-related disorders, and death.[78-81]

Inappropriate Eating Behaviors

The following thoughts are frequently associated with weight gain:

"I deserve it."
"It's just no use. I have no willpower."
"I'm bored."
"I'm off that rotten diet now."

Each of these thoughts have a direct bearing on the individual's propensity to gain weight. Nutrition counselors must be aware of a variety of thought processes as well as overt eating behaviors. It is important to try to identify antecedents and consequences of inappropriate eating behaviors.

Many present or future clients begin thinking about weight loss in terms of going on and off diets: "I go on a diet to lose weight. Usually I can't stand the diet. I just wait until I lose 10 or 15 pounds and then go back to eating those really good foods I'm accustomed to." This syndrome frequently is associated with alternating increases and decreases in weight.

Nutrition counselors might consider trying to avoid the term "diet" in their instructions to describe a means toward weight loss. The rationale is that along with the word "diet", the two negative words, "going off", tend to follow. Many clients will suggest that food is a kind of reward: "When I finish the house work (or reach the 3 PM break at my job), I feel like I deserve a reward, so I just go to the refrigerator (or vending machines or cafeteria). Right there in front of me are all the rewards I need. I really deserve to eat in payment for my hard work."

Signals or cues to eat are everywhere. Counselors should study each client's environment and note specific cues that trigger inappropriate eating behaviors. At home, candy near the television set can trigger snacking responses that might not occur otherwise. TV commercials may provide a stimulus to go to the kitchen for potato chips, candy bars, beverages, etc. Hu indicates that one-third of television watching can be attributed to increase in weight gain due to inactivity, but two-thirds is the suggestion to eat given by commercials advertising food.[82]

Many clients admit that boredom can cause inappropriate eating behaviors: "I eat because there is nothing else to do." Counselors can suggest many substitutes for eating to eliminate bore-dom and possibly increase activity. In some cases, hobbies or chores can serve as substitutes for eating while watching TV.

Some inappropriate behaviors involve rapid eating. It appears that the client is saying, "How fast can I clear this plate?" Along with this behavior is the inability to listen when the body provides signals of fullness or satiety. Booth states that satiety may not orig-inate solely from gastric motility and distention or a physiological state, and that the power of suggestion also may play a large role in providing signals of fullness.[83]

In the eating-chain syndrome as described by Ferguson, activi-ties can be used to break up patterns that lead to inappropriate behaviors.[84] Ferguson says that eating occurs at one end of a chain of responses. If the nutrition counselor works backward from the terminal behavior of eating, events or cues in the environment that started the chain of events leading to it can be identified. Wardle focuses on cueing in research that has shown positive results in weight control.[85]

Much of what goes on in the client's head, such as negative thoughts, can trigger inappropriate eating behaviors. The client who is thinking, "I'm really a rotten person for eating that piece of candy. It's no use. I might as well eat until I'm stuffed," probably will overeat out of despair. Mahoney describes the reversal of this process as "cognitive ecology."[86] By substituting positive thoughts for negative ones, clients can develop a built-in self-reward sys-tem.[87,88] Wing and Hill describe maintainers as persons who have skills to cope with negative thoughts. Instead of coming home after a bad day and binging on comfort foods, they use behaviors appro-priate for the feelings of anger, i.e., crying, going for a long walk, or writing thoughts down in a journal. [34]

In some cases, lack of exercise can be a problem. Some clients may complain, "I just don't feel like moving." Studies have shown that decreased caloric intake plus exercise can be beneficial.[56,89,90] In fact, more fat tissue is reduced (as opposed to muscle tissue) if exercise programs are included with lowered caloric intake.

In general, inappropriate eating behaviors and lack of exercise may contribute to weight gain. The first step in achieving weight loss is to identify accurately the inappropriate eating behaviors.

Assessment of Eating Behaviors

The nutrition counselor must assess clients' eating behaviors. The first step is to try to identify the general problem from the many that may surface in a general interview. In reality, overweight clients may not want to lose weight but appear for a counseling session because their spouse or doctor has sent them. In some cases the major problem may be psychological, and referral to a specialist in that field may be the best course of action.[91]

If referral does not seem necessary, the next step is data collection. Six factors related to weight gain should be emphasized:

1. eating patterns
2. food quantities
3. food quality
4. activity levels
5. food-related thoughts
6. food-related cues

Exhibit 4–1 presents instructions and a form to use in gathering information in each of these categories, and Exhibit 4–2 is a sample already filled out. Adherence Tool 4–1 is a questionnaire for clients to fill out, and a simplified monitoring device for use with goal attainment is provided in Adherence Tool 4–2. Brownell states that when assessing obese clients, it is important to cover the following categories:[92]

- physiology
- eating behaviors
- physical activity
- psychological and social adjustment

In assessing physical status, several categories should be considered: endocrine, hypothalamic, cardiopulmonary, orthopedic, genetic, weight, and family history. Bray and Teague provide an algorithm for medical assessment and delineate the steps necessary in diagnosing medical problems of an obese client.[93–96]

In the physiologic analysis, counselors should be concerned about body fat, which can be assessed through a variety of tests. The one most commonly used is skinfold thickness, using a caliper.

Exhibit 4–1   Data Collection Chart

INSTRUCTIONS FOR FILLING OUT THE FOOD DIARY

Time: Starting time for a meal or snack

Minutes spent eating: Length of the eating episode in minutes

M/S: Meal or snack (Indicate type of eating by the appropriate letter)

H: Hunger on a scale of 0 to 3, with 0 = no hunger, 3 = extreme hunger

Body position: 1 = walking; 2 = standing; 3 = sitting; 4 = lying down

Activity while eating: Record any activity you carry out while eating, such as watching television, reading, functioning in a workplace, or sweeping the floor.

Location of eating: Record each place you eat, such as your car, workplace, kitchen table, living room couch, or bed.

Food type and quantity: Indicate the content of your meal or snack by kind of food and quantity. Choose units of measurement that you will be able to reproduce from week to week. Accuracy is not as important as consistency.

Eating with whom: Indicate with whom you are eating or whether you are eating that meal or snack alone.

Feelings before and during eating: Record your feelings or mood immediately before (B) or while (W) eating. Typical feelings are anger, boredom, confusion, depression, frustration, sadness, etc.

Minutes spent exercising today: Record the total number of minutes you spent exercising, followed by the type of exercise (walking, jogging, running, riding a bicycle or a horse, dancing, skiing, swimming, bowling, etc.).

FOOD DIARY

Day of Week _____ Name _____

Time	Minutes Spent Eating	M/S	H	Body Position	Activity While Eating	Location of Eating	Food Type and Quantity	Eating with Whom	Feeling Before (B) and While (W) Eating	Minutes Spent Exercising Today
6:00										
11:00										
4:00										

M = Meal; S = Snack

H: Degree of Hunger (0 = None; 3 = Maximum)

Body Position: 1 = Walking, 2 = Sitting, 3 = Standing, 4 = Lying Down

(B): Before (W): While

Source: Adapted from *Habits Not Diets* by J.M. Ferguson, pp. 13–14, with permission of Bull Publishing Company, © 1976.

Exhibit 4–2 Example of Completed Food Diary Form

SAMPLE

Day of Week: Monday   Name: _____   R.S.T. _____

Time	Minutes Spent Eating	M/S	H	Body Position	Activity While Eating	Location of Eating	Food Type and Quantity	Eating With Whom	Feeling Before (B) and While (W) Eating	Minutes Spent Exercising Today
6:00										
7:20–30	10 min	M	0	3	Paper	Kitchen	8 oz. coffee, 1 cup cereal	Wife	Happy	40 minutes walking
8:15–20	5 min	S	0	2	Talking	Work	4 oz. whole milk, 1 cake doughnut	Friends	Tired (B)	
10:30–?	5 min	S	1	1	Walking	Hall	8 oz. coffee, 1 cake doughnut	Alone	Late (W)	
11:00										
12:30	1 min	S	2	2	Work	Desk	1–1.5 oz. Snicker	Alone	Late (W)	
3:30–3:40	10 min	M	3	3	Reading	Restaurant	1–8 oz. Coke, 3 oz. chd. Hamburger patty, 1 hamburger bun	Alone	Tired (B)	
4:00										
5:30–6:00	30 min	S	3 TV	3	Paper, 1/4 c. peanuts	L.R.	1 oz. Scotch	Family	Tired (B)	
6:00–7:00	1 hour	M	2	3	TV	D.R.	Beef TV dinner, 1 c. ice cream	Family	Angry (B)	
9:00										
10:30–10:45	15 min	S	0	2	TV	L.R.	1/2 c. ice cream	Wife	Bored (B)	

M/S: Meal or Snack H: Degree of Hunger (0 = None, 3 = Maximum)

Body Position: 1 = Walking, 2 = Standing, 3 = Sitting, 4 = Lying Down; (B): Before; (W): While

Source: Adapted from Habits Not Diets by J.M. Ferguson, pp. 13–14, with permission of Bull Publishing Company, © 1976.

Body fat is an indicator of physical status. Appendix C provides information on physiological measures of nutritional status.

Assessing eating behaviors is very important to eventual treatment. The most frequently used assessment method is a diet record. This can provide details on food preferences, eating style, environmental cues to eating, and amounts eaten.

Physical activity is an important component in any weight-loss program. Nutrition counselors should check on the client's exercise during both working and nonworking hours. Equally important is psychological and social functioning. Psychological functioning can include positive and negative monologues as described earlier; social functioning deals with responses by spouse, children, coworkers, or friends to weight loss and eating behaviors.

Treatment Strategies

All theories, behavioral modification, cognitive-behavioral theory, health-beliefs model, social learning theory, and the transtheoretical model/stages of change, are important in changing behaviors toward weight reduction.

Treatment strategies for obesity include self-management, self-monitoring, stimulus-control methods, reinforcement techniques, and motivational interviewing. Current programs have incorporated cognitive restructuring approaches, exercise, and social support in the achievement of long-term weight loss. Brownell provides a detailed list of many specific techniques that may be of value in the treatment of obesity.[31] The treatment strategies described below deal with the following three problems: lack of knowledge, lack of planning, and lack of commitment.

Strategies Dealing with Lack of Knowledge

At baseline, the client needs a clear understanding of information pertinent to weight gain. Adherence Tool 4–1 elicits information on current eating disorders. Baseline data should be compared with information collected during strategy implementation (Adherence Tool 4–2). Adherence Tool 4–3 provides suggestions on facilitating weight loss.

Within cognitive-behavioral theory are strategies to combat inappropriate eating behaviors that may begin with the concept of stimulus control. Many specific suggestions follow. One is substitution of non–food-related activities. With this method, it is necessary to work with the clients in developing a list of enjoyable activities, particularly those requiring substantial expenditure of energy. The information obtained in the Data Collection Chart (Exhibit 4–1) can suggest a starting point. It is preferable to select activities that fit into the clients' daily routine, based on their suggestions as to which ones would work best. This is a time when counselors' listening skills and encouragement for clients can generate solutions that will lead to optimum results. Instead of eating, clients can substitute other activities such as those in Exhibit 4–3.

Interposing time between eating episodes is a second method for diminishing the urge. This strategy may require the use of a cooking timer, alarm clock, etc. Clients are asked to delay a snack

---

Exhibit 4–3   *Activity Substitutes for Eating*

Clients can resort to numerous activities as alternatives to overeating. They can:
- Rearrange furniture.
- Spend extra time with a friend.
- Play cards or a game with someone—chess, Monopoly, bridge, etc.
- Go to a movie, play, or concert.
- Do something for charity.
- Go to a museum.
- Take a quiet walk.
- Take a long, leisurely bubble bath.
- Balance their checkbook.
- Write a letter.
- Make a phone call to a friend or relative.
- Wash their hair.
- Start a garden.
- Do home repairs.
- Write a creative poem or story.
- Do some sewing or creative stitchery.
- Do a crossword puzzle.
- Go jogging.
- Play golf.
- Join a softball team.
- Jump rope.
- Take up weight lifting.
- Go hiking.
- Take up, or increase participation in, a sport.

for a certain number of minutes. Gradually they will be able to increase the time between the urge to snack and the actual act of eating to 10 or 15 minutes. During this interlude, they should be encouraged to perform some other activity. Clients usually are amazed at how well this strategy curbs their appetites.

The third strategy is cue elimination. Exhibit 4–1 can help in determining which cues lead to improper eating. For example, by looking at a rough house plan and identifying where eating episodes are occurring, clients can set up roadblocks to those cues. Many clients will find their snacking locations show up in clusters around the television set, favorite chairs, or in the kitchen by the refrigerator or sink (or the cafeteria or vending machines at work). They may be shocked to find they eat in more places than they believed.

Ferguson has designed an exercise to help eliminate eating cues:[84]

1. Ask the clients to select a specific room in the house in which all eating should occur. This place should be regarded as relatively comfortable. They should be cautioned to avoid eating while working to break the chain of association between eating and other activities. The nutrition counselor could suggest that every designated eating place be special. For example, if clients must eat while working, if at all feasible a place mat and silverware should be set, with a real (not plastic) cup for coffee or tea. At home, candlelight, flowers, and attractive plates and silverware can make the designated place "special."
2. Ask the clients to separate eating from other activities—to avoid combining eating with telephone conversations, watching TV, reading, working, etc. The emphasis should be on food with others and on making eating enjoyable by focusing on the taste and texture of the ingredients.
3. Ask clients to remove food from all places (particularly visible ones) except appropriate storage areas in the kitchen and to keep stored food out of sight by placing it in cupboards, in opaque containers, or in the refrigerator.
4. Suggest that clients keep fresh fruits and vegetables for snacks in attractive containers.
5. Request that clients remove serving containers from the table during mealtimes.

Once nutrition counselors have helped clients eliminate cues, the strategy can turn to decreasing serving size slowly. The use of smaller plates and smaller portions will decrease total caloric consumption. Nouvelle cuisine, with its very small portions arranged artistically in the center of large plates, is an attractive alternative. The regular menu can simply be restaged in a fancier setting at no additional cost.

Many of the strategies that were just described might include social support to involve spouse, family, and/or friends. Clients should be told to explain the strategies to anyone seen regularly. Closest friends' understanding of the program rationale can provide moral support. Through teaching others, clients may grasp strategies more clearly. Appendixes D and E provide useful tools for recording eating behaviors.

Strategies Dealing with Lack of Planning

In the Women's Health Initiative (WHI), a group of women were asked about their success with eating behavior change. They indicated that the one strategy that helped most in achieving adherence to the low-fat dietary pattern was planning for eating situations. Planning ahead can make a social situation a success when following a more healthful dietary pattern.

At social events planning ahead can provide stimulus control in avoiding inappropriate eating behaviors. A note on the refrigerator can remind the client of an upcoming event, "Don't forget to plan for Jan's party." Planning may involve calling the hostess on the phone to obtain a list of party foods to be served. This same idea can help clients plan for problem times such as eating out, weddings, or anniversaries. The cues should be simple and visible, such as "Remember your restaurant engagement Friday at noon!" posted on the bathroom mirror.

Strategies that have helped research participants follow a more healthful dietary pattern include bringing a healthy and flavorful dish to a potluck. Sitting and talking with a friend is one way of avoiding the banquet table during dessert time. One client described asking a relative to go for a walk after eating a large Thanksgiving meal. Each of these activities is helpful in avoiding overeating and should be a part of planning ahead for a healthy lifestyle.

Many problems occur when people act spontaneously and

either unknowingly or by choice fall into old habits. Planning ahead can give clients the time they need to avoid situations that lead to inappropriate eating behaviors.

Strategies to Deal with Lack of Commitment

When clients know what is causing inappropriate behaviors and have used planning ahead without success, they may be entering a phase in which altering their lifestyle to make changes in body weight no longer seems important—the relapse phase. At this point, a review of the client's initial list of reasons for wanting to lose weight may be valuable in identifying why commitment is waning. Both steps 1 and 3 of the nutrition care process require the identification of behavioral problems and potential solutions to those problems. In this text Part II describes the two steps, assessment and intervention, in the nutrition care process that focus on behavioral strategies.

Step 3 of the intervention focuses on behavioral theories or approaches as described in Chapter 3 and strategies that will help in implementing the theories or approaches. Below are examples of potential uses of both theories and strategies.

The strategy of motivational interviewing uses the stages of change to assist in reestablishing motivation. While the stages of change description includes five stages, the text that follows collapses them into three.[97]

Pre-contemplation will be assigned the label of unready to change. Contemplation is equivalent to unsure about change. Preparation and action stages will be the ready to change group.

In a relapse situation, it is important to emphasize that slips are normal. They are expected whenever changes in long-standing behaviors occur. Slips can be positive because they provide lessons in dealing with problems associated with eating behavior changes. The nutrition counselor's goal is to help the client avoid discouragement and continue change in eating behaviors (cognitive restructuring). This includes the use of concepts in cognitive-behavioral theory. Use the adherence thermometer as described in Chapter 3 (Figure 3-2) and the readiness-to-change thermometer (Figure 3-3) to scale behavior into a stage as described in the strategy of motivational interviewing. Scaling provides a way of quantifying a behavior so that both the client and counselor can describe the degree of movement toward or away from meeting a goal. Following scaling a dialogue helps to identify barriers to change and strategies to eliminate them.

One strategy involves exploring negative thoughts. In some cases negative thoughts result from repeated indiscretions. Positive thinking is a useful strategy to deal with negative thoughts. Appendix F gives examples of ways in which record-keeping (self-monitoring) can help uncover negative thoughts associated with inappropriate eating behaviors. Getting clients to see how often negative thoughts force excessive food consumption can be a first step to weight control (cognitive restructuring). This change from negative to positive thinking is an activity in which clients are very much in charge. An example of a negative thought is: "I'm such a failure. I can't do anything right. I might as well give up. Who cares if I stuff myself with this cake?"

This negative monologue can be transformed to more positive thinking: "I ate one piece of cake, and even though it is high in calories I can stop with that one piece. I'm really feeling good about being able to stop without going ahead and eating the entire cake." From that point on, the clients can formulate positive self-thoughts to replace their negative ones (cognitive restructuring) (see Appendix G).

For most people, increasing exercise in combination with decreasing calories is helpful. Exhibit 4-1 is used to determine baseline activity levels. Many of the suggestions listed as substitutes for eating in Exhibit 4-3 involve an increase in activity. Nutrition counselors should encourage clients to enroll in exercise programs but caution them to check with a physician first.

Client progress is evaluated by comparing current and past data (use of self-monitoring records), as in Exhibit 4-4. Graphs of weight loss over time associated with specific eating behaviors (i.e., fat intake) may provide valuable feedback. Also, tables or graphs will show when successes occurred so that the client can reflect on what specifically happened at those positive weight loss points. Clients can be asked to extend a strategy, possibly by increasing negative-to-positive thought transformations (cognitive restructuring). If a strategy is not working, it should be revised. For example, if finding a designated eating place at work poses problems (stimulus control/contingency management), the nutrition counselor may need to discuss other means of cue elimination (e.g., finding a

Exhibit 4–4 Eating Pattern Maintenance Data Collection

Day of Week _____ Name _____

Time	M/S	H	Food type and Quantity	Minutes Spent Exercising and Type of Exercise
6:00 AM				
11:00 AM				
4:00 PM				
9:00 PM				

M/S: Meal or Snack
H: Degree of Hunger (0 = none; 3 = maximum)
Source: Adapted from *Habits Not Diets* by J.M. Ferguson, pp. 87, with permission of Bull Publishing Company, © 1976.

specific place to eat with a plate and silverware). In some cases, a new strategy may be appropriate. If clients find it impossible to substitute non-eating activities for routine snacking, it may be necessary first to work to eliminate negative monologues (cognitive restructuring), and then to add other activities as monologues are transformed to a more positive mode.

Preparation and Action (Ready to Change)

For clients who are ready to change, the process of negotiating a goal is a process that occurs easily. The overall goal is to present a reasonable plan for 5–10% weight loss from the client's initial weight with gradual movement toward a reasonable weight goal.

Counselor: Daniel, how are things going with the eating pattern we discussed last time?

Client: I just think that I need a bit more information on how to find substitutes for snacks. I have been able to reach my goal of last time to cut down on total calories at night but during lunch time I am in a hurry and often eat foods too high in saturated fat.

Counselor: Would you like to set a new goal?

Client: Yes.

Counselor: Do you have a suggestion?

Client: I could eat a bag of low-fat pretzels, I remember they were a low-calorie alternative to chips that we discussed several visits ago.

Counselor: Yes, great idea.

Client: Great, I will eat pretzels at lunch instead of the chips I am now eating.

Contemplation (Unsure About Change)

In this scenario the client is contemplating change. The counselor's goal is to move toward preparation and action. To accomplish this goal, a very client-focused approach is necessary. Initially the client is asked why he/she does not want to change. This is followed with the positive reasons for wanting to change. Within motivational intervening as a strategy, this pro/con discussion about reasons for change can often result in movement toward a more positive focus on making lifestyle behavioral changes.

Client: I just feel that everyone is forcing me to make a change in my eating habits, and I really want everything to stay the same (not ready for dietary change).

Counselor: Would it be OK to talk about some of the reasons for not making changes and just keeping everything the same?

Client: I really feel that reducing my weight is too much work.

Counselor: Any other reasons?

Client: I just want to forget about my weight and not worry about it anymore.

Counselor: Other reasons?

Client: I have tried in the past and always failed. I reduce my weight and something happens and I go right back to where I started. Why even try?

Counselor: Very good! I appreciate your openness. Let's look at this from the other side. What are some reasons that make you feel you should reduce your weight?

Client: My doctor says I would be healthier.

Counselor: Other reasons?

Client: I would have more energy.

Counselor: Any other reasons?

Client: I really love to play with my grandchildren. Being overweight really makes that impossible. Being able to do things with them is really the joy of my life.

Counselor: Thank you so much for sharing this with me. So you have several reasons for wanting to keep your weight the same: it is too much work; you just don't want to worry about it anymore; and you always fail, why keep trying. On the other side, you have some positive thoughts: you would be healthier; you would have more energy; and you could play with your grandchildren. So what are your thoughts? What is most important to you now and how are the scales tipped in terms of the positive and negative of changing your eating pattern?

Client: There really is no contest. My grandchildren mean the world to me, and I want to spend quality time with them.

The scenarios above show a way of listing the positives and negatives of making a dietary change. It is best to review the positives last and first to allow the client to vent about some of the frustrations of making dietary changes.

Precontemplation (Not Ready to Change)

In this stage, we have a person who is not ready to change and sees the change as being something that is desired by others but not him/her. Below is an example of a scenario where the client may be moved to make a change despite the desire to keep things the same. For this client, goal setting will only result in feelings of failure for both client and counselor. The goal is to allow the client to feel in control. The counselor might say, "You know best what will work for you now. Please go home and think about the possibility of working on a change. You do not need to focus on details now. Just think carefully about beginning a discussion on changing your lifestyle in a very manageable and minor way. I am always here to help you. You have my e-mail address and phone number. I am here for you whenever you want to talk."

This process of redirecting actual change to the client allows for a level of client control and changes the counseling from one of "do what I say" to "your feelings and thoughts on change matter." This method immediately results in a mutual respect. For the client who is on the defensive because he/she really is not ready to make major life changes, at least initially, this opens a door of opportunity. Clients begin thinking, "This counselor really isn't here to force changes. I do have a say in what I might do to make lifestyle changes. Maybe by starting slowly this will work."

Facilitating the desire for commitment may require more intensive counselor–client interaction. This may involve periodic phone calls set up to assess compliance with behaviors identified in a contract such as the one shown in Exhibit 4–5. Many psychologists who use the stages of change methodology may not use contracting. The use of a contract will depend on the receptivity of the client. For example, a contract often involves a reward. Some clients may feel uncomfortable rewarding themselves. If the scaling process above is used, a contract may not be necessary.

Although individual counseling is important and is effective initially in tailoring the diet, additionally group sessions can be very helpful in facilitating maintenance of a low-calorie eating

---

Exhibit 4-5   Sample Contract

I will reward myself each day for avoiding a high-calorie snack from 8:00 AM to 12:00 noon. I will avoid those foods I frequently use:
- 3 doughnuts or
- 2 Hostess Twinkies or
- 24 chocolate drops

I will substitute instead one of the following low-calorie foods from home:
- 5 saltine crackers with reduced sugar fruit jam
- Sugar-free gum
- 5 pretzel sticks

If I accomplish this goal in three out of five working days, I will reward myself with one of the following:
- shopping spree
- visit to my best friend who lives 20 miles away
- a night out at the theater

If I do not achieve the above goal, I will receive no rewards.

Every Friday at 10:00 AM (nutrition counselor) will call to check on my progress.

Client_____

Friend or Spouse_____

Nutrition Counselor_____

pattern. Groups provide support, ideas, chastisement, and concern. They can be very potent factors in achieving behavior change. The following are some basic group process guidelines:

- Ask open questions to begin sessions and start conversations on successes or failures with weight loss.
- Use the group members as a source for problem-solving ideas.
- Place yourself, the counselor, in the role of facilitator.
- Make eye contact with less verbal class members to draw them out.
- Use more positive group members to keep other members' negative thoughts at a minimum.
- Use basic interviewing and counseling skills.

Group counseling is more a matter of skill mastery than concept memorization. To gain skill in this area, counselors should request to observe any group-process meeting that requires members' active participation.

Conclusion

In summary, nutrition counseling for weight loss requires a knowledge of cues that promote overeating, suggestions for planning ahead, and theories and related behavioral strategies to increase commitment to dietary change once readiness to change is determined.

Review of Chapter 4

1. In the following examples, identify the inappropriate eating behaviors associated with weight gain:

   "I have followed this diet so religiously, I'm really proud of myself. The agony of passing up cocktails and opting for the diet drink at a party, the embarrassment of refusing my friend's seven-layer torte, the pain of refusing the birthday cake my kids made especially for me, and on and on. Those days are behind me now. I lost 20 pounds and now I'm home free."

What syndrome is this sort of thinking leading to?

"What is wrong with me? Don't I have any willpower? I look like a fat slob and yet I continue to eat. I'm just a hopeless case."

What syndrome does this sort of self-talk tell you as a counselor that the client is struggling with?

2. List three steps in assessing individual eating behaviors.

   a.

   b.

   c.

3. List six strategies with their corresponding theories that might be used to facilitate weight loss in the following two clients.

   Jan, a 30-year-old female, is nearly 20 pounds overweight. She is very upset over this and has tried many ways toward quick and easy weight control—diet pills, fasting, fad diets, etc. Jan has a family of four and works from 8 AM to 5 PM at a dress shop. She prepares breakfast for her family each morning, eats at a cafeteria for lunch, and fixes dinner for the family each evening. Her major problem, she indicates, is evening snacking.

   Dan, a 40-year-old male, is 30 pounds overweight. He frequently is depressed over his weight and has tried many lose-weight-quick treatments. All have failed. He lives alone and works nights on a line in a factory. He sleeps during the day and eats all of his meals away from home.

   a.

   b.

   c.

   d.

   e.

   f.

4. Describe one situation in which you would use one or more of those six strategies. Indicate your rationale.

References

1. Ogden CL, Carroll MD, Curtin LR, McDowell MA, Tabak CJ, Flegal KM. Prevalence of overweight and obesity in the United States, 1999–2004. *JAMA* 2006;295(13):1549–1555.
2. National Center for Health Statistics. *Obesity Still a Major Problem.* February 12, 2007. Available at: http://www.cdc.gov/nchs/press-room/06facts/obesity03_04.htm. Accessed July 17, 2007.
3. Pi-Sunyer FX. Health implications of obesity. *Am J Clin Nutr* 1991;53(6 Suppl):1595S–1603S.
4. Calle EE, Thun MJ, Petrelli JM, Rodriguez C, Heath CW, Jr. Body-mass index and mortality in a prospective cohort of U.S. adults. *N Engl J Med* 1999;341(15):1097–1105.
5. Field AE, Coakley EH, Must A, et al. Impact of overweight on the risk of developing common chronic diseases during a 10-year period. *Arch Intern Med* 2001;161(13):1581–1586.
6. Sturm R, Wells KB. Does obesity contribute as much to morbidity as poverty or smoking? *Public Health* 2001;115(3):229–235.
7. Doyle R. Sizing up. *Sci Am* 2006;294(2):32.
8. Heshka S, Buhl K, Heymsfield SB. Clinical evaluation of body composition and energy expenditure. In: Blackburn GL, Kanders BS, eds. *Obesity: Pathophysiology, Psychology, and Treatment.* New York: Chapman and Hall, 1994:39–56, 61–62.
9. Kyle UG, Bosaeus I, De Lorenzo AD, et al. Bioelectrical impedance analysis—part I: review of principles and methods. *Clin Nutr* 2004;23(5):1226–1243.
10. Brodie D, Moscrip V, Hutcheon R. Body composition measurement: a review of hydrodensitometry, anthropometry, and impedance methods. *Nutrition* 1998;14(3):296–310.
11. Simple Online Data Archive for POPulation Studies. Penn State. Available at: http://sodapop.pop.psu.edu/data-collections/nhanes/nhanes03. Accessed July 3, 2007.
12. National Institutes of Health, National Heart, Lung and Blood Institute, Obesity Education Initiative (OEI). The practical guide: Identification, evaluation, and treatment of overweight and obesity in adults. Bethesda, MD: NIH, 2000. NIH Publication number 00-4084.
13. Kissebah AH, Freedman DS, Peiris AN. Health risks of obesity. *Med Clin North Am* 1989;73(1):111–138.
14. Vague J. Diabetogenic and atherogenic fat. In: Oomura Y, Tarui S, Inoue S, Shimazu T, eds. *Progress in Obesity Research.* London: John Libbey, 1991:343–358.
15. Ostlund RE, Jr., Staten M, Kohrt WM, Schultz J, Malley M. The ratio of waist-to-hip circumference, plasma insulin level, and glucose intoler-

ance as independent predictors of the HDL2 cholesterol level in older adults. *N Engl J Med* 1990;322(4):229–234.

16. Björntorp P. Criteria of Obesity. In: Oomura Y, Tarui S, Inoue S, Shimazu T, eds. *Progress in Obesity Research.* London: John Libbey, 1990, 1991:655–658.

17. Canada H. Body Mass Index (BMI) Nomogram. Available at: http://www.hc-sc.gc.ca/fn-an/nutrition/weights-poids/guide-ld-adult/bmi_chart_java-graph_imc_java_e.html. Accessed April 17, 2007.

18. Institute of Medicine of the National Academies. Dietary reference intakes: Essential guide to nutrient requirements. Washington, D.C.: The National Academies Press, 2006.

19. Whitney E, Hamilton E. *Understanding Nutrition*, 5th ed. Eagen, MN: West Publishing Company, 1990.

20. Howard BV, Manson JE, Stefanick ML, et al. Low-fat dietary pattern and weight change over 7 years: the Women's Health Initiative Dietary Modification Trial. *JAMA* 2006;295(1):39–49.

21. National Institutes of Health. Clinical guidelines on the identification, evaluation, and treatment of overweight and obesity in adults—the evidence report. *Obes Res* 1998;6 Suppl 2:51S–209S.

22. Westerlind KC. Physical activity and cancer prevention—mechanisms. *Med Sci Sports Exerc* 2003;35(11):1834–1840.

23. Brownell K, Kramer F. Behavioral management of obesity. In: Blackburn GL, Kanders BS, eds. *Obesity: Pathophysiology, Psychology and Treatment.* New York: Chapman and Hall, 1994:231–236.

24. Brownell K, Jeffery R. Improving long-term weight loss: pushing the limits of treatment. *Behav Ther* 1987(18):353–374.

25. Kramer FM, Jeffery RW, Forster JL, Snell MK. Long-term follow-up of behavioral treatment for obesity: patterns of weight regain among men and women. *Int J Obes* 1989;13(2):123–136.

26. Wadden TA, Stunkard AJ, Liebschutz J. Three-year follow-up of the treatment of obesity by very low calorie diet, behavior therapy, and their combination. *J Consult Clin Psychol* 1988;56(6):925–928.

27. Agras WS, Telch CF, Arnow B, Eldredge K, Marnell M. One-year follow-up of cognitive-behavioral therapy for obese individuals with binge eating disorder. *J Consult Clin Psychol* 1997;65(2):343–347.

28. Anderson JW, Konz EC, Frederich RC, Wood CL. Long-term weight-loss maintenance: a meta-analysis of US studies. *Am J Clin Nutr* 2001;74(5):579–584.

29. Wadden TA, Frey DL. A multicenter evaluation of a proprietary weight loss program for the treatment of marked obesity: a five-year follow-up. *Int J Eat Disord* 1997;22(2):203–212.

30. Wilson G, Brownell K. Behavior therapy for obesity: an evaluation of treatment outcome. *Adv Behav Res Therap* 1980(3):49.

31. Brownell KD. *The LEARN Program for Weight Management*, 10th ed. Dallas, TX: American Health Publishing Company, 2004.

32. Klauer J, Aronne LJ. Managing overweight and obesity in women. *Clin Obstet Gynecol* 2002;45(4):1080–1088.

33. Wing RR. Behavioral strategies to improve long-term weight loss and maintenance. *Med Health RI* 1999;82(4):123.
34. Wing RR, Hill JO. Successful weight loss maintenance. *Annu Rev Nutr* 2001;21:323–341.
35. Dietz W. Current trends in obesity: clinical impact and interventions that work. *Ethn Dis* 2002;12(1):S2-17-20.
36. Jeffrey D. Prevalence of overweight and weight loss behavior in a metropolitan adult population: The Minnesota Heart Survey Experience. *Addict Behav* 1975;1:23–26.
37. Leon GR. Current directions in the treatment of obesity. *Psychol Bull* 1976;83(4):557–578.
38. Stunkard AJ. From explanation to action in psychosomatic medicine: the case of obesity. *Psychosomatic Med* 1975;37:195–236.
39. Hall S, Hall R, Hanson R, Borden B. Permanence of two self-managed treatments of overweight in university and community populations. *J Consult Clin Psychol* 1974;42(6):781–786.
40. Beneke WM, Paulsen BK. Long term efficacy of a behavior modification weight loss program: a comparison of two follow-up maintenance strategies. *Behav Therap* 1978;10:8–13.
41. Wing RR. Behavioral treatment of severe obesity. *Am J Clin Nutr* 1992;55(2 Suppl):545S–551S.
42. Kingsley RG, Wilson GT. Behavior therapy for obesity: a comparative investigation of long-term efficacy. *J Consult Clin Psychol* 1977;45(2):288–298.
43. Stuart RB. Behavior control of overeating. *Behav Res Ther* 1967;5:357–365.
44. Miller PM, Sims KL. Evaluation and component analysis of a comprehensive weight control program. *Int J Obes* 1981;5(1):57–65.
45. Brownell KD, Stunkard AJ. Behavior therapy and behavior change: uncertainties in programs for weight control. *Behav Res Ther* 1978;16(4):301.
46. Anderson JW, Grant L, Gotthelf L, Stifler LT. Weight loss and long-term follow-up of severely obese individuals treated with an intense behavioral program. *Int J Obes (Lond)* 2007;31(3):488–493.
47. Riebe D, Blissmer B, Greene G, et al. Long-term maintenance of exercise and healthy eating behaviors in overweight adults. *Prev Med* 2005;40(6):769–778.
48. Foster GD, Phelan S, Wadden TA, Gill D, Ermold J, Didie E. Promoting more modest weight losses: a pilot study. *Obes Res* 2004;12(8):1271–1277.
49. Raynor HA, Jeffery RW, Phelan S, Hill JO, Wing RR. Amount of food group variety consumed in the diet and long-term weight loss maintenance. *Obes Res* 2005;13(5):883–890.
50. Mahoney MJ. Treatment of obesity: a clinical exploration. In: Williams BJ, Sander M, Foreyt JP, eds. *Obesity: Behavioral Approaches to Dietary Management.* New York: Brunner/Mazel; 1976:30–39.
51. Teixeira PJ, Going SB, Houtkooper LB, et al. Pretreatment predictors of

attrition and successful weight management in women. *Int J Obes Relat Metab Disord* 2004;28(9):1124–1133.

52. Wilmore JH. Body composition in sport and exercise: directions for future research. *Med Sci Sports Exerc* 1983;15(1):21–31.

53. Zuti WB, Golding LA. Comparing diet and exercise as weight reduction tools. *Phys Sports Med* 1976;4:49.

54. Gwinup G. Weight loss without dietary restriction: efficacy of different forms of aerobic exercise. *Am J Sports Med* 1987;15(3):275–279.

55. Meijer GAL. *Physical Activity: Implications for Human Energy Metabolism.* Doctoral dissertation, University of Limburg at Maastricht, 1990.

56. Hill JO, Sparling PB, Shields TW, Heller PA. Effects of exercise and food restriction on body composition and metabolic rate in obese women. *Am J Clin Nutr* 1987;46(4):622–630.

57. Borg P, Kukkonen-Harjula K, Fogelholm M, Pasanen M. Effects of walking or resistance training on weight loss maintenance in obese, middle-aged men: a randomized trial. *Int J Obes Relat Metab Disord* 2002;26(5):676–683.

58. Miller WC. How effective are traditional dietary and exercise interventions for weight loss? *Med Sci Sports Exerc* 1999;31(8):1129–1134.

59. Treatment of obesity in adults. Council on Scientific Affairs. *JAMA* 1988;260(17):2547–2551.

60. Pavlou KN, Steffee WP, Lerman RH, Burrows BA. Effects of dieting and exercise on lean body mass, oxygen uptake, and strength. *Med Sci Sports Exerc* 1985;17(4):466–471.

61. Jeffery RW, Linde JA, Finch EA, Rothman AJ, King CM. A satisfaction enhancement intervention for long-term weight loss. *Obesity (Silver Spring)* 2006;14(5):863–869.

62. Malone M, Alger-Mayer SA, Anderson DA. The lifestyle challenge program: a multidisciplinary approach to weight management. *Ann Pharmacother* 2005;39(12):2015–2020.

63. Tate DF, Wing RR, Winett RA. Using Internet technology to deliver a behavioral weight loss program. *JAMA* 2001;285(9):1172–1177.

64. Brownell KD, Heckerman CL, Westlake RJ, Hayes SC, Monti PM. The effect of couples training and partner co-operativeness in the behavioral treatment of obesity. *Behav Res Ther* 1978;16(5):323–333.

65. McLean N, Griffin S, Toney K, Hardeman W. Family involvement in weight control, weight maintenance and weight-loss interventions: a systematic review of randomised trials. *Int J Obes Relat Metab Disord* 2003;27(9):987–1005.

66. Mahoncy MJ. The obese eating style: bites, beliefs, and behavior modification. *Addict Behav* 1975;1(1):47–53.

67. Adams N, Ferguson J, Stunkard AJ, Agras S. The eating behavior of obese and nonobese women. *Behav Res Ther* 1978;16(4):225–232.

68. Rolls BJ, Morris EL, Roe LS. Portion size of food affects energy intake in normal-weight and overweight men and women. *Am J Clin Nutr* 2002;76(6):1207–1213.

69. McCrory MA, Fuss PJ, Saltzman E, Roberts SB. Dietary determinants of

energy intake and weight regulation in healthy adults. *J Nutr* 2000;130(2S Suppl):276S–279S.

70. Lluch A, Herbeth B, Mejean L, Siest G. Dietary intakes, eating style and overweight in the Stanislas Family Study. *Int J Obes Relat Metab Disord* 2000;24(11):1493–1499.
71. Honig JF, Blackburn GL. The problem of obesity: an overview. In: Blackburn GL, Kanders BS, eds. *Obesity: Pathophysiology, Psychology and Treatment.* New York: Chapman and Hall, 1994:1–8.
72. Heshka S, Anderson JW, Atkinson RL, et al. Weight loss with self-help compared with a structured commercial program: a randomized trial. *JAMA* 2003;289(14):1792–1798.
73. Djuric Z, DiLaura NM, Jenkins I, et al. Combining weight-loss counseling with the weight watchers plan for obese breast cancer survivors. *Obes Res* 2002;10(7):657–665.
74. Rippe JM, Price JM, Hess SA, et al. Improved psychological well-being, quality of life, and health practices in moderately overweight women participating in a 12-week structured weight loss program. *Obes Res* 1998;6(3):208–218.
75. Van Itallie TB. Dietary approaches to the treatment of obesity. In: Stunkard AJ, ed. *Obesity.* Philadelphia: Saunders; 1980:249–261.
76. Shikora SA, Benorri PN, Norse RA. Surgical treatment of obesity. In: Blackburn GL, Kanders BS, eds. *Obesity: Pathophysiology, Psychology and Treatment.* New York: Chapman and Hall, 1994:264–282.
77. Staten MA. Pharmacologic therapy for obesity. In: Blackburn GL, Kanders BS, eds. *Obesity: Pathophysiology, Psychology and Treatment.* New York: Chapman and Hall, 1994:283–299.
78. Despres JP, Golay A, Sjostrom L. Effects of rimonabant on metabolic risk factors in overweight patients with dyslipidemia. *N Engl J Med* 2005;353(20):2121–2134.
79. Maggard MA, Shugarman LR, Suttorp M, et al. Meta-analysis: surgical treatment of obesity. *Ann Intern Med* 2005;142(7):547–559.
80. Abenhaim L, Moride Y, Brenot F, et al. Appetite-suppressant drugs and the risk of primary pulmonary hypertension. International Primary Pulmonary Hypertension Study Group. *N Engl J Med* Aug 29 1996;335(9):609–616.
81. Connolly HM, Crary JL, McGoon MD, et al. Valvular heart disease associated with fenfluramine-phentermine. *N Engl J Med* Aug 28 1997;337(9):581–588.
82. Hu FB, Li TY, Colditz GA, Willett WC, Manson JE. Television watching and other sedentary behaviors in relation to risk of obesity and type 2 diabetes mellitus in women. *JAMA* 2003;289(14):1785–1791.
83. Booth DA. Acquired behavior controlling energy input and output. In: Stunkard AJ, ed. *Obesity.* Philadelphia: W.B. Saunders Company, 1980:102.
84. Ferguson JM. *Habits Not Diets.* Palo Alto, CA: Bull Publishing Co., 1976.
85. Wardle J. Conditioning processes and cue exposure in the modification of excessive eating. *Addict Behav* 1990;15(4):387–393.

86. Mahoney MJ, Mahoney K. *Permanent Weight Control, A Solution to the Dieter's Dilemma.* New York: W.W. Norton & Company, 1976.

87. Telch CF, Agras WS, Rossiter EM, Wilfley D, Kenardy J. Group cognitive-behavioral treatment for the nonpurging bulimic: an initial evaluation. *J Consult Clin Psychol* 1990;58(5):629–635.

88. Dimatteo MR, DiNicola DD. *Achieving Patient Compliance: The Psychology of the Medical Practitioner's Role.* New York: Pergamon Press, 1982.

89. Woo R, Garrow JS, Pi-Sunyer FX. Effect of exercise on spontaneous calorie intake in obesity. *Am J Clin Nutr* 1982;36(3):470–477.

90. Miller WC, Koceja DM, Hamilton EJ. A meta-analysis of the past 25 years of weight loss research using diet, exercise or diet plus exercise intervention. *Int J Obes Relat Metab Disord* 1997;21(10):941–947.

91. Russell ML. *Behavioral Counseling in Medicine: Strategies for Modifying At-Risk Behavior.* New York: Oxford University Press, 1986.

92. Brownell KD. Assessment of eating disorders. In: Barlow D, ed. *Assessment of Adult Disorders.* New York: Guilford Press; 1981:366–374.

93. Bray BA, Teague RJ. An algorithm for the medical evaluation of obese patients. In: Bray GA, ed. *Obesity.* Philadelphia: W.B. Saunders Company, 1980:240–248.

94. Kanders BS, Blackburn GL. In: Rakel RE, ed. *Conns Current Therapy.* Philadelphia: W.B. Saunders Company; 1981:524–531.

95. Frankel RT, Yang MY. *Obesity and Weight Control: The Health Professional's Guide to Understanding and Treatment.* Gaithersburg, MD: Aspen Publishers, Inc., 1988.

96. Pi-Sunyer FX. Obesity. In: Shils ME, Young VR, eds. *Modern Nutrition in Health and Disease.* Philadelphia: Lea & Febiger, 1988:795–816.

97. Berg-Smith SM, Stevens VJ, Brown KM, et al. A brief motivational intervention to improve dietary adherence in adolescents. The Dietary Intervention Study in Children (DISC) Research Group. *Health Educ Res* 1999;14(3):399–410.

Adherence Tool 4–1   Client Questionnaire for Low-Calorie Eating Patterns in Treating Obesity

---

The following questionnaire is a monitoring device that has been designed to efficiently collect patient information in clinical weight control programs. It has several functions.

Initially, it is a useful screening device or test of motivation. Individuals who will not take time to fill it out probably will not take time to participate fully in the behavioral weight-control program.

Second, the answers to these questions can be of great use to the therapist during the initial interviews and later during the weight-control sessions. The weight history allows the therapist to look systematically at the clients' own views of their weight problems, and at some of the environmental influences they feel are important to their weight problems. The history of past attempts to lose weight, the lengths of time they have stayed in weight-loss programs, and the reasons for past failure can all be useful. Also, clients' reports of mood changes during previous periods of weight loss can help you anticipate and deal with problems that might arise during treatment.

A brief medical history is included to give you a basis for referral. For example, if someone indicates he or she is a diabetic, and does not have a physician, you might suggest contacting a doctor before the weight-control program begins. Similarly, if someone indicates a history of heart disease, you may want to check with that person's physician before dealing with increased activity and exercise.

The questions about social and family history provide additional information that is of use medically (for example, the cause of parental death and the family weight history).

In most states, the information contained in this questionnaire is confidential. Without *written* approval from the clients, this information cannot be divulged to interested individuals, physicians, insurance companies, or law enforcement agencies.

Source: Adapted with permission from J.M. Ferguson, *Learning To Eat, Behavior Modification for Weight Control,* © 1975, Bull Publishing Company.

continued

Adherence Tool 4–1 *(continued)*

Name: _____ Sex: M   F   Age: _____ Birthdate: _____

Address: _____ Home phone: _____
_____ Office phone: _____

_____

WEIGHT HISTORY

1. Your present weight _____ Height _____

2. Describe your present weight (check one)
   _____ Very overweight _____ About average
   _____ Slightly overweight

3. Are you dissatisfied with the way you look at this weight? (check one)
   _____ Completely satisfied _____ Dissatisfied
   _____ Satisfied _____ Very dissatisfied
   _____ Neutral

4. At what weight have you *felt* your best or do you think you would feel your best? _____

5. How much weight would you like to lose? _____

6. Do you feel your weight affects your daily activities?
   _____ No effect _____ Often interferes
   _____ Some effect _____ Extreme effect

7. Why do you want to lose weight at this time? _____
   _____

8. Do these attitudes affect your weight loss or gain?   Yes   No (circle response)
   If yes, please describe: _____
   _____
   _____

9. How *physically* active are you? (check one)
   _____ Very active _____ Inactive _____ Average
   _____ Active _____ Very inactive

10. Which method did you use for the longest period of time? _____
    _____

11. What usually goes wrong with your weight-loss programs? _____
    _____

MEDICAL HISTORY

12. When did you last have a complete physical examination? _____

continued

Adherence Tool 4–1   *(continued)*

13. Who is your current doctor? _____

14. What medical problems do you have at the present time? _____

_____

_____

15. What medications or drugs do you take regularly?   _____

_____

SOCIAL HISTORY

16. Circle the last year of school attended:

    1 2 3 4 5 6 7 8   9 10 11 12   1 2 3 4   M.A.   Ph.D.
     Grade School   High School   College
     Other _____

17. Describe your present occupation_____

_____

18. How long have you worked for your present employer?   _____

19. Present marital status (check one):

    _____ Single

    _____ Married

    _____ Widowed

    _____ Divorced

    _____ Separated

    _____ Engaged

20. Answer the following questions for each marriage:

    Date of marriage   _____   _____   _____

    Date of termination   _____   _____   _____

    Reason (death, divorce, etc.)   _____   _____   _____

    Number of children   _____   _____   _____

21. Spouse's Age _____ Weight _____ Height _____

22. Describe your spouse's occupation _____

23. Describe your spouse's weight (check one):

    _____ Very overweight

    _____ Slightly overweight

    _____ About average

    _____ Slightly underweight

    _____ Very underweight

24. Who lives at home with you? _____

continued

Adherence Tool 4–1   *(continued)*

FAMILY HISTORY

25. Is your father living?   Yes No   Father's age now, or age at and cause of death _____

    _____

26. Is your mother living?   Yes No   Mother's age now, or age at and cause of death _____

27. Describe your father's occupation _____

28. Describe your mother's occupation _____

29. Describe your father's weight while you were growing up (check one).

    _____ Very overweight

    _____ Slightly overweight

    _____ About average

    _____ Slightly underweight

    _____ Very underweight

30. Describe your mother's weight while you were growing up (check one).

    _____ Very overweight

    _____ Slightly overweight

    _____ About average

    _____ Slightly underweight

    _____ Very underweight

31. What are the attitudes of the following people about your attempt(s) to lose weight?

	Negative (They disapprove or are resentful)	*Indifferent* (They don't care or don't help)	*Positive* (They encourage me and are understanding)
Husband			
Wife			
Children			
Parents			
Employer			
Friends			

continued

Adherence Tool 4–1   *(continued)*

32. Indicate on the following table the periods in your life when you have been overweight. *Where appropriate*, list your maximum weight for each period and number of pounds you were overweight. Briefly describe any methods you used to lose weight in that five-year period (e.g., diet, shots, pills). Also list any significant life events you feel were related to either your weight gain or loss (e.g., college tests, marriage, pregnancies, illness).

Age	Maximum Weight	Pounds Overweight	Methods Used To Lose Weight	Significant Events Related to Weight Change
Birth				
0–5				
6–10				
11–15				
16–20				
21–25				
26–30				
31–35				
36–40				
41–45				
46–50				
51–55				
56–60				
61–65				

33. What do you do for physical exercise and how often do you do it?

ACTIVITY (for example, swimming, jogging, dancing)	FREQUENCY (daily, weekly, monthly)

continued

Adherence Tool 4–1   *(continued)*

34. A number of different ways of losing weight are listed below. Please indicate which methods you have used by filling the appropriate blanks.

	Ages Used	Number of Times Used	Maximum Weight Lost	Comments (Length of Time Weight Loss Maintained; Successes; Difficulties)
TOPS (Take Off Pounds Sensibly)				
Weight Watchers				
Pills				
Supervised Diet				
Unsupervised Diet				
Starvation				
Behavior Modification				
Psychotherapy				
Hypnosis				
Other				

35. Have you had a major mood change during or after a significant weight loss? Indicate any mood changes on the following checklist.

	Not at All	A Little Bit	Moderately	Quite a Bit	Extremely
a. Depressed, sad, feeling down, unhappy, the blues	____	____	____	____	____
b. Anxious, nervous, restless, or uptight all the time	____	____	____	____	____
c. Physically weak	____	____	____	____	____
d. Elated or happy	____	____	____	____	____
e. Easily irritated, annoyed, or angry	____	____	____	____	____
f. Fatigued, worn out, tired all the time	____	____	____	____	____
g. A lack of self-confidence	____	____	____	____	____

36. List any medications, drugs, or foods to which you are allergic. ____

_____

_____

continued

Adherence Tool 4–1   *(continued)*

37. List any hospitalizations or operations. Indicate how old you were at each hospital admission.

    Age   Reason for hospitalization

    _____   _____

    _____   _____

    _____   _____

    _____   _____

38. List any serious illnesses you have had that have not required hospitalization. Indicate how old you were during each illness.

    Age   Reason for hospitalization

    _____   _____

    _____   _____

    _____   _____

    _____   _____

39. Describe any of your medical problems that are complicated by excess weight.

    _____

    _____

    _____

    _____

    _____

40. How much alcohol do you usually drink per week? _____

41. List any psychiatric contact, individual counseling, or marital counseling that you have had or are now having.

    Age   Reason for contact and type of therapy

    _____   _____

    _____   _____

    _____   _____

    _____   _____

continued

Adherence Tool 4–1 *(continued)*

42. List your children's ages, sex, heights, weights, and circle whether they are overweight, average, or underweight. Include any children from previous marriages, whether they are living with you or not.

Age	Sex	Height	Weight	Overweight			Underweight	
___	___	___	___	very	slightly	average	slightly	very
___	___	___	___	very	slightly	average	slightly	very
___	___	___	___	very	slightly	average	slightly	very
___	___	___	___	very	slightly	average	slightly	very
___	___	___	___	very	slightly	average	slightly	very

43. List your brothers' and sisters' ages, sex, present weights, heights, and circle whether they are overweight, average, or underweight.

Age	Sex	Height	Weight	Overweight			Underweight	
___	___	___	___	very	slightly	average	slightly	very
___	___	___	___	very	slightly	average	slightly	very
___	___	___	___	very	slightly	average	slightly	very
___	___	___	___	very	slightly	average	slightly	very
___	___	___	___	very	slightly	average	slightly	very

44. Please add any additional information you feel may be relevant to your weight problem. This includes interactions with your family and friends that might sabotage a weight-loss program, and additional family or social history that you feel might help us understand your weight problem.

_____

_____

_____

_____

_____

_____

_____

Adherence Tool 4-2   Goal Attainment Chart (Monitoring Device)

Action Plan for Goal Attainment

Name:_____   Date: _____

1. Goal: _____
    _____
    _____
    _____

2. Was goal achieved? _____

Week	1	2	3	4	5	6	7
1							
2							
3							
4							

Days

☆ = Yes, goal was achieved

○ = No, goal was not achieved

3. Significant events that helped or hindered goal attainment:_____
    _____
    _____

4. Rewards given for achieving goal: _____
    _____
    _____
    _____

5. Comments/suggestions:_____
    _____

6. Next contact date and time: _____
    _____

Adherence Tool 4–3   Don't Be Caught in the Trees (Informational and Cueing Device)

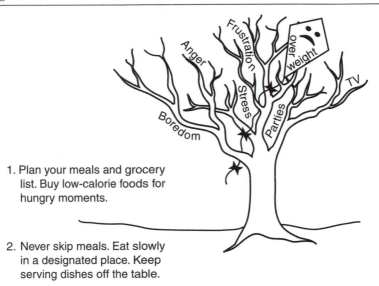

1. Plan your meals and grocery list. Buy low-calorie foods for hungry moments.

2. Never skip meals. Eat slowly in a designated place. Keep serving dishes off the table.

3. Ask friends and family to help.

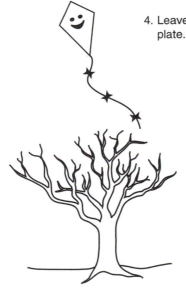

4. Leave a bit of everything on your plate. Eat from smaller plates.

5. Store food only in the kitchen.

6. When preparing foods, taste only once.

7. Let other people clean their own plates after eating.

CHAPTER 5

NUTRITION COUNSELING IN PREVENTION AND TREATMENT OF CORONARY HEART DISEASE

Chapter Objectives

1. Identify common dietary misconceptions about saturated fat-modified patterns that lead to inappropriate eating behaviors.

2. Identify common dietary excesses that contribute to inappropriate eating behaviors associated with diets low in saturated fat.

3. Identify specific nutrients that should be emphasized in assessing (step 1) a baseline eating pattern before providing dietary instruction and intervention as a part of step 3.

4. As a part of step 3, intervention, identify theories and approaches to treat inappropriate behaviors associated with saturated fat-modified eating patterns.

5. As a part of step 3, negotiate strategies to deal with clients following low saturated fat eating patterns.

6. Recommend dietary adherence tools for clients on low saturated fat-modified eating patterns.

Saturated Fat and Coronary Heart Disease

Coronary heart disease (CHD) is the leading cause of death among adult Americans.[1] Based on this fact, in 2001 the National Heart, Lung, and Blood Institute sponsored a Second Report of the Expert Panel on Detection, Evaluation, and Treatment of High Blood Cholesterol in Adults (Adult Treatment Panel III, or ATP III). The results of this group's deliberations were the National Cholesterol Education Program's (NCEP's) updated recommendations for cholesterol management.[2]

The NCEP report identifies low-density lipoproteins (LDL) as the primary target of cholesterol-lowering therapy. Dietary therapy remains the first line of treatment of high blood cholesterol, and drug therapy is reserved for patients who are considered to be at high risk for CHD. This report focuses on CHD risk status and serves as a guide to type and intensity of cholesterol-lowering therapy. High-density lipoprotein (HDL) is targeted as reducing CHD risk. The NCEP report emphasizes physical activity and weight loss as components of the dietary therapy for high blood cholesterol. The ATP III recommends that patients with high-risk LDL-cholesterol (>160 mg/dL), those with borderline high-risk LDL cholesterol (130–159 mg/dL) who have two or more risk factors, and those with CHD or other clinical atherosclerotic disease and an LDL-cholesterol >100 mg/dL should enter into a program of therapy. The first two groups qualify for primary prevention and the latter for secondary prevention. In primary prevention, most patients should receive dietary therapy and should increase physical activity. For patients with CHD or other clinical atherosclerotic disease, the target goal for LDL-cholesterol reduction is 100 mg/dL or lower with diet therapy initiated in these patients (see Tables 5–1 through 5–4. Table 5–5 provides the nutrient composition of the Therapeutic Lifestyle Change (TLC) Diet. Table 5–6 shows LDL-cholesterol goals and cutpoints for diet and drug therapy.

This chapter provides counseling strategies for low saturated fat-modified eating patterns to help prevent coronary disease. Good basic nutrition plays a primary role in devising a saturated fat-modified diet pattern. The Institutes of Medicine of the National Academies has not established an Estimated Average Requirement (EAR), Recommended Dietary Allowances (RDA) or an Adequate Intake (AI) for total and saturated fat in individuals age 1 and older. It does recommend that adequate lipids be incorporated into the diet to provide the body with essential fatty acids and carriers of fat-soluble vitamins. The Acceptable Macronutrient Distribution Ranges (AMDRs) for total fat are estimated to be 20–35% of energy for adults and children ages 4 and older with 30–40% for children ages 1 to 3 years.[3]

Table 5–1 Serum Total Cholesterol (mg/dL) Levels for Persons 20 Years of Age and Older, United States, 1988–1994

Sex, Age, and Race/Ethnicity	Number of Examined Persons	Mean	Selected Percentile									
			5th	10th	15th	25th	50th	75th	85th	90th	95th
Men*											
20 years and older	7,531	202	139	151	160	173	200	226	244	255	273
20–34	2,298	186	131	142	148	161	183	209	223	233	253
35–44	1,323	206	143	154	163	180	205	232	247	257	267
45–54	904	216	154	167	178	191	214	242	255	266	283
55–64	1,004	216	154	167	174	189	214	243	258	270	282
65–74	1,058	212	149	163	175	186	209	237	248	263	284
75+	944	205	145	155	164	176	203	230	246	255	273
Women*											
20 years and older	8,531	206	143	153	161	175	201	233	251	265	284
20–34	2,651	184	132	141	148	158	181	205	219	231	248
35–44	1,645	195	144	153	160	171	192	215	234	243	257
45–54	1,013	217	157	166	174	187	212	243	259	274	298
55–64	1,045	235	167	184	191	204	229	261	276	286	307
65–74	1,075	233	170	181	189	204	232	258	276	289	308
75+	1,102	229	161	174	185	198	228	258	274	286	305
Mexican American											
Men	2,175	199	137	150	157	171	197	224	241	253	272
Women	2,165	198	139	148	156	167	193	223	238	249	274
Non-Hispanic Black											
Men	1,923	198	136	147	155	169	195	222	239	251	275
Women	2,360	201	136	148	157	170	196	226	246	261	284
Non-Hispanic White											
Men	3,161	203	141	153	162	174	201	229	244	256	272
Women	3,645	208	144	155	163	177	203	235	252	267	284

*Total sample of men and women includes racial/ethnic groups other than those shown.

Source: National Institutes of Health, *Third Report of the National Cholesterol Education Program (NCEP) Expert Panel on Detection, Evaluation, and Treatment of High Blood Cholesterol in Adults (Adult Treatment Panel III) Final Report*, September 2002, NIH Publication No. 02-5215, B-I-B-II.

Table 5-2 Serum LDL Cholesterol (mg/dL) Levels for Persons 20 Years of Age and Older, United States, 1988–1994

Sex, Age, and Race/Ethnicity	Number of Examined Persons	Mean	Selected Percentile								
			5th	10th	15th	25th	50th	75th	85th	90th	95th
Men*											
20 years and older	3,154	130	76	87	93	105	128	153	166	177	194
20-34	970	119	72	81	87	97	119	139	151	156	170
35-44	546	135	82	91	96	111	132	156	171	186	205
45-54	388	140	76	95	106	117	140	164	178	188	195
55-64	428	138	82	90	99	115	135	162	174	182	200
65-74	468	136	83	92	103	113	133	158	171	182	196
75+	354	132	86	92	97	109	128	151	167	177	194
Women*											
20 years and older	3,641	125	69	81	89	98	121	147	162	172	190
20-34	1,190	111	63	71	79	90	109	130	142	152	170
35-44	741	118	70	83	90	96	115	137	147	159	171
45-54	444	131	70	85	93	106	129	153	166	177	190
55-64	457	144	80	93	107	121	143	167	184	192	209
65-74	417	143	76	95	106	119	144	166	182	188	203
75+	392	145	83	102	106	119	144	167	186	196	209
Mexican American											
Men	913	124	71	78	85	98	121	144	160	171	188
Women	943	117	67	75	83	93	115	137	152	161	178
Non-Hispanic Black											
Men	802	127	71	79	86	100	124	149	165	179	200
Women	1,012	122	63	77	84	97	119	145	161	172	193
Non-Hispanic White											
Men	1,317	131	79	88	95	106	129	154	167	179	194
Women	1,539	126	70	81	89	98	122	149	164	173	189

*Total sample of men and women includes racial/ethnic groups other than those shown.

Source: National Institutes of Health, *Third Report of the National Cholesterol Education Program (NCEP) Expert Panel on Detection, Evaluation, and Treatment of High Blood cholesterol in Adults (Adult Treatment Panel III) Final Report*, September 2002, NIH Publication No. 02-5215, B-I–B-II.

Table 5-3 Serum HDL Cholesterol (mg/dL) Levels for Persons 20 Years of Age and Older, United States, 1988–1994

Sex, Age, and Race/Ethnicity	Number of Examined Persons	Mean	Selected Percentile									
			5th	10th	15th	25th	50th	75th	85th	90th	95th
Men*											
20 years and older	7,473	46	28	30	34	37	44	53	58	62	72
20–34	2,285	46	28	32	34	38	45	53	59	62	69
35–44	1,306	45	28	30	32	36	43	52	57	61	73
45–54	893	45	26	30	32	35	42	52	58	66	75
55–64	999	45	28	31	34	36	42	51	57	61	71
65–74	1,052	46	28	30	32	36	43	54	58	64	73
75+	938	47	28	31	34	37	44	54	61	66	75
Women*											
20 years and older	8,478	55	34	38	41	44	53	64	70	75	83
20–34	2,640	55	34	38	41	45	53	64	69	74	83
35–44	1,628	54	34	38	41	44	53	64	68	72	79
45–54	1,004	56	36	38	41	45	55	65	72	77	84
55–64	1,039	56	33	37	40	44	53	65	73	78	89
65–74	1,071	56	33	37	40	45	54	65	71	76	84
75+	1,096	56	32	37	40	44	55	65	71	76	86
Mexican American											
Men	2,151	46	28	32	34	37	44	52	58	61	67
Women	2,156	52	33	36	38	42	51	60	66	71	77
Non-Hispanic Black											
Men	1,916	52	32	35	37	41	50	60	68	74	85
Women	2,348	57	35	39	42	46	55	66	73	79	86
Non-Hispanic White											
Men	3,138	45	27	30	33	36	43	52	57	61	71
Women	3,615	56	34	38	41	45	54	64	70	76	84

*Total sample of men and women includes racial/ethnic groups other than those shown.

Source: National Institutes of Health, Third Report of the National Cholesterol Education Program (NCEP) Expert Panel on Detection, Evaluation, and Treatment of High Blood cholesterol in Adults (Adult Treatment Panel III) Final Report, September 2002, NIH Publication No. 02-5215, B-I–B-II.

Table 5–4   Serum Triglyceride (mg/dL) Levels for Persons 20 Years of Age and Older, United States, 1988–1994

Sex, Age, and Race/Ethnicity	Number of Examined Persons	Mean	Selected Percentile								
			5th	10th	15th	25th	50th	75th	85th	90th	95th
Men*											
20 years and older	3,251	148	53	62	69	83	118	173	218	253	318
20–34	987	118	46	55	60	70	94	139	171	204	256
35–44	570	150	53	62	70	82	126	180	213	242	307
45–54	415	182	62	72	82	100	135	201	269	296	366
55–64	446	176	64	80	87	101	144	228	276	311	396
65–74	476	160	64	76	83	99	137	190	226	256	319
75+	357	144	64	71	82	96	125	175	200	220	304
Women*											
20 years and older	3,707	128	48	56	61	72	102	152	193	226	273
20–34	1,201	101	43	49	55	61	84	117	147	177	226
35–44	754	123	46	53	57	67	93	132	170	215	288
45–54	457	136	49	59	66	76	114	163	201	239	277
55–64	470	166	62	72	82	96	135	203	251	313	396
65–74	426	157	70	76	85	99	134	182	228	253	283
75+	399	150	64	74	79	94	130	178	211	235	274
Mexican American											
Men	955	152	53	60	69	83	120	184	225	259	361
Women	962	140	55	63	72	85	118	170	210	237	293
Non-Hispanic Black											
Men	815	114	45	51	56	64	89	135	164	192	245
Women	1,021	96	41	46	51	58	79	113	142	162	207
Non-Hispanic White											
Men	1,357	152	55	64	71	85	123	181	223	258	319
Women	1,573	130	49	56	63	75	104	156	196	229	274

*Total sample of men and women includes racial/ethnic groups other than those shown.

Source: National Institutes of Health, *Third Report of the National Cholesterol Education Program (NCEP) Expert Panel on Detection, Evaluation, and Treatment of High Blood Cholesterol in Adults (Adult Treatment Panel III) Final Report*, September 2002, NIH Publication No. 02-5215, B-I–B-II.

Table 5–5   Nutrient Composition of the TLC Diet

Nutrient	Recommended Intake
Saturated fat*	Less than 7% of total calories
Polyunsaturated fat	Up to 10% of total calories
Monounsaturated fat	Up to 20% of total calories
Total fat	25–35% of total calories
Carbohydrate**	50–60% of total calories
Fiber	20–30 g/day
Protein	Approximately 15% of total calories
Cholesterol	Less than 200 mg/day
Total calories (energy)***	Balance energy intake and expenditure to maintain desirable body weight/prevent weight gain

*Trans fatty acids are another LDL-raising fat that should be kept at a low intake.
**Carbohydrate should be derived predominantly from foods rich in complex carbohydrates including grains, especially whole grains, fruits, and vegetables.
***Daily energy expenditure should include at least moderate physical activity (contributing approximately 200 Kcal/day).

Source: National Institutes of Health, *Third Report of the National Cholesterol Education Program (NCEP) Expert Panel on Detection, Evaluation, and Treatment of High Blood Cholesterol in Adults (Adult Treatment Panel III) Final Report*, September 2002, NIH Publication No. 02-5215, B-I–B-II.

The AMDRs for essential fatty acids is 5–10% of the total caloric intake provided by linolenic acid and 0.6–1.2% provided by alpha-linolenic acid.[3] The Tolerable Upper Intake Level (UL) for *cis* monounsaturated and polyunsaturated (n-6 and n-3) fatty acids was not set due to insufficient evidence.[3]

Achieving the AMDR for essential fatty acids is accomplished easily by using vegetable oils in cooking and salad dressing. Corn, soy, and cottonseed oils each contain 6 to 8 grams of linolenic acid per tablespoon, mayonnaise 6 grams, and margarine 1 to 5 grams.

Table 5–6   Cholesterol Goals and Cutpoints for TLC and Drug Therapy

Risk Category	LDL Goal	LDL Level at Which to Initiate Therapeutic Lifestyle Changes (TLC)	Level at Which to Consider Drug Therapy
CHD or CHD Risk Equivalents (10-year risk > 20%)	< 100 mg/dL	≥ 100 mg/dL	≥130 mg/dL (100–129 mg/dL; drug optional)*
2+ Risk Factors (10-year risk ≤ 20%)	< 130 mg/dL	≥ 130 mg/dL	10-year risk 10–20%; ≥ 130 mg/dL 10-year risk <10%; ≥ 160 mg/dL
0–1 Risk Factor**	< 160 mg/dL	≥ 160 mg/dL	≥ 190 mg/dL (160–189 mg/dL; LDL-lowering drug optional)

*Some authorities recommend use of LDL-lowering drugs in this category if an LDL cholesterol < 100 mg/dL cannot be achieved by therapeutic lifestyle changes. Others prefer use of drugs that primarily modify triglycerides and HDL, e.g., nicotinic acid or fibrate. Clinical judgment also may call for deferring drug therapy in this subcategory.

**Almost all people with 0–1 risk factor have a 10-year risk < 10%, thus 10-year risk assessment in people with 0–1 risk factor is not necessary.

Source: National Institutes of Health, *Third Report of the National Cholesterol Education Program (NCEP) Expert Panel on Detection, Evaluation, and Treatment of High Blood Cholesterol in Adults (Adult Treatment Panel III) Final Report,* September 2002, NIH Publication No. 02-5215, B-I–B-II.

Theories and Facts About Nutrition and Coronary Heart Disease

Eating large amounts of saturated fat can cause an elevation in various lipid-carrying particles in the blood, a condition called dyslipidemia. There is clinical interest in dyslipidemia because of its close association with CHD. Although the etiology of CHD involves a multitude of factors, past epidemiological studies have conclusively shown that dyslipidemia is a major risk factor for coronary heart disease.[4-13] Many of these studies use a single value of cholesterol at the time of entry into the study. However, multiple measurements of plasma cholesterol concentrations increase the power to identify premature risk for CHD.

Research on Lipoproteins

Although total plasma cholesterol serves as an indicator of CHD, identifying the risk associated with specific particles that carry cholesterol provides even greater diagnostic information. The transport of cholesterol in lipoprotein particles is discussed below.

Before insoluble cholesterol is transported out of the liver cell into the plasma, it must be solubilized by special mechanisms. The liver has developed the capacity to "package" cholesterol into macromolecular complexes in which specific proteins, called apoproteins, interact with phospholipids to bring lipids into soluble form. The resultant particles are called lipoproteins. They contain lipids in their core with unesterified cholesterol (free cholesterol or FC), phospholipids (PL), and apoproteins (aP) in their membrane-like coats.[14]

The major lipoprotein secreted by the liver is very-low-density lipoprotein (VLDL). Newly secreted VLDL contains triglyceride (TG) in its core. Immediately upon entrance into plasma, the basic structure of VLDL begins to alter. First, it acquires more cholesterol esters (CE) in the core. High-density lipoprotein (HDL) appears to transfer CE directly into VLDL, which is altered by lipolysis of triglyceride through the action of lipoprotein lipase. As hydrolysis proceeds, free fatty acids (FFA) are released, the size of VLDL is reduced, and density increases, resulting in a new category of lipoprotein, designated intermediate-density lipoprotein (IDL). IDL appears to be transformed to LDL, a lipoprotein of lower density. In tissue culture studies, when lipoproteins are added to media cells they can derive most of their cholesterol from uptake of these IDL particles. Figure 5–1 illustrates schematically the mechanisms for cholesterol transport.[14,15]

One of the protective effects of HDL involves reverse cholesterol transport where cholesterol removal from the peripheral cells is promoted. Cholesterol is transported from the peripheral tissues to the liver. Additionally, HDL is also an antioxidant that inhibits phospholipid oxidation of LDL, minimizing fatty acid streaks in the arterial walls.[16-19]

Research on Fatty Acids and Their Effect on Lipoproteins

Researchers have found that dietary saturated fat and cholesterol are related to morbidity and mortality from coronary heart dis-

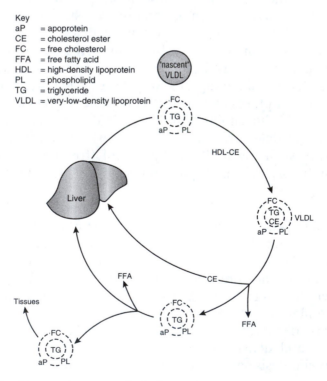

FIGURE 5–1   Plasma Transport of Cholesterol

ease.[7,20–24] A number of investigators have examined the effect of various fatty acids on lipoprotein levels. All have concluded that a significant portion of the saturated fatty acids should be removed to lower total cholesterol significantly.[25] The investigations have raised questions about what source of energy should replace the saturated fatty acids, with the three major candidates being carbohydrate, polyunsaturated fatty acids, and monounsaturated fatty acids.

In most people, when carbohydrates are substituted for saturated fats, the LDL-cholesterol level will fall about as much as with monounsaturated or polyunsaturated fats.[26–28] If fats are restricted to much below 30% of calories and are replaced by carbohydrates, there is a tendency for HDL-cholesterol levels to fall and VLDL-triglyceride levels to rise.[26,29–31] Many authorities consider these latter changes to be harmless, although there is still some disagreement on this question.[14]

There are two major categories of polyunsaturated fat, commonly referred to as omega-6 and omega-3 fatty acids. The major omega-6 fatty acid is linolenic acid. Substitution of foods rich in linoleic acid for those high in saturated fats results in a fall in LDL-cholesterol levels.[32–34] Oils rich in linoleic acid include: soybean oil, corn oil, and high-linoleic acid forms of safflower and sunflower seed oils. Fish is the major source of omega-3 fatty acid. At high intakes, it reduces serum triglycerides substantially.[35,36]

The Mediterranean diet and its positive effects on cardiovascular disease (CVD) may partially be attributed to the large amounts of omega-3 fatty acids in this diet. The Mediterranean diet is targeted as having a positive effect on reduction in overall mortality and coronary heart disease events. The American Heart Association (AHA) provides an advisory recommending that a Mediterranean-style diet has positive effects on cardiovascular disease and that clients with CVD might benefit in reducing blood LDL-cholesterol if components of the Mediterranean diet were combined with existing AHA recommendations.[37,38] The beneficial nutrients in the Mediterranean diet include beta-carotene, vitamins C and E, polyphenols, fiber, antioxidants, and many important minerals.[39] The fatty acid content of the Mediterranean diet is a clue to the reason it may have positive cardio-protective effects.[40,41]

Table 5–7 shows how the Mediterranean diet compares to diets of other cultures. The ratio of omega-6 to omega-3 essential fatty

Table 5–7   Ratio of Omega-6 Compared to Omega-3 Fatty Acids in Different Areas of the World

Type of Diet	Omega-6	Omega-3
Mediterranean	1–2	1
Western and Northern European	15	1
US	16.7	1

acids is much lower than those in the westernized world.[41] Additionally the Mediterranean diet is characterized by locally grown, whole foods purchased from markets devoid of highly processed foods that often are also high in trans-fatty acids.[42] Unlike those fats in highly processed foods, this diet is high in monounsaturated fat. Researchers believe that the major component of monounsaturated fat, oleic acid, may cause almost as much of a decrease in LDL-cholesterol levels as the polyunsaturated linoleic acid when either is substituted for trans and/or saturated fat in the diet.[34, 43–45]

Research on American Diet Quality Over Time

The Minnesota Heart Study compared American eating habits within two time periods, 1980–1982 and 2000–2002. In this study that included 5,369 men and 6,070 women, an index of scores was used to provide indications of the quality of eating patterns using adherence to the current American Heart Association (AHA) Dietary Guidelines. Over the past two decades, the index scores have increased, showing better compliance with the AHA Dietary Guidelines. In terms of foods eaten, this study provided evidence that grains and whole grains were consumed at a higher rate. Index scores showed that positive cardiovascular effects may have been the result of decreases in saturated fats, trans fats, cholesterol, and total fat. The negative side to this was the fact that increases occurred in sodium and energy balance with decreases in fish intake. Of concern to the investigators in this study was the fact that for some periods of time, a plateau was reached, with no improvement in the index scores occurring.[46]

Research on Compliance with Eating Patterns Modified in Fat and Cholesterol

Studies aimed at changing dietary habits to include modified fat eating patterns are summarized below.

In the Multiple Risk Factor Intervention Trial (MRFIT), intervention focused on the subjects' developing healthier lifelong shopping, cooking, and eating patterns rather than specifying a structured diet.[47] Individual nutrition counseling with periodic monitoring resulted in significant cholesterol reductions, although risk also declined in the control group.[48] A comprehensive community health–promotion program in North Karelia, Finland, yielded significant reductions in cholesterol in comparison with a reference county where no intervention was implemented.[49] However, the North Karelia Project's design precluded knowledge of which aspects of the health education program instigated the change.

In an evaluation of nutrition education for persons with post-myocardial infarction, Karvetti and Hamalainen found significant improvements with both lecture-discussion and food preparation demonstration strategies. Although neither approach was significantly more effective for stimulating behavior change, this study pointed out the possible importance of organized nutrition education programs for persons with CHD.[50] Several studies have compared the use of educational materials and mass media with interventions augmented by personal contact or counseling by a health professional.[51-62] In each instance, educational programs that included interpersonal methods were more successful.

Several of the programs designed for delivery to groups have engaged social support. For example, Witschi et al. found that family participation improved the magnitude of cholesterol reductions, although the study subjects did not maintain the reductions after the intervention was discontinued.[63] In fact, it has been found repeatedly that improved eating habits and reduced lipid levels do not persist when an intervention is not sustained.[53,63,64] Bruno et al. were able to attain high continuous participation rates (81%) in a worksite program that included six monthly maintenance meetings.[65] The achievement of long–term benefits from dietary interventions on lipids requires further development of booster sessions, self-monitoring techniques, and reinforcement techniques. Glanz summarizes the elements needed to maintain dietary compliance to low-cholesterol, fat-modified diets: enlist social support, maintain periodic contact, encourage self-monitoring, and provide feedback about adherence.[66]

Kris-Etherton describes the current state of our efforts in public health nutrition to maintain the declining rates in Coronary Heart Disease (CHD) incidence and death. She states that while we have a good understanding of lifestyle factors, including diet, that contribute to CHD, we must continue to focus on effective behavior change interventions to sustain these healthful behaviors.[38]

Several studies have focused on lifestyle change. Berg-Smith and registered dietitians working in the Diet Intervention Study in Children (DISC) used motivational interviewing techniques when dietary adherence in teens became a problem. Results showed that it is possible to reverse negative dietary behaviors in teens who know the appropriate eating behaviors necessary to reduce LDL-cholesterol, but do not use them.[67]

Likewise, in the Women's Health Initiative (WHI) where one of the outcomes targeted was coronary heart disease, dietary adherence in the 12-year diet intervention arm of the study began to drop after two to three years of diet intervention. To stop the decline in dietary adherence rates, motivational interviewing was implemented in a pilot study in three WHI centers to determine whether it should be used in all 40 centers. Once again, in this study, similar to DISC, adherence to diet took a sharp turn upward when all centers began this behavioral technique to reestablish dietary adherence.[68]

More recently, a major NIH study, PREMIER, evaluated different interventions for blood pressure reduction. The interventions focused on lifestyle changes including healthy diet patterns, exercise and weight loss. The results showed that after an 18-month intervention, blood pressure was reduced using behavioral strategies.[69,70]

These are just a few of the studies where long-term dietary maintenance in large groups of participants was achieved using behavioral change methods focused on healthy eating patterns. The examples that follow provide concrete ways of using the strategies that were successful in DISC, WHI, and PREMIER.

Inappropriate Eating Behaviors

False information about eating patterns modified for fat and cholesterol can lead to inappropriate eating behaviors.

A common problem many clients face is determining how commercial products fit into appropriate eating behavior. Keeping abreast of information on the fat content of new products must be a continuing effort by both nutrition counselors and their clients. Clients and counselors can develop and use a shopping guide to determine whether new products are low or high in fat, as in Exhibit 5–1. This information is based on labels; more specific data can be obtained by writing or emailing to the manufacturers.

Some clients feel that certain foods possess strange powers to eliminate cholesterol and therefore lower its concentration in the blood. They see single foods as a panacea. A client might claim: "I eat large amounts of fruits and vegetables, so I don't worry about my dietary intake." The total diet must be considered when assessing fat intake. Single foods do not eliminate the effect of fat on the diet.

Still another erroneous idea is that total fat content does not really matter. As long as a high-fat item is cholesterol free, clients may believe mistakenly that it can be eaten in unlimited quantities. A client might state proudly: "I eat large amounts of peanut butter because it is cholesterol free." The client is correct, but large quantities of fat elevate the caloric level of the diet and can lead to weight gain.

These misconceptions are just a few examples that clients voice and are common sources of problem eating behaviors. Nutrition counselors see only a small sampling of daily eating behaviors if short-term self-reporting methods such as three-day diet diaries are used, so it is possible that clients can consume commercial products containing saturated fat without detection for long periods of time.

Clients following fat-modified eating patterns wrestle with problems of excess. Social pressures can lead clients to eat something they know increases cholesterol, with the familiar alibi: "I just couldn't stop with one bite of that cheesecake at the party last night." These modified eating patterns also may mean a drastic reduction in the amounts of foods clients are accustomed to eating.

Exhibit 5–1   Low-Fat and Fat-Free Commercial Soups

Below is a list of lower-fat and fat-free commercial soups. Be sure to check the label for the most up-to-date fat gram information.

Healthy Choice

Broth-based soups

- Bean and Ham
- Beef and Potato
- Chicken with Pasta
- Chicken with Rice
- Country Vegetable
- Hearty Chicken
- Lentil
- Minestrone
- Split Pea with Ham
- Old Fashioned Chicken Noodle
- Vegetable Beef

Cream-based soups

- Chicken Corn Chowder
- Chicken Noodle
- Cream of Mushroom
- New England Clam Chowder
- Turkey with White & Wild Rice

Tomato-based soups

- Chili Beef
- Garden Vegetable
- Tomato Garden

Campbell's

Campbell's Healthy Request Soups

- Tomato

READY-TO-SERVE SOUPS

- Bean with Bacon
- Hearty Minestrone
- Chicken Corn Chowder
- Hearty Chicken Noodle
- Hearty Chicken Vegetable
- Hearty Vegetable
- Hearty Vegetable Beef
- New England Clam Chowder
- Southwest Style Vegetable
- Split Pea with Ham
- Tomato Vegetable with Pasta
- Turkey Vegetable with White and Wild Rice

Progresso

- Healthy Classics Chicken Noodle
- Healthy Classics Lentil
- Healthy Classics New England Clam Chowder
- Healthy Classics Tomato Garden Vegetable
- Vegetable
- Chicken Minestrone
- Ham and Bean
- Macaroni and Bean

Pritikin Soups

- Chicken and Rice
- Hearty Vegetable
- Lentil

- Minestrone
- Split Pea
- Three Bean Chili
- Vegetarian Vegetable

Hain Soups (No Salt Added)

- Chicken Vegetable
- Beef Vegetable
- Garlic and Pasta
- Lentil
- Home Style Naturals Cream of Mushroom
- Split Pea
- Tomato Garden Vegetable

Health Valley

- Black Bean and Vegetables
- Lentil and Carrots
- Bean Vegetable
- Split Pea and Carrots

Pepperidge Farm

- Chicken with Wild Rice
- French Onion

Exhibit 5–1   Low-Fat and Fat-Free Commercial Soups

Fantastic Foods

Hearty Soups
- Cha-Cha Chili
- Country Lentil
- Couscous with Lentils
- Five Bean
- Minestrone
- Jumpin' Black Bean
- Split Pea
- Vegetable Barley

Creamy Soups
- Broccoli & Cheddar
- Corn and Potato Chowder
- Mushroom
- Tomato Rice Parmesano

"Just a Pinch" Cups
- Couscous with Lentils
- Spanish Rice and Beans

Rice and Beans (brown rice/legumes/vegetables and spices):
- Bombay Curry
- Cajun

Campbell's
- Chicken Noodle
- Manhattan Clam Chowder

Campbell's Healthy Request:
(Soups that can be used to create an entrée or a one-dish meal. Recipe ideas are provided on the can label).

DRY/INSTANT SOUP MIXES

- Caribbean
- Northern Italian
- Szechuan
- Tex Mex

Couscous Cups (couscous/spices):
- Black Bean Salsa
- Sweet Corn
- Nacho Cheddar
- Creole Vegetable

Lipton's

Lipton Recipe Secrets
(Mixes can be used to create an entree or complete one dish meal; recipe ideas are included on the packaging)
- Golden Herb with Lemon Soup
- Onion Soup
- Fiesta Herb with Red Pepper Soup
- Savory Herb with Garlic Soup
- Beefy Onion Soup
- Onion-Mushroom Soup
- Beefy-Mushroom Soup

Lipton's Kettle Creations
- Split Pea

- Chicken with Wild Rice

Lipton's Cup-A-Soup
- Chicken Noodle with Meat
- Cream of Chicken or Mushroom
- Chicken Vegetable
- Tomato
- Ring Noodle
- Green Pea
- Spring Vegetable

Knorr

Broth-based soups
- Chicken Flavor Vegetable

Hearty soups
- Hearty Lentil
- Navy Bean

Cream-based soups
- Potato Leek

Other low-fat varieties
- Black Bean
- Hearty Minestrone

CONDENSED SOUPS

Creative Chef Soups
- Cream of Roasted Chicken with Savory Herbs
- Cream of Mushroom with Roasted Garlic and Herbs
- Tomato with Garden Herbs

Campbell's 98% Fat Free Soups
- Reduced Fat Cream of Mushroom
- Reduced Fat Cream of Broccoli
- Reduced Fat Broccoli Cheese

Courtesy of the Women's Health Initiative, 1996, Seattle, Washington.

They may comment: "No one can live on this small amount of meat." Inappropriate eating behaviors may be a direct result of childhood excesses. The stalwart farmer may declare: "I grew up eating three eggs every morning."

Manufacturers have come to the aid of clients who must follow fat-modified diets by providing either "filled" products or nearly fat-free substitutes. The "filled" products are those that may, for example, have animal fat removed and a polyunsaturated fat added. Others may have all animal fat removed, with no polyunsaturated fat replacement. This can leave the product virtually fat free. Unfortunately, in many cases clients anticipate that these new products will be identical in taste to the originals, so frustration and even anger may result when those expectations are not met. In desperation, clients may revert to old eating habits, including products high in animal fat.

Clients equate excesses with the prevention of medical problems: "I use large amounts of oil and margarines extremely high in monounsaturated fat because I know that type of fat lowers cholesterol." These inappropriate eating behaviors can lead to excess calories. Clients must learn first to examine ways to reduce saturated fats.

Assessment of Eating Behaviors

As in counseling about other eating patterns, knowledge of what the client is currently eating is extremely important. By learning how restricted the client's present dietary pattern is, the nutrition counselor can tailor dietary intake to lower blood cholesterol. For example, learning that a client currently consumes 50 grams of saturated fat a day through a three-day food record may mean that a dietary prescription lowering intake to 20 grams of saturated fat per day will lower blood cholesterol dramatically. In contrast, for a client whose intake is 30 grams of saturated fat per day, an eating pattern containing 15 grams of saturated fat per day may be necessary to lower blood cholesterol. Ideally, a seven-day record along with a quantified food frequency gives excellent information on current dietary patterns. The NCEP guidelines recommend 25–35% of calories from total fat and 7% of calories from saturated fat.[2]

When time is short, Exhibit 5–2 may serve as a quick means of estimating fat and cholesterol intake. The list can be increased or abbreviated, depending on the information needed in formulating a dietary pattern.

The review of the dietary data should indicate where a major problem is occurring. Identification of where the major excess lies will lead to a plan for dietary change focused on strategies to help eliminate the inappropriate patterns.

If nutrition counselors use the brief food frequency monitor in Exhibit 5–2 and the overall nutritional quality of the diet is in question, clients might fill out a more detailed, all-inclusive food frequency questionnaire to assess the nutrient content of their diet. Adherence Tool 5–1 is a questionnaire that focuses on food preparation and food patterns, with an emphasis on fat and cholesterol intake.

The fat-related misinformation in the media makes it important to assess the amount of misinformation a client currently has by asking, "Is this statement true or false? All vegetable oil helps lower cholesterol." An instrument with a variety of short true-or-false questions could serve as a basis for discussions of misinformation. Adherence Tool 5–2, Fat Facts, is a short, fun way to discuss misconceptions about the low-saturated, fat-controlled eating pattern. This tool should not be used as a test but as a way of opening a discussion about incorrect ideas the media may have promoted.

As with other eating patterns, assessment of adherence to the saturated fat-controlled eating pattern is important. It may involve seven-day diet records or very simple check-off systems, as in Adherence Tool 5–3. A check in the box would indicate adherence with the recommendation of two ounces of meat at lunch. Analysis of dietary intake from diet diaries can provide valuable information on adherence. Adherence Tools 5–4 and 5–5 provide graphs that illustrate the client's level of dietary adherence. A survey of food items in the kitchen can reveal inappropriate cueing that triggers inappropriate eating behaviors. Adherence Tool 5–6 is an example of a monitoring device that helps identify foods high in saturated fat that are in the client's kitchen. Clients write down the food and check the column corresponding to the type of fat present in the largest quantity.

Exhibit 5–2 Fat and Cholesterol Intake Monitor

Name _____ Visit No. _____ Date _____

	Amount	Cholesterol (mg)	Total Fat (g)	Saturated Fat (g)	Polyunsaturated Fat (g)	Monounsaturated Fat (g)	Minimum Significant Amount
Eggs							½/mo
Bacon							4 strips/mo
Sausage							2 oz/mo
Meat, Lunch							
Dinner							
Luncheon Meat							See sausage
Shrimp							2 oz/mo
Liver, Pork, or Beef							3 oz/6 mo
Liver, Chicken							1 oz/2 mo
Gravy							1 cup/mo
Milk, whole ____							½ cup/wk
2% ____							1 cup/wk
Cheese							1 oz/2 wks
Cottage Cheese							½ cup/2 wks
Cream—Light, Sour							1 Tbsp/wk
Heavy							1 Tbsp/mo
Half and Half							1 Tbsp/wk
Nondairy							1 Tbsp/wk
Creamer							
Ice Cream							½ cup/mo
Ice Milk							1 cup/mo
Butter							1 tsp/2 wks
Margarine (as spread)							1 tsp/wk
Oil (in cooking)							1 tsp/wk

continued

Exhibit 5–2 *(continued)*

	Amount	Cholesterol (mg)	Total Fat (g)	Saturated Fat (g)	Polyunsaturated Fat (g)	Monounsaturated Fat (g)	Minimum Significant Amount
Salad Dressing							1 tsp/wk
*Breaded Fried Foods							1 Tbsp/wk
*Fried Potatoes							1 tsp/wk
*Baked Products							1 sv/mo
*Snack Foods							1 sv/mo
Chocolate							½ oz/wk
Peanut Butter							1 Tbsp/wk
Nuts							4 Tbsp/mo
Total							

Polyunsaturated fat ÷ saturated fat (P/S) = _____

*For use in calculating:

	Yields
3–4" diameter pancakes	1 tsp fat
1 fried egg	1 tsp fat
1 Tbsp of salad dressing	1½ tsp fat
1 oz pan-fried meat, fish, and poultry	½ tsp fat
1 oz breaded and fried meat, fish, and poultry	1 tsp fat
15 pieces of French fried potatoes (1½" × ½" × ½")	2 tsp fat

	Yields
½ cup pan-fried potatoes	2 tsp fat
Cake with frosting (1 piece, 2" × 3" × 2")	3 tsp fat
Pie (1 piece, 1/7th of 9")	4 tsp fat
Cookies (4 pieces, 3" diam.)	3 tsp fat
Doughnuts and sweet rolls (1 piece, 4" diam.)	2 tsp fat
Crackers and chips (excluding low-fat crackers) (12 pieces)	3 tsp fat

Courtesy of Joan Bickel, Karen Smith, Linda G. Snetselaar, and Laura Vailas.

Treatment Strategies

Treatment strategies involve three aspects of compliance: lack of knowledge, lack of planning, and lack of commitment.

Strategies to Address Lack of Knowledge

Meal planning is one way to avoid last-minute decisions and to ensure that clients consistently adhere to the basics of a low-cholesterol, fat-modified diet. Adherence Tool 5–7 provides a format for planning menus. Showing clients how to select foods low in saturated fat is crucial to their eventual success. Counselors might indicate the total cholesterol, saturated fat, polyunsaturated fat, and monounsaturated fat in the original high-fat eating pattern. The client's eating pattern can then be compared with one that includes preferred foods but follows a prescription low in saturated fat. Adherence Tool 5–8 is a short list of suggestions for use when dining out, and Adherence Tool 5–9 provides examples of meals eaten at home and in restaurants that are both high and low in cholesterol and fat. Adherence Tool 5–10 shows ranges of P/S ratios for various fats and oils. Demonstrations of the fat content of meals using food models, pats of model margarine and sticks of real margarine provide graphic examples that are lasting images in a client's mind.

With a clear description of the problem, counselors can tailor the diet to specific client needs. Tailoring involves more than simply adapting a standard low-cholesterol, fat-modified diet instruction sheet. A major element is calculating a pattern compatible with the prescription and the client's previous daily eating behavior. A hypothetical example of how tailoring might work in one situation follows:

Mrs. S. eats fourteen eggs each week and six ounces of meat a day, drinks only skim milk, and uses four teaspoons of margarine (soft, tub, non-diet) with approximately two teaspoons of Mazola oil. She loves eggs and eats only high-fat meats such as bologna, salami, traditional high-fat wieners, etc. Based on her blood values and past health history, the dietary prescription agreed upon by the medical team is 200 milligrams of cholesterol, saturated fat 7 and total fat 20 to 25% of total calories.

Table 5–8 offers a possible dietary pattern designed to incorporate this basic information and still meet the prescription. The table shows how to design a regimen to give success initially because it is tailored to past eating habits. Clients should be cautioned that there always will be compromises and changes necessary to meet a specific prescription. For example, an alteration in Mrs. S.'s diet may involve eliminating some of the fourteen eggs she eats each week. She may need to experiment with low-saturated fat breakfast items such as cereal and English muffins.

Once clients and counselors agree on the pattern, instruction on the diet can begin. This consists of planned steps, beginning with tasks accomplished most easily, and working up to the more difficult ones, a process called staging the diet instruction. For example, Mrs. S. is not a dairy-product lover and eats high-saturated fat dairy products only occasionally. Her program would begin by working to eliminate all such products and arranging substitutes. The next step would be changing the amounts and types of meats eaten. Finally, eggs are her "first love" and it will be difficult to eliminate them or to substitute alternate foods. Each of these three changes can be accomplished gradually during separate interviews

Table 5–8   Example of a Tailoring Pattern

	Cholesterol*	Total Fat[†]	Saturated Fat[†]	Polyun-saturated Fat[†]	Monoun-saturated Fat[†]
3 eggs/week	91	2.27	.69	.30	.86
4 oz. meat/day	119	15.90	9.00	1.12	5.78
0 dairy (fat)	—	—	—	—	—
3 tsp Fleischmann's tub margarine/day		11.20	1.90	3.90	5.20
3 tsp Mazola oil/day		14.00	2.00	8.00	4.00
Total	210	43.37	13.59	13.32	15.84
(% of 1,500 calories)		(26%)	(8%)	(8%)	(10%)

*Figures are calculated to the nearest whole number.
[†]Figures are calculated to the nearest hundredth.

Source: Values were calculated using data from Pennington JAT and Douglas JS, *Bowes and Church's Food Values of Portions Commonly Used* (Eighteenth Edition, Philadelphia: Lippincott Williams & Wilkins, 2005). The meat values are a composite score including red meats, poultry, and fish.

or telephone conversations. Either way, time should be allowed for the client to experiment with ideas in daily life before moving on to more difficult changes.

Lack of knowledge or confusion from past learning can play a major part in the client's ability to lower blood cholesterol. For example, a man who is asked to lose weight may initially switch from foods that provide monounsaturated fat to those lower in calories, such as from regular French dressing to low-calorie, fat-free French dressing and from large amounts of margarine to small amounts of diet margarine (which is lower in monounsaturated fat per teaspoon than regular margarine). The result may be an elevation in blood cholesterol due to a lowering of monounsaturated fat intake. Several diet diaries may be needed to identify this type of information. The change to small amounts of regular dressing and regular margarine can help in lowering blood cholesterol.

In addition to lack of knowledge, counselors should address misconceptions. A few were covered earlier in this chapter. Others include the following:

- "All beef should be avoided because it is too high in saturated fat." Breeding methods have resulted in low-fat beef cuts that can be used in moderation.
- "All pork is forbidden on low-cholesterol diets." In reality, lean pork is lower in saturated fat than beef.
- "If I fry commercial pork sausage until it's brown, all of the fat is removed." It is impossible to remove all fat from high-fat meats such as pork sausage.

To help clear up misconceptions, counselors can provide a list of commercial and noncommercial foods such as that in Exhibit 5–1.

Strategies Addressing Lack of Planning

While information on manufactured products is valuable, clients also need to know how to alter old eating habits on social occasions. In the past, food was considered a symbol of gratitude, love, and celebration on special occasions—associations that can make changing old eating habits at such events very unpleasant or difficult. Telephoning the host prior to a social function can help to determine which foods would be best to eat and can aid in avoiding major deviations from the diet prescription.

Reminders to eat low-saturated, fat-modified foods can take the form of a change in the types of foods clients keep in the refrigerator. Substituting low-fat cheeses and dips for high-fat can serve as a cueing device always to eat appropriately. A reminder on the cupboard door saying, "Don't forget to eat low-fat foods!" can also serve as a cueing device. Notes on the refrigerator to remind the client to call the host before a party are valuable cues, too.

Clients for whom diet alone is not enough to bring blood cholesterol levels to within normal range may be prescribed medications by a physician. Statins are used frequently to change blood cholesterol levels in addition to lifestyle change. A calendar that indicates when medication is taken can also serve as a reminder to take it. Adherence Tool 5–3 provides examples of a one-month and a one-week calendar. This tool can be used to find patterns in the day and time in a week that a client forgets to take medication. For example, Friday lunches may preclude taking medication, resulting in missed doses. A note on the refrigerator saying, "Don't forget to take your medication on Friday" may help. The monthly calendar might be used to observe whether this strategy increases adherence.

Strategies Addressing Lack of Commitment

Frequent expressions of waning commitment include: "I have more difficulty eating in restaurants than I used to," or "I miss all the 'good' food I used to eat," or "I'm tired of worrying about the fat in foods." Responding to these comments with more than information requires careful assessment of the actual problem. Why is commitment declining? Changes in clients' lives can lead to declines in adherence. Is the family in financial hardship? If the family is in danger of losing financial stability, that problem will become a priority. The family that goes through the turmoil of divorce, marriage, remarriage, the addition of a new family member, or the death of a close relative may be at risk for declining adherence and lack of commitment to the medical regimen. Other adherence problems may stem from losing a job or starting a new job.

Streamlining dietary regimen requirements may be necessary for a time to help the client through the difficulties of the life change. Exhibit 5–3 is a contract that provides an example of how to address this type of problem. Relapse should be discussed with the client as a usual step in the process of behavioral change. Ask the client to be specific in discussing what the slip or slips are. It is

Exhibit 5–3   Contract

I will not take my cholestyramine for the two days that I am in divorce court (January 21–22, 2007). On January 23, I will begin to take the full dose of medication again and will reward myself by going to a movie on that night. The nutrition counselor will contact me on January 24 at 7:00 PM to check on reestablishing the medication regimen.

If I do not take the full dose of medication on January 23, I forfeit the reward of going to a movie.

Client _____

Nutrition Counselor _____

Physician _____

helpful to use past data to show how well the client has done over time. Emphasize that current life events will pass, and life will go back to its normal phase.

Positive monologues can be important in increasing adherence when commitment is low (cognitive-behavioral theory with cognitive restructuring as the strategy). By assessing thought processes before and following eating, counselors can observe negative monologues and teach clients to change them to positive monologues. Appropriate improvements in adherence may result. For example, the client who eats a small piece of cheddar cheese may say, "That's it. I blew the diet. It is no use! I just can't stay on this diet. I give up!" With this comment, the client may go into a binge that includes eating three more pieces of cheese. A change from negative to positive might have resulted in this: "I had one small piece of cheese. I know that it is high in saturated fat. I will only have this one piece. I feel great that I was able to stop with this one piece. I will be careful the rest of the day and can still be within the limits of my diet." Most positive thinking involves positive self-rewards. This type of self-rewarding system can be embellished with positive reinforcement from others.

The support of the family or significant others is crucial to adherence (social support). Sometimes family members become upset if eating habits must focus on lowering saturated fat. This negative attitude may have an equally negative effect on client adherence. Changes in eating behavior are easier if clients can tell friends and relatives why the new pattern is necessary. For example, clients can explain that cutting down on cholesterol and saturated fats can help prevent coronary heart disease. Such a rationale can encourage helping others who are hosting parties to serve foods that are low in saturated fat. On their own, clients will find that a positive step is to learn to avoid foods that are high in saturated fat and to limit their intake to those that are lower in this element. Exhibit 5–4 shows a food list that allows for holiday treats.

Families can do much to help clients adhere to a saturated fat-modified diet. Nutrition counselors might involve family members in sessions in which the clients are taught food preparation and receive dietary recommendations. However, too much family involvement can pose problems. For example, a quiet teenager may have a mother who volunteers all information and allows no verbal contact between client and counselor. The nutrition counselor may decide to see the client alone for parts of the interview or use subtle extinction techniques and nonverbal gestures (e.g., no eye contact) to curb too much involvement by the mother. The counselor might state at the beginning of the interview, "Mrs. J., during today's session I would like to find out from your son what his eating habits are at school. When he has finished, I will ask you to help him in describing eating habits at home." It is important to keep good eye contact with the son to encourage his responses rather than his mother's.

Counselors might instruct the client's friends and other family members (if possible) on how to provide positive reinforcement as a way to improve the individual's adherence to a saturated fat-modified diet. The following is a checklist that family members might use for positive reinforcement techniques:

- Praise efforts at decreasing serving sizes of meat, cheese, eggs, and other high-fat, high-cholesterol products (rewards/reinforcement)
- Avoid teasing or tempting with high-fat, high-cholesterol foods (social support).
- Record the number of positive and negative comments the

Exhibit 5–4   Watch the Lights for Eating at Parties

Go Ahead!

Finger Foods
Carrot sticks
Celery sticks
Cauliflower
Radishes
Lettuce
Cabbage
Tomatoes
Mushrooms
Pickles
Artichokes
Avocado

Low-Fat Munchies
Pretzels
Rye crisps
Saltines
Popcorn, no butter
Bread, white, rye,
   and pumpernickel
Oyster crackers
Graham crackers
Melba toast
Bread sticks

Sauces and Spreads
Cocktail sauce
Sweet and sours
Peanut butter

Candy
Gumdrops
Hard candies
Peanut brittle

Fruits
All kinds:
   Fresh
   Frozen
   Canned

Beverages
Soft drinks
Fruit punches
Alcoholic beverages
   (without egg or cream)

Proceed Slowly

Meat Appetizers
Shrimp
Crab
Chicken and ham salad
Sweet and sour pork
Fish

Party Munchies
Potato chips
Cheese nibbles
Corn chips
Party crackers

Dips and Nibbles
(Use only skim milk the rest
   of the day)
Low-fat yogurt dips

Pizza Hors D'oeuvres

Fruit Breads and Cakes

Stop!

Chicken livers
Hors d'oeuvres wrapped in bacon
Cocktail wieners and sausages
Braunschweiger
Chopped liver, liver pâté
Cheese and chocolate fondues (unless
   you can stop at one bite)
Chocolate candies
Commercial snacks containing high-
   fat crust (eggrolls, tarts, etc.)
Cream cheese appetizerrs
Sour cream dips

Courtesy of Karen Smith and Linda G. Snetselaar.

client makes about the diet and try to increase the positive and decrease the negative ones (self-monitoring).

Use of the transtheoretical model in counseling those with elevated lipids may be a very positive step and has been used in two large clinical trials, DISC and WHI. Again the stages of change are divided into three groups rather than five.

The client with elevated LDL-cholesterol is frequently in the precontemplation stage before a major event, i.e., myocardial infarction, has occurred. This not-ready-to-change stage occurs because elevated lipids are often painless and dietary change does not relieve noticeable symptoms. The impetus to change is forced upon the client by the physician and well-meaning family members. The following example is one possible scenario involving a client who has just learned about his elevated lipids.

Counselor: I was just wondering about your thoughts on making dietary changes.

Client: I just don't see a need to make changes. I feel fine. The only reason I am here is that my doctor and family forced me to come. Again, I feel fine. I am at an age where I just want to spend the rest of my days having fun, not worrying about a number that doesn't make me feel badly. I know my doctor and the nurse say I am at risk for a heart attack, but at my age I am willing to take chances. (Precontemplation)

Counselor: You know the facts about risks of a heart attack. You need to make decisions about what to do now. I will not force you to do anything about changing your lifestyle until you have thought about this carefully.

Client: [Looks surprised] You mean that I don't have to stop eating everything I love?

Counselor: I would not force you to eat totally differently from the way you eat now, but rather help you with more healthy substitutes. We would start gradually.

Client: Well, maybe I could make one or two changes. (Contemplation)

Counselor: What would be an easy first step for you?

Client: [Looks surprised] You mean I can choose something on my own?

Counselor: Yes.

Client: I thought I would be totally revamping my life. But if I can just do just one or two things maybe this won't be difficult.

Counselor: Do you have a suggestion?

Client: Here is my food record, and I know that I eat too much fat. Work is the worst. I would like to change some of the high fat foods I eat at lunch without making that meal tasteless. (Preparation)

Counselor: Great! Let's look at your lunches and identify the changes you feel would work best. (Headed Toward Action)

In this counseling session, the client moved through several stages. This happened because all of a sudden he was given the power to make decisions. Notice how the counselor was not rushing to give advice or demeaning the client by refuting his initial argument that it just was not necessary to change dietary habits. This session did not become a confrontation. It was focused on the client's ability to problem solve and make decisions. As counselors, we often work very hard to solve the client's problems. The goal should be to facilitate the client's *own* problem-solving by using reflective listening to redirect the client toward making his or her own decisions about what is the best direction for change. The above example shows how reflective listening helped the client reach a decision to make a change toward a more healthful lifestyle.

Conclusion

In summary, facilitating adherence to low-cholesterol, fat-modified eating patterns requires clients to have a thorough knowledge of the fat and cholesterol content of foods. Along with increasing clients' knowledge, the nutrition counselor facilitates adherence by providing suggestions for more appropriate cueing devices that help with planning appropriate meals. Lack of commitment to this eating pattern can cause lapses in dietary adherence. The nutrition counselor has many behavioral strategies available to increase commitment to dietary change.

Review of Chapter 5

1. List six dietary misconceptions and excesses related to low-saturated fat-modified eating patterns that lead to inappropriate eating behaviors.

   a.

   b.

   c.

   d.

   e.

   f.

2. List three of five specific dietary components of a baseline diet that must be assessed before instructing a client on a saturated fat-modified dietary pattern.

   a.

   b.

   c.

3. List a theory and three strategies that might help the client follow a saturated-fat modified dietary pattern.

   a.

   b.

   c.

4. The following is an exercise (based on data collected using Exhibit 5–3) to help you apply the ideas just discussed.

   Jim is a 48-year-old mailman who eats all meals at home except for social occasions, in which he participates frequently. He loves meat and rarely eats eggs or dairy products. Tailor an eating pattern to his needs and explain one theory and two counseling strategies that might be used to help his dietary adherence on social occasions. The dietary prescription is 15 grams of saturated fat.

References

1. American Heart Association, American Stroke Association. *Heart Disease and Stroke Statistics 2007: Updates At-a-Glance*. American Heart Association, 2007.
2. Executive Summary of The Third Report of The National Cholesterol Education Program (NCEP) Expert Panel on Detection, Evaluation, and Treatment of High Blood Cholesterol In Adults (Adult Treatment Panel III). *JAMA* 2001;285(19):2486–2497.
3. Institutes of Medicine of the National Academies. *Dietary Reference Intakes (DRI), the Essential Guide to Nutrient Requirements*. Washington, D.C.: The National Academies Press, 2006.
4. Renaud S, de Lorgeril M. Dietary lipids and their relation to ischaemic heart disease: from epidemiology to prevention. *J Intern Med* 1989;731(Suppl):39–46.
5. Stamler J, Shekelle R. Dietary cholesterol and human coronary heart disease. The epidemiologic evidence. *Arch Pathol Lab Med* 1988;112(10):1032–1040.
6. Shekelle RB, Stamler J. Dietary cholesterol and ischaemic heart disease. *Lancet* 1989;1(8648):1177–1179.
7. Grundy SM, Barrett-Connor E, Rudel LL, Miettinen T, Spector AA. Workshop on the impact of dietary cholesterol on plasma lipoproteins and atherogenesis. *Arteriosclerosis* 1988;8(1):95–101.
8. Hegsted DM, Ausman LM. Diet, alcohol and coronary heart disease in men. *J Nutr* 1988;118(10):1184–1189.
9. Liu K, Stamler J, Trevisan M, Moss D. Dietary lipids, sugar, fiber and mortality from coronary heart disease. Bivariate analysis of international data. *Arteriosclerosis* 1982;2(3):221–227.
10. Kromhout D, Bosschieter EB, de Lezenne Coulander C. The inverse relation between fish consumption and 20-year mortality from coronary heart disease. *N Engl J Med* 1985;312(19):1205–1209.
11. Ulbricht TL, Southgate DA. Coronary heart disease: seven dietary factors. *Lancet* 1991;338(8773):985–992.
12. Steinberg D. Antioxidants in the prevention of human atherosclerosis. Summary of the proceedings of a National Heart, Lung, and Blood Institute Workshop: September 5–6, 1991, Bethesda, Maryland. *Circulation* 1992;85(6):2337–2344.
13. Gey KF, Puska P, Jordan P, Moser UK. Inverse correlation between plasma vitamin E and mortality from ischemic heart disease in cross-cultural epidemiology. *Am J Clin Nutr* 1991;53(1 Suppl):326S–334S.
14. National Institutes of Health. *Third Report of the National Cholesterol Education Program (NCEP) Expert Panel on Detection, Evaluation, and*

Treatment of High Blood Cholesterol in Adults (Adult Treatment Panel III). Final Report, September 2002, NIH Publication No. 02-5215, B-I-B-II.

15. Brewer HBJ. Lipid and lipoprotein metabolism. In: Rifkind BM, ed. *Drug Treatment of Hyperlipidemia*. New York: Marcel Dekker, 1991:1–15.

16. Assmann G, Gotto AM. HDL cholesterol and protective factors in atherosclerosis *Circulation* 2004;109 [suppl III]: III-8–III-14.

17. Ansell BJ, Watson KE, Fogelman AM, Navab M, Fonarow GC. High-density lipoprotein function. *J Am Coll Cardiol* 2005;46:1792–1798.

18. Brewer HBJ. High density lipoproteins: an overview. In: Lippel K, ed. *Report of the High-Density Lipoprotein Methodology Workshop*. Washington, D.C.: U.S. Department of Health, Education and Welfare, 1979:29–42.

19. Eisenberg S. High density lipoprotein metabolism. *J Lipid Res* 1984;25(10):1017–1058.

20. Clifton PM, Kestin M, Abbey M, Drysdale M, Nestel PJ. Relationship between sensitivity to dietary fat and dietary cholesterol. *Arteriosclerosis* 1990;10(3):394–401.

21. Katan MB, Beynen AC. Characteristics of human hypo- and hyperresponders to dietary cholesterol. *Am J Epidemiol* 1987;125(3):387–399.

22. Katan MB, Berns MA, Glatz JF, Knuiman JT, Nobels A, de Vries JH. Congruence of individual responsiveness to dietary cholesterol and to saturated fat in humans. *J Lipid Res* 1988;29(7):883–892.

23. Katan MB, van Gastel AC, de Rover CM, van Montfort MA, Knuiman JT. Differences in individual responsiveness of serum cholesterol to fat-modified diets in man. *Eur J Clin Invest* 1988;18(6):644–647.

24. Connor SL, Connor WE. The importance of dietary cholesterol in coronary heart disease. *Prev Med* 1983;12(1):115–123.

25. Grundy SM, Denke MA. Dietary influences on serum lipids and lipoproteins. *J Lipid Res* 1990;31(7):1149–1172.

26. Grundy SM. Comparison of monounsaturated fatty acids and carbohydrates for lowering plasma cholesterol. *N Engl J Med* 1986;314(12):745–748.

27. Grundy SM, Florentin L, Nix D, Whelan MF. Comparison of monounsaturated fatty acids and carbohydrates for reducing raised levels of plasma cholesterol in man. *Am J Clin Nutr* 1988;47(6):965–969.

28. Ginsberg HN, Barr SL, Gilbert A, et al. Reduction of plasma cholesterol levels in normal men on an American Heart Association Step 1 diet or a Step 1 diet with added monounsaturated fat. *N Engl J Med* 1990;322(9):574–579.

29. Knuiman JT, West CE, Katan MB, Hautvast JG. Total cholesterol and high density lipoprotein cholesterol levels in populations differing in fat and carbohydrate intake. *Arteriosclerosis* 1987;7(6):612–619.

30. Brinton EA, Eisenberg S, Breslow JL. A low-fat diet decreases high density lipoprotein (HDL) cholesterol levels by decreasing HDL apolipoprotein transport rates. *J Clin Invest* 1990;85(1):144–151.

31. West CE, Sullivan DR, Katan MB, Halferkamps IL, van der Torre HW.

Boys from populations with high-carbohydrate intake have higher fasting triglyceride levels than boys from populations with high-fat intake. *Am J Epidemiol* 1990;131(2):271–282.

32. Keys A, Parlin RW. Serum cholesterol response to changes in dietary lipids. *Am J Clin Nutr* 1966;19(3):175–181.

33. Hegsted DM, McGandy RB, Myers ML, Stare FJ. Quantitative effects of dietary fat on serum cholesterol in man. *Am J Clin Nutr* 1965;17(5):281–295.

34. Mensink RP, Katan MB. Effect of dietary fatty acids on serum lipids and lipoproteins. A meta-analysis of 27 trials. *Arterioscler Thromb* 1992;12(8):911–919.

35. Harris WS. Fish oils and plasma lipid and lipoprotein metabolism in humans: a critical review. *J Lipid Res* 1989;30(6):785–807.

36. Connor WE. Hypolipidemic effects of dietary omega-3 fatty acids in normal and hyperlipidemic humans: effectiveness and mechanisms. In: Simopoulos AP, Kifer RR, Martin RE, eds. *Health Effects of Polyunsaturated Fatty Acids in Seafoods.* Orlando, FL: Academic Press, 1986:173–210.

37. Bautista MC, Engler MM. The Mediterranean diet: is it cardioprotective? *Prog Cardiovasc Nurs* 2005;20(2):70–76.

38. Kris-Etherton PM. The Minnesota heart survey: nutrition successes pave the way for strategic opportunities for food and nutrition professionals. *J Am Diet Assoc* 2007;107(2):209–212.

39. Panagiotakos DB, Pitsavos C, Polychronopoulos E, Chrysohoou C, Zampelas A, Trichopoulou A. Can a Mediterranean diet moderate the development and clinical progression of coronary heart disease? A systematic review. *Med Sci Monit* 2004;10(8):RA193–198.

40. Din JN, Newby DE, Flapan AD. Omega 3 fatty acids and cardiovascular disease—fishing for a natural treatment. *BMJ* 2004;328(7430):30–35.

41. Simopoulos AP. The Mediterranean diets: What is so special about the diet of Greece? The scientific evidence. *J Nutr* Nov 2001;131(11 Suppl):3065S–3073S.

42. Curtis BM, O'Keefe JH, Jr. Understanding the Mediterranean diet. Could this be the new "gold standard" for heart disease prevention? *Postgrad Med* 2002;112(2):35–38, 41–35.

43. Dreon DM, Vranizan KM, Krauss RM, Austin MA, Wood PD. The effects of polyunsaturated fat vs monounsaturated fat on plasma lipoproteins. *JAMA* 1990;263(18):2462–2466.

44. Berry EM, Eisenberg S, Haratz D, et al. Effects of diets rich in monounsaturated fatty acids on plasma lipoproteins—the Jerusalem Nutrition Study: high MUFAs vs high PUFAs. *Am J Clin Nutr* 1991;53(4):899–907.

45. Caggiula AW, Christakis G, Farrand M, et al. The multiple risk intervention trial (MRFIT). IV. Intervention on blood lipids. *Prev Med* 1981;10(4):443–475.

46. Lee S, Harnack L, Jacobs DR, Jr., Steffen LM, Luepker RV, Arnett DK. Trends in diet quality for coronary heart disease prevention between

1980–1982 and 2000–2002: The Minnesota Heart Survey. *J Am Diet Assoc* 2007;107(2):213–222.

47. Dolecek TA, Milas NC, Van Horn LV, et al. A long-term nutrition intervention experience: lipid responses and dietary adherence patterns in the Multiple Risk Factor Intervention Trial. *J Am Diet Assoc* 1986;86(6):752–758.

48. Multiple risk factor intervention trial. Risk factor changes and mortality results. Multiple Risk Factor Intervention Trial Research Group. *JAMA* 1982;248(12):1465–1477.

49. McAlister A, Puska P, Salonen JT, Tuomilehto J, Koskela K. Theory and action for health promotion illustrations from the North Karelia Project. *Am J Public Health* 1982;72(1):43–50.

50. Karvetti RL, Hamalainen H. Long-term effect of nutrition education on myocardial infarction patients: a 10-year follow-up study. *Nutr Metab Cardiovasc Dis* 1993;3:185–192.

51. Buller AC. Improving dietary education for patients with hyperlipidemia. *J Am Diet Assoc* 1978;72(3):277–281.

52. Heller RF, Knapp JC, Valenti LA, Dobson AJ. Secondary prevention after acute myocardial infarction. *Am J Cardiol* 1993;72(11):759–762.

53. Stern MP, Farquhar JW, McCoby N, Russell SH. Results of a two-year health education campaign on dietary behavior. The Stanford Three Community Study. *Circulation* 1976;54(5):826–833.

54. European collaborative trial of multifactorial prevention of coronary heart disease: final report on the 6-year results. World Health Organisation European Collaborative Group. *Lancet* 1986;1(8486):869–872.

55. Rose G. European collaborative trial of multifactorial prevention of coronary heart disease. *Lancet* 1987;1(8534):685.

56. Wilhelmsen L, Berglund G, Elmfeldt D, et al. The multifactor primary prevention trial in Göteborg, Sweden. *Eur Heart J* 1986;7(4):279–288.

57. Farquhar JW, Fortmann SP, Flora JA, et al. Effects of communitywide education on cardiovascular disease risk factors. The Stanford Five-City Project. *JAMA* 1990;264(3):359–365.

58. Tuomilehto J, Geboers J, Salonen JT, Nissinen A, Kuulasmaa K, Puska P. Decline in cardiovascular mortality in North Karelia and other parts of Finland. *Br Med J (Clin Res)* 1986;293(6554):1068–1071.

59. Engblom E, Hietanen EK, Hamalainen H, Kallio V, Inberg M, Knuts LR. Exercise habits and physical performance during comprehensive rehabilitation after coronary artery bypass surgery. *Eur Heart J* 1992;13(8):1053–1059.

60. Schuler G, Hambrecht R, Schlierf G, et al. Regular physical exercise and low-fat diet. Effects on progression of coronary artery disease. *Circulation* 1992;86(1):1–11.

61. Barnard ND, Scherwitz LW, Ornish D. Adherence and acceptability of a low-fat, vegetarian diet among patients with cardiac disease. *J Cardiopulmonary Rehab*1992;12:423–431.

62. Haskell WL, Alderman EL, Fair JM, et al. Effects of intensive multiple risk factor reduction on coronary atherosclerosis and clinical cardiac

events in men and women with coronary artery disease. The Stanford Coronary Risk Intervention Project (SCRIP). *Circulation* Mar 1994;89(3):975–990.

63. Witschi JC, Singer M, Wu-Lee M, Stare FJ. Family cooperation and effectiveness in a cholesterol-lowering diet. *J Am Diet Assoc* 1978;72(4):384–389.

64. Reeves RS, Foreyt JP, Scott LW, Mitchell RE, Wohlleb J, Gotto AM, Jr. Effects of a low cholesterol eating plan on plasma lipids: results of a three-year community study. *Am J Public Health* 1983;73(8):873–877.

65. Bruno R, Arnold C, Jacobson L, Winick M, Wynder E. Randomized controlled trial of a nonpharmacologic cholesterol reduction program at the worksite. *Prev Med* 1983;12(4):523–532.

66. Glanz K. Nutrition education for risk factor reduction and patient education: a review. *Prev Med* Nov 1985;14(6):721–752.

67. Berg-Smith SM, Stevens VJ, Brown KM, et al. A brief motivational intervention to improve dietary adherence in adolescents. The Dietary Intervention Study in Children (DISC) Research Group. *Health Educ Res* 1999;14(3):399–410.

68. Bowen D, Ehret C, Pedersen M, et al. Results of an adjunct dietary intervention program in the Women's Health Initiative. *J Am Diet Assoc* 2002;102(11):1631–1637.

69. Appel LJ, Champagne CM, Harsha DW, et al. Effects of comprehensive lifestyle modification on blood pressure control: main results of the PREMIER clinical trial. *JAMA* 2003;289(16):2083–2093.

70. Elmer PJ, Obarzanek E, Vollmer WM, et al. Effects of comprehensive lifestyle modification on diet, weight, physical fitness, and blood pressure control: 18-month results of a randomized trial. *Ann Intern Med* 2006;144(7):485–495.

Adherence Tool 5–1   Client Questionnaire for Cholesterol- and
Fat-Controlled Eating Patterns

The following questionnaire is a monitoring device that has been
designed to efficiently collect patient information in clinical nutrition
programs. It has several functions.

Initially, it is a useful screening device or test of motivation. Individuals who may not take time to fill it out probably won't take time to participate fully in the behavioral diet and cholesterol modification
programs.

Secondly, the answers to these questions can be of great use to the
therapist during the initial interviews and later during the nutrition sessions. The weight history allows a systematic look at the clients' own
views of their weight problems (if there are any), and at some of the
environmental influences they feel are important to their eating habits.
The history of past attempts to make changes in eating patterns, the
lengths of time they have stayed in dietary modification programs, and
the reasons for past failure can all be useful. Also, their report of mood
changes during previous periods of dieting can help you anticipate and
address problems that might arise during treatment.

The questions about social and family history provide additional
information that is of use medically: for example, the cause of parental
death and the family weight history.

In most states the information contained in this questionnaire is confidential. Without *written* approval from the clients, this information
cannot be divulged to interested individuals, physicians, insurance companies, or law enforcement agencies.

Sources: Adapted from J. M. Ferguson, *Learning To Eat: Behavior Modification for Weight Control*, with permission of Bull Publishing Company,
© 1975. Questions 50–56 are reprinted from "Food Preparation Questionnaire" with permission of Nutrition Coordinating Center, University of
Minnesota.

continued

Adherence Tool 5–1   *continued*

Name:_____ Sex: M F Age:___ Birthdate:_____
Address: _____ Home phone: _____
_____ Office phone: _____

WEIGHT HISTORY

1. Your present weight _____   Height _____
2. Describe your present weight (check one)
    _____ Very overweight
    _____ Slightly overweight
    _____ About average
3. Are you dissatisfied with the way you look at this weight? (check one)
    _____ Completely satisfied
    _____ Satisfied
    _____ Neutral
    _____ Dissatisfied
    _____ Very dissatisfied
4. At what weight have you *felt* your best or do you think you would feel your best? _____
5. How much weight would you like to lose? _____
6. Do you feel your weight affects your daily activities? (check one)
    _____ No effect
    _____ Some effect
    _____ Often interferes
    _____ Extreme effect
7. Why do you want to lose weight at this time? _____
    _____
8. Do these attitudes affect your weight loss or gain? Yes _____
    No _____
    If yes, please describe: _____
    _____
9. Which method did you use for the longest period of time? _____
    _____
10. What usually goes wrong with your weight-loss programs? _____
    _____
    _____
    _____

continued

Adherence Tool 5–1 *continued*

11. How physically active are you? (check one)

_____ Very active   _____ Average   _____ Very inactive

_____ Active   _____ Inactive

MEDICAL HISTORY

12. When did you last have a complete physical examination? _____

13. Who is your current doctor? _____

14. What medical problems do you have at the present time?_____

_____

_____

15. What medications, vitamins or mineral preparations, or drugs do you take regularly? _____

_____

_____

Attach label if available.

16. List any medications, drugs, or foods you are allergic to: _____

_____

_____

_____

17. List any hospitalizations or operations. Indicate how old you were at each hospital admission.

Age   Reason for hospitalization

_____   _____

_____   _____

_____   _____

18. List any serious illnesses you have had that have not required hospitalization. Indicate how old you were during each illness.

Age   Illness

_____   _____

_____   _____

_____   _____

19. Describe any of your medical problems that are complicated by excess weight.

_____

_____

_____

continued

Adherence Tool 5–1   *continued*

20. How much alcohol do you usually drink per week? _____

21. List any psychiatric contact, individual counseling, or marital counseling that you have had or are now having.

    Age   Reason for contact and type of therapy

    _____   _____

    _____   _____

    _____   _____

SOCIAL HISTORY

22. Circle the last year of school attended:

    1 2 3 4 5 6 7 8   9 10 11 12   1 2 3 4   M. A.   Ph.D.

       Grade School   High School   College

    Other _____

23. Describe your present occupation_____

    _____

24. How long have you worked for your present employer? _____

25. Present marital status (check one):

    _____ Single

    _____ Married

    _____ Divorced

    _____ Widowed

    _____ Separated

    _____ Engaged

26. Answer the following questions for each marriage:

    Date of marriage   _____ _____ _____

    Date of termination   _____ _____ _____

    Reason (death, divorce, etc.) _____ _____ _____

    Number of children   _____ _____ _____

27. Spouse's Age _____ Weight _____ Height _____

28. Describe your spouse's occupation _____

    _____

29. Describe your spouse's weight (check one):

    _____ Very overweight   _____ Slightly underweight

    _____ Slightly overweight   _____ Very underweight

    _____ About average

30. Who lives at home with you? _____

    _____

continued

Adherence Tool 5–1 *continued*

FAMILY HISTORY

31. Is your father living?___ Yes___ No   Father's age now, or age at
    and cause of death _____

    _____

32. Is your mother living?___ Yes___ No   Mother's age now, or age at
    and cause of death _____

    _____

33. Describe your father's occupation _____

34. Describe your mother's occupation _____

35. Describe your father's weight while you were growing up (check
    one). If you have never been overweight, skip to question 50.

    _____ Very overweight   _____ Slightly underweight

    _____ Slightly overweight   _____ Very underweight

    _____ About average

36. Describe your mother's weight while you were growing up (check
    one).

    _____ Very overweight   _____ Slightly underweight

    _____ Slightly overweight   _____ Very underweight

    _____ About average

FOOD PREPARATION HABITS

37. Do you salt your food at the table? (check one)

    _____ always

    _____ occasionally

    _____ never

38. If you add salt, how would you rate yourself in terms of amount of
    salt added at the table? (check one)

    _____ light

    _____ moderate

    _____ heavy

39. Do you use a salt substitute at the table such as Lite, Lo-Salt, or
    No-salt? (check one)

    _____ always

    _____ occasionally

    _____ never

    If used, specify brand name: _____

    continued

Adherence Tool 5–1 *continued*

40. Do you regularly use other salt seasonings at the table such as Accent, onion salt, or garlic salt? (check one)

_____ Yes

_____ No   Specify kind(s): _____

41. Check whether salt or salt substitute is usually added in *preparing* the following foods:

	Salt	Salt Substitute	Seasoning Salts	None
Pasta, such as noodles, macaroni	[ ]	[ ]	[ ]	[ ]
Rice	[ ]	[ ]	[ ]	[ ]
Potatoes	[ ]	[ ]	[ ]	[ ]
Other vegetables	[ ]	[ ]	[ ]	[ ]
Meat	[ ]	[ ]	[ ]	[ ]
Fruit	[ ]	[ ]	[ ]	[ ]
Other (e.g., coffee)	[ ]	[ ]	[ ]	[ ]
specify_____	[ ]	[ ]	[ ]	[ ]
_____	[ ]	[ ]	[ ]	[ ]

If salt substitute, specify kind/brand _____

42. Are the following table and cooking fats used (check one)?

Butter   _____ yes   (Specify: _____regular, _____unsalted)

                   _____ no

Margarine   _____ yes   (Specify: _____regular, _____unsalted)

                   _____ no

Specify brand(s):

_____   _____ stick_____ tub _____ diet _____ spread

_____   _____ stick_____ tub _____ diet _____ spread

_____   _____ stick_____ tub _____ diet _____ spread

Vegetable oil (such as corn, soy, safflower, sunflower, etc.) (circle one)

_____ yes   (Specify types and/or brands used:)   _____

_____ no   _____

_____

Spray shortening (such as Pam)

_____ yes   (Specify brand:)_____

_____ no   _____

_____

continued

Adherence Tool 5–1   *continued*

Solid shortening (such as Crisco, Spry, Fluffo, etc.) (circle one)

_____ yes   (Specify types and/or brands used:) _____

_____ no   _____

_____

Other cooking fats (such as lard, bacon drippings, salt pork, poultry fat, etc.) (circle one)

_____ yes   (Specify)_____

_____ no   _____

_____

43. Do you use gravy on meats? (check one)

_____ Yes   _____ No

44. If you prepare gravies, do you usually use (check one):

_____ cornstarch   _____ flour

Is the liquid usually (check one): _____ milk   _____ water

_____ other

(Specify:)_____

45. Indicate how much fat is usually trimmed from the meat before cooking or eating (check one):

_____ trim most   _____ trim some   _____ usually don't trim

46. Indicate on the following table the periods in your life when you have been overweight. *If you have never been overweight, skip to question 15.* Where appropriate, list your maximum weight for each period and number of pounds you were overweight. Briefly describe any methods you used to lose weight in that five-year period (e.g., diet, shots, pills). Also list any significant life events you feel were related to either your weight gain or loss (e.g., college tests, marriage, pregnancies, illness).

Age	Maximum Weight	Pounds Overweight	Methods Used To Lose Weight	Significant Events Related to Weight Change
Birth				
0–5				
6–10				
11–15				
16–20				
21–25				

continued

Adherence Tool 5–1   *continued*

Age	Maximum Weight	Pounds Overweight	Methods Used To Lose Weight	Significant Events Related to Weight Change
26–30				
31–35				
36–40				
41–45				
46–50				
51–55				
56–60				
61–65				

47. What are the attitudes of the following people about your attempt(s) to lose weight?

	Negative (They disapprove or are resentful)	Indifferent (They don't care or don't help)	Positive (They encourage me and are understanding)
Husband			
Wife			
Children			
Parents			
Employer			
Friends			

48. A number of different ways of losing weight are listed below. Please indicate which methods you have used by filling the appropriate blanks.

	Ages Used	Number of Times Used	Maximum Weight Lost	Comments (Length of Time Weight Loss Maintained; Successes; Difficulties)
TOPS (Take Off Pounds Sensibly)				
Weight Watchers				
Pills				
Supervised Diet				
Unsupervised Diet				

continued

Adherence Tool 5–1 *continued*

	Ages Used	Number of Times Used	Maximum Weight Lost	Comments (Length of Time Weight Loss Maintained; Successes; Difficulties)
Starvation				
Behavior Modification				
Psychotherapy				
Hypnosis				
Other				

49. Have you had a major mood change during or after a significant weight loss? Indicate any mood changes on the following checklist.

	Not at All	A Little Bit	Moderately	Quite a Bit	Extremely
a. Depressed, sad, feeling down, unhappy, the blues					
b. Anxious, nervous, restless, or uptight all the time					
c. Physically weak					
d. Elated or happy					
e. Easily irritated, annoyed, or angry					
f. Fatigued, worn out, tired all the time					
g. A lack of self-confidence					

50. What do you do for physical exercise and how often do you do it?

Activity (for example, swimming, jogging, dancing)	Frequency (daily, weekly, monthly)

continued

Adherence Tool 5–1   *continued*

51. List your children's ages, sex, heights, weights, and circle whether they are overweight, average, or underweight. Include any children from previous marriages, whether they are living with you or not.

			Weight				
Age	Sex	Height	Overweight				Underweight
			very	slightly	average	slightly	very
			very	slightly	average	slightly	very
			very	slightly	average	slightly	very
			very	slightly	average	slightly	very
			very	slightly	average	slightly	very

52. List your brothers' and sisters' ages, sex, present weights, heights, and circle whether they are overweight, average, or underweight.

			Weight				
Age	Sex	Height	Overweight				Underweight
			very	slightly	average	slightly	very
			very	slightly	average	slightly	very
			very	slightly	average	slightly	very
			very	slightly	average	slightly	very
			very	slightly	average	slightly	very

53. Please add any additional information you feel may be relevant to your current eating habits. This includes interactions with your family and friends that might sabotage a dietary modification program, and additional family or social history that you feel might help us understand your dietary habits.

continued

54. Check the fat most often used in preparing each of the following foods:

	Butter	Margarine	Spray shortening	Oil, such as Wesson, Mazola	Vegetable shortening such as Crisco, Fluffo, Spry	Bacon fat	Lard	Chicken fat	Beef suet	None
Eggs, fried	[ ]	[ ]	[ ]	[ ]	[ ]	[ ]	[ ]	[ ]	[ ]	[ ]
Eggs, scrambled	[ ]	[ ]	[ ]	[ ]	[ ]	[ ]	[ ]	[ ]	[ ]	[ ]
French toast	[ ]	[ ]	[ ]	[ ]	[ ]	[ ]	[ ]	[ ]	[ ]	[ ]
Cornbread	[ ]	[ ]	[ ]	[ ]	[ ]	[ ]	[ ]	[ ]	[ ]	[ ]
Potatoes, mashed	[ ]	[ ]	[ ]	[ ]	[ ]	[ ]	[ ]	[ ]	[ ]	[ ]
Potatoes, french fried	[ ]	[ ]	[ ]	[ ]	[ ]	[ ]	[ ]	[ ]	[ ]	[ ]
Potatoes, pan fried	[ ]	[ ]	[ ]	[ ]	[ ]	[ ]	[ ]	[ ]	[ ]	[ ]
Greens	[ ]	[ ]	[ ]	[ ]	[ ]	[ ]	[ ]	[ ]	[ ]	[ ]
Other vegetables	[ ]	[ ]	[ ]	[ ]	[ ]	[ ]	[ ]	[ ]	[ ]	[ ]
White beans, pinto	[ ]	[ ]	[ ]	[ ]	[ ]	[ ]	[ ]	[ ]	[ ]	[ ]
Gravy	[ ]	[ ]	[ ]	[ ]	[ ]	[ ]	[ ]	[ ]	[ ]	[ ]
White sauce	[ ]	[ ]	[ ]	[ ]	[ ]	[ ]	[ ]	[ ]	[ ]	[ ]
Pie crust	[ ]	[ ]	[ ]	[ ]	[ ]	[ ]	[ ]	[ ]	[ ]	[ ]

55. Indicate the most usual method of preparing each of the following. If you fry any of them, comment on whether the item is dipped in flour or batter or breaded before frying and what fat is used for frying. Also check whether gravy is prepared.

Item	Method of Cooking (e.g., pan frying, broiling, deep frying)	Kind of Fat Used (if any)
Hamburger		
Steaks		
Chops		
Poultry		
Fish		
Shellfish (shrimp, etc.)		
Liver		
Other, specify		

continued

Adherence Tool 5–1   *continued*

56. Check the salad dressing *most often* used with the following salads: (Specify brand)

	Mayonnaise-Type (Such as Miracle Whip, Spin Blend)	Regular Mayonnaise (Such as Hellmann's, Kraft)	Imitation Mayonnaise (Such as Bright Day)	Weight Watchers' Mayonnaise	Other—Specify as French, Italian, Ranch-style, etc. Also Specify Creamy, Clear, Lo-Cal, etc.
Potato salad					
Cole slaw					
Tossed salad					
Macaroni salad					
Other (specify)					

Adherence Tool 5–2   Fat Facts or Misfacts (Monitoring Device)

	True	False
1. All vegetable oil helps lower cholesterol.	____	____
2. Saturated fat is found only in animal products.	____	____
3. Hydrogenation is a beneficial process that makes fat less saturated.	____	____
4. Cholesterol is found in some peanut butter.	____	____
5. Cholesterol is found in all animal products.	____	____
6. All foods that are high in saturated fat are also high in cholesterol.	____	____

Adherence Tool 5–3   One-Month and One-Week Calendar (Monitoring Device)

ONE–MONTH CALENDAR

Sun.	Mon.	Tues.	Wed.	Thur.	Fri.	Sat.
1	2	3	4	5	6	7
8	9	10	11	12	13	14
15	16	17	18	19	20	21
22	23	24	25	26	27	28
29	30	31	1	2	3	4

month of _____ 20_____. If you have any questions, please call: _____

ONE–WEEK CALENDAR

NAME: _____

ATTN: _____   THANK YOU!

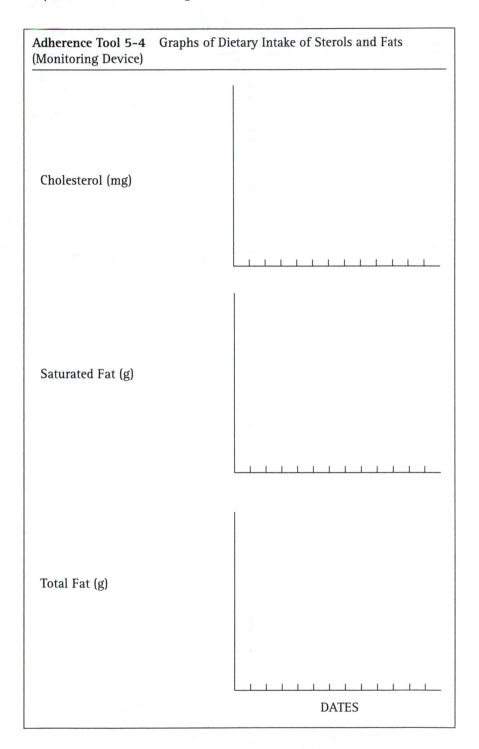

Adherence Tool 5-4   Graphs of Dietary Intake of Sterols and Fats
(Monitoring Device)

Cholesterol (mg)

Saturated Fat (g)

Total Fat (g)

DATES

Adherence Tool 5-5   Graphs of Serum Lipid Values (Monitoring Device)

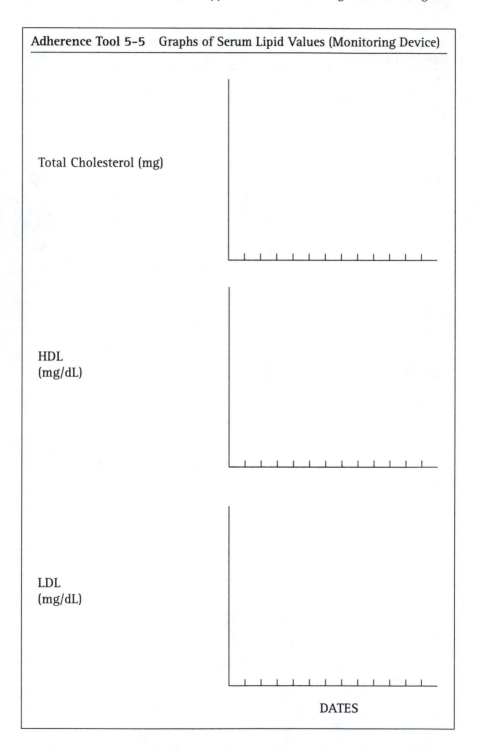

Total Cholesterol (mg)

HDL
(mg/dL)

LDL
(mg/dL)

DATES

Adherence Tool 5-6   Pantry Survey (Monitoring Device)

Food	Saturated Fat (Hydrogenated Vegetable Fat)	Poly-unsaturated Fat	Mono-unsaturated Fat

Adherence Tool 5-7   Client Meal Planning Chart (Informational Device)

Meal planning can help you in keeping your fat and cholesterol intake low. Before your next visit, plan three days of meals that avoid foods high in fat and cholesterol.

	Day 1	Day 2	Day 3
Breakfast			
Snack			
Lunch			
Snack			
Dinner			
Snack			

Adherence Tool 5-8   Tips for Dining in Restaurants (Informational Device)

Select from the following suggestions:

Appetizers
Clear soup (bouillon, fat-free consomme), fruits or vegetables, juices, seafood cocktail (except shrimp), oysters, or clams on the half-shell. (Be sure to count the seafood as part of your meat allowance.)

Salads
Lettuce and other vegetables, fruits, fruit and cottage cheese (use as part of milk allowance), gelatin. Use lemon juice, vinegar and oil, French dressing, or mayonnaise as your dressing.

Entree
Baked, broiled, or roasted fish, poultry, lean meat, cottage cheese.

Vegetables
All vegetables prepared without butter, meat fat, or cream sauce.

Potatoes and Substitutes
Baked or broiled without dressing, mashed if made without butter, plain rice, macaroni, or spaghetti.

Desserts
Fresh or canned fruits, fruit compotes, sherbet, gelatin, unfrosted angel food cake.

Beverages
Coffee or tea (without cream), carbonated beverages, fruit juices, milk (as allowed), and alcoholic beverages (unless not allowed because of medical problems).

Breakfast Cereals
All cereals without coconut, served with allowed milk.

Miscellaneous
Nuts (except walnuts and filberts), honey, jam, syrup, hard candy, marshmallows, gumdrops, hard fruit drops, jellybeans, mints (no chocolate or bon bons), condiments, and seasoning, as allowed.

Avoid
Combination dishes, fried or creamed foods, foods made with whole milk products, butter, cheese, or gravy. Do not eat pastries (sweet rolls, pies, cakes, cookies, doughnuts, waffles), fatty meats (bacon, sausage, luncheon meats), cream soups, or potato or corn chips.

Inquire about the fat and other ingredients used in menu items. Then give specific instructions regarding the methods of preparation of your selection.

Adherence Tool 5-9   Comparing High-Cholesterol, High-Fat Menus with Low-Cholesterol, Low-Fat Menus (Informational Device)

HIGH-CHOLESTEROL, HIGH-FAT MENU (AT HOME)

Breakfast 1	Lunch 1
Egg (1)	Bologna (1 ounce)
Bacon (2 strips)	Bread (2 slices)
Toast (2 slices)	Mayonnaise (1 tablespoon)
Blue Bonnet Stick Margarine	Blue Bonnet Stick Margarine
(2 teaspoons)	(2 teaspoons)
Milk, Whole (8 ounces)	Potato Chips (1 cup)
Orange Juice (4 ounces)	Mr. Goodbar (1 bar)
	Milk, whole (8 ounces)

Dinner 1
Roast Beef (5 ounces)
Mashed Potatoes ($^1/_2$ cup)
Corn ($^1/_2$ cup)
Bread (2 slices)
Blue Bonnet Stick Margarine (6 teaspoons)
Cherry Cobbler (1 cup)
Ice Cream ($^1/_2$ cup)
Milk, whole (8 ounces)

Note: Nutrient values are taken from a variety of sources including Pennington JAT and Douglas JS, Bowes and Church's *Food Values of Portions Commonly Used* (Eighteenth Edition, Philadelphia: Lippincott Williams & Wilkins, 2005) labels; and Nutrient Data System (NDS), University of Minnesota. Actual calculations for individual eating patterns could include a variety of data tables currently available to the nutrition counselor.

continued

Adherence Tool 5-9 *continued*

Breakfast 1

	Amount	Cholesterol (mg)	Total Fat (g)	Saturated Fat (g)	Polyunsaturated Fat (g)	Monounsaturated Fat (g)	P/S Ratio
Egg	1	213	5.30	1.60	.70	2.00	
Bacon	2 strips	11	6.24	2.20	.74	3.30	
Toast	2 slices	–	–	–	–	–	
Blue Bonnet Stick Margarine	2 tsp.	–	5.33	1.00	1.00	1.33	
Milk, whole	8 oz.	34	8.15	5.08	.29	2.78	
Orange juice	4 oz.	–	–	–	–	–	
TOTAL		258	25.02	9.88	2.73	9.41	.28

Lunch 1

	Amount	Cholesterol (mg)	Total Fat (g)	Saturated Fat (g)	Polyunsaturated Fat (g)	Monounsaturated Fat (g)	P/S Ratio
Bologna	1 slice (23 g)	13	6.52	2.68	.24	3.60	
Bread	2 slices	–	–	–	–	–	
Mayonnaise	1 Tbsp.	8	10.96	1.60	5.70	3.10	
Blue Bonnet Stick Margarine	2 tsp.	–	5.33	1.00	1.00	1.33	
Potato Chips	1 cup	8	8.60	3.42	1.02	4.16	
Mr. Goodbar	1 bar	10	16.10	9.00	0.80	5.70	
Milk, whole	8 oz.	34	8.15	5.08	.29	2.78	
TOTAL		73	55.66	22.78	9.05	20.67	.40

continued

Adherence Tool 5-9 *continued*

Dinner 1

	Amount	Cholesterol (mg)	Total Fat (g)	Saturated Fat (g)	Polyunsaturated Fat (g)	Monounsaturated Fat (g)	P/S Ratio
Roast Beef (medium fat)	5 oz.	130	21.10	9.15	5.50	6.45	
Mashed Potatoes*	1/2 cup	–	–	–	–	–	
Corn*	1/2 cup	–	–	–	–	–	
Bread	2 slices	–	–	–	–	–	
Blue Bonnet Stick Margarine	6 tsp.	–	16.00	3.00	3.00	4.00	
Cherry Cobbler*	1 cup	–	–	–	–	–	
Ice Cream	1/2 cup	30	7.16	4.46	.27	2.43	
Milk, whole	8 oz.	34	8.15	5.08	.29	2.78	
TOTAL		194	52.41	21.69	9.06	15.66	.42

*Fat used in these recipes was figured into the amount of Blue Bonnet margarine.

Total Daily Intake—Diet 1

	Cholesterol (mg)	Total Fat (g)	Saturated Fat (g)	Polyunsaturated Fat (g)	Monounsaturated Fat (g)	P/S Ratio
Diet 1	525	133.09	54.35	20.84	45.74	.38
Percent of 2,770 Calories*		43%	18%	7%	15%	
Recommendations	200	25%	8.3%	8.3%	8.3%	1.00

*All calorie values here and on the following pages are estimates and may include fat-free foods not listed.

continued

Adherence Tool 5-9   *continued*

HIGH-CHOLESTEROL, HIGH-FAT MENU (IN A RESTAURANT)

Breakfast 2
Egg McMuffin (1)
Orange Juice (4 ounces)
Milk, whole (8 ounces)

Lunch 2
Big Mac (1)
Fries (regular)
Milk, whole (8 ounces)
Apple Pie (1)

Dinner 2
Tenderloin (1)
Fries (regular)
Milk, whole (8 ounces)

continued

Adherence tool 5-9   *continued*

Breakfast 2

	Amount	Cholesterol (mg)	Total Fat (g)	Saturated Fat (g)	Polyunsaturated Fat (g)	Monounsaturated Fat (g)	P/S Ratio
Egg McMuffin	1	226	11.20	3.80	1.30	6.10	
Orange Juice	4 oz.	–	–	–	–	–	
Milk, whole	8 oz.	34	8.15	5.08	.29	2.78	
TOTAL		260	19.35	8.88	1.59	8.88	.18

Lunch 2

	Amount	Cholesterol (mg)	Total Fat (g)	Saturated Fat (g)	Polyunsaturated Fat (g)	Monounsaturated Fat (g)	P/S Ratio
Big Mac	1	103	32.40	10.10	1.50	20.90	
Fries, regular	1	12	17.10	7.20	.70	9.20	
Milk, whole	8 oz.	34	8.15	5.08	.29	2.78	
Apple Pie	1	12	14.80	4.80	.90	9.10	
TOTAL		161	72.45	27.18	3.39	41.98	.12

continued

Adherence tool 5-9 *continued*

Dinner 2

	Amount	Cholesterol (mg)	Total Fat (g)	Saturated Fat (g)	Polyunsaturated Fat (g)	Monounsaturated Fat (g)	P/S Ratio
Tenderloin	1	90	24.99	6.42	5.55	13.02	
Fries, regular	1	12	17.10	7.20	.70	9.20	
Milk, whole	8 oz.	34	8.15	5.08	.29	2.78	
TOTAL		136	50.24	18.70	6.54	25.00	.35

Total Daily Intake–Diet 2

	Cholesterol (mg)	Total Fat (g)	Saturated Fat (g)	Polyunsaturated Fat (g)	Monounsaturated Fat (g)	P/S Ratio
Diet 2	557	142.04	54.76	11.52	75.86	.21
Percentage of 2,500 Calories		51%	20%	4%	27%	–
Recommendations	200	25%	8.3%	8.3%	8.3%	1.00

continued

Adherence Tool 5-9   *continued*

LOW-CHOLESTEROL, LOW-FAT MENU (AT HOME)

Breakfast 3
English Muffin (1)
Canadian Bacon (1 ounce)
Milk, skim (8 ounces)
Fleischmann's Tub Margarine (2 teaspoons)
Orange Juice (4 ounces)

Lunch 3
Turkey (1 ounce)
Bread (2 slices)
Miracle Whip (1 teaspoon)
Chips ($^1/_2$ cup)
Zucchini Cake (1 serving)
Milk, skim (8 ounces)

Dinner 3
Fish (5 ounces)
Mashed Potatoes ($^1/_2$ cup)
Corn ($^1/_2$ cup)
Tossed Salad (1 cup)
Dressing (1 tablespoon)
Fleischmann's Tub Margarine (1 teaspoon)
Sherbet ($^1/_2$ cup)
Milk, skim (8 ounces)

continued

Adherence Tool 5-9   *continued*

Breakfast 3

	Amount	Cholesterol (mg)	Total Fat (g)	Saturated Fat (g)	Polyunsaturated Fat (g)	Monounsaturated Fat (g)	P/S Ratio
English Muffin	1	–	–	–	–	–	
Canadian Bacon	1 oz.	25	2.84	.87	.28	1.69	
Milk, skim	8 oz.	5	.44	.29	.02	.13	
Fleischmann's Tub Margarine	2 tsp.	–	6.00	1.00	2.67	1.67	
Orange Juice	4 oz.	–	–	–	–	–	
TOTAL		30	9.28	2.16	2.97	3.49	1.4

Lunch 3

	Amount	Cholesterol (mg)	Total Fat (g)	Saturated Fat (g)	Polyunsaturated Fat (g)	Monounsaturated Fat (g)	P/S Rati
Turkey	1 oz.	22	1.10	.33	.26	.51	
Bread	2 slices	–	–	–	–	–	
Miracle Whip	1 tsp.	1	1.63	.24	.88	.51	
Chips	1/2 cup	–	4.67	.59	2.72	1.36	
Zucchini Cake	1 sv.	–	4.67	.59	2.72	1.36	
Milk, skim	8 oz.	5	.44	.29	.02	.13	
TOTAL		28	12.51	2.04	6.60	3.87	3.2

continued

Adherence Tool 5-9 *continued*

Dinner 3

	Amount	Cholesterol (mg)	Total Fat (g)	Saturated Fat (g)	Polyunsaturated Fat (g)	Monounsaturated Fat (g)	P/S Ratio
Fish (6%)	5 oz.	113	5.70	1.50	1.32	2.88	
Mashed Potatoes	1/2 cup	–	3.78	.69	1.68	1.41	
Corn	1/2 cup	–	3.78	.69	1.68	1.41	
Tossed Salad	1 cup	–	–	–	–	–	
Dressing Fleischmann's	1 Tbsp.		4.67	.61	1.87	2.19	
Tub Margarine	1 tsp.		3.00	.50	1.33	.83	
Sherbet	1/2 cup	–	–	–	–	–	
Milk, skim	8 oz.	5	.24	.14	.00	.10	
TOTAL		118	21.17	4.13	7.88	8.82	1.91

Total Daily Intake–Diet 3

	Cholesterol (mg)	Total Fat (g)	Saturated Fat (g)	Polyunsaturated Fat (g)	Monounsaturated Fat (g)	P/S Ratio
Diet 3	176	42.96	8.33	17.45	16.18	2.09
Percent of 1,923 Calories		20%	4%	8%	8%	
Recommendations	200	25%	8.3%	8.3%	8.3%	1.00

continued

Adherence Tool 5-9 *continued*

LOW-CHOLESTEROL, LOW-FAT MENU (IN A RESTAURANT)

Breakfast 4
Apple Danish (1)
Orange Juice (4 ounces)
Milk, skim (8 ounces)

Lunch 4
McChicken (1)
Orange Drink (12 ounces)
Strawberry Sundae (1)

Dinner 4
Broiled Cod (13 ounces)
Baked Potato (1)
Tossed Salad (2 cups)
Dressing (1 tablespoon)
Fleischmann's Tub Margarine (2 teaspoons)
Fresh Fruit Compote (1 cup)
Milk, skim (8 ounces)

Adherence Tool 5-9 *continued*

Breakfast 3

	Amount	Cholesterol (mg)	Total Fat (g)	Saturated Fat (g)	Polyunsaturated Fat (g)	Monounsaturated Fat (g)	P/S Ratio
Apple Danish	1	25	17.90	3.50	2.00	10.80	
Orange Juice	4 oz.	–	–	–	–	–	
Milk, skim	8 oz.	5	.44	.29	.02	.13	
TOTAL		30	18.34	3.79	2.02	10.93	.58

Lunch 4

	Amount	Cholesterol (mg)	Total Fat (g)	Saturated Fat (g)	Polyunsaturated Fat (g)	Monounsaturated Fat (g)	P/S Ratio
McChicken	1	43	28.60	5.40	11.60	11.40	
Orange Drink	12 oz.	–	–	–	–	–	
Strawberry Sundae	1	5	1.10	.60	–	.40	
TOTAL		48	29.70	6.00	11.60	11.80	1.93

continued

Adherence Tool 5-9 *continued*

Dinner 4

	Amount	Cholesterol (mg)	Total Fat (g)	Saturated Fat (g)	Polyunsaturated Fat (g)	Monounsaturated Fat (g)	P/S Ratio
Broiled Cod (6%)	3 oz.	68	3.84	.87	1.26	1.71	
Baked Potato	1	—	—	—	—	—	
Tossed Salad	2 cups	—	—	—	—	—	
Fleischmann's Dressing	1 Tbsp.	—	4.54	.71	2.60	1.23	
Tub Margarine	2 tsps.	—	6.00	1.00	2.67	1.67	
Fresh Fruit Compote	1 cup	—	—	—	—	—	
Milk, skim	8 oz.	5	.44	.29	.02	.13	
TOTAL		73	14.82	2.87	6.55	4.74	2.28

Total Daily Intake—Diet 4

	Cholesterol (mg)	Total Fat (g)	Saturated Fat (g)	Polyunsaturated Fat (g)	Monounsaturated Fat (g)	P/S Ratio
Diet 4	151	62.86	12.66	20.35	27.47	1.60
Percent of 2,455 Calories		23%	5%	8%	10%	
Recommendations	200	25%	8.3%	8.3%	8.3%	1.00

Adherence Tool 5–10   P/S Ratios of Various Fats and Oils (Informational Device)

	Oils and Margarines	*Nuts*	*Other Fats*
	8. 0 ┬ Safflower oil	8.0 ┬	8.0 ┬ Safflower mayonnaise
	7. 0 ┼ Sunflower oil / Walnut oil	7.0 ┼	7.0 ┼
	6. 0 ┼	6.0 ┼ Sunflower seeds / Walnuts	6.0 ┼
Helps Raise P/S Ratio	5. 0 ┼ / Corn oil	5.0 ┼	5.0 ┼ Sandwich spread
	4. 0 ┼ Soybean/ Cottonseed oil (Wesson, Crisco, etc.)	4.0 ┼	4.0 ┼ Mayonnaise / Salad dressing (Miracle Whip type)
	3. 0 ┼ Soybean oil / Sesame oil	3.0 ┼ Pecans, Pumpkin seeds, Chest-nuts, Almonds	3.0 ┼ Imitation mayonnaise
Has Little Effect on P/S Ratio	2. 0 ┼ Peanut oil	2.0 ┼ Peanuts, Mixed nuts, Brazil nuts, Filberts,	2.0 ┼ Peanut butter
	1. 0 ┼ / Olive oil	1.0 ┼ Hazelnuts Pistachio nuts Cashews	1.0 ┼ Crisco shortening, Avocado, Olives
Has Negative Effect on P/S Ratio	Palm oil / 0. 0 ┼ Coconut oil	Macadamia 0.0 ┼ nuts	Carob coated candy, 0.0 ┼ Bacon, Butter, Chocolate, Coconut

Note: P/S = polyunsaturated fat ÷ saturated fat.
Courtesy of Pat Pace, R. D., M. S., Baylor University.

CHAPTER 6

NUTRITION COUNSELING IN TREATMENT OF DIABETES

Chapter Objectives

1. Identify factors that contribute to common inappropriate behaviors associated with carbohydrate-, protein-, and fat-controlled eating patterns.

2. As a part of step 1, assessment, identify specific nutrients to emphasize in assessing a baseline eating pattern before providing dietary instruction.

3. Identify theories to help combat inappropriate eating behaviors as a part of step 3, intervention.

4. Also as a part of step 3, intervention, generate strategies to deal with clients following carbohydrate-, protein-, and fat-controlled eating patterns.

5. Recommend dietary adherence tools for clients on carbohydrate-, protein-, and fat-controlled eating patterns.

Nutrition and Diabetes

Diabetes affects a large segment of the U.S. population, with 20.8 million Americans diagnosed with the disease.[1] The prevalence increases with age and is higher in nonwhite racial and ethnic populations.[2,3]

The publication of results from the Diabetes Control and Complications Trial (DCCT) has pointed to the importance of intensive therapy, including dietary eating pattern control, in delaying progression of diabetic retinopathy, nephropathy, and neuropathy in patients with insulin-dependent diabetes mellitus.[4] Providing appropriate and tailored eating patterns for clients with diabetes can be a challenge. All dietary factors, both amount and content, must be carefully controlled, yet the client must be allowed a reasonable selection of foods. This chapter is designed to provide potential solutions to problems encountered in working with clients with both type 1 and type 2 diabetes.

The American Diabetes Association provides the following basic goals for medical nutrition therapy in persons with diabetes[5,6]:

- Attain and maintain optimal metabolic outcomes, including:
  1. Blood glucose levels in the normal range or as close to normal as is safely possible to prevent or reduce the risk for complications of diabetes.
  2. A lipid and lipoprotein profile that reduces the risk for macrovascular disease.
  3. Blood pressure levels that reduce the risk for vascular disease.
- Prevent and treat the chronic complications of diabetes. Modify nutrient intake and lifestyle as appropriate for the prevention and treatment of obesity, dyslipidemia, cardiovascular disease, hypertension, and nephropathy.
- Improve health through healthy food choices and physical activity.
- Address individual nutritional needs taking into consideration personal and cultural preferences and lifestyle while respecting the individual's wishes and willingness to change.

In tailoring goals, many situations require individualization[5,6]:

- For youth with type 1 diabetes, to provide adequate energy to ensure normal growth and development, integrate insulin regimens into usual eating and physical activity habits.
- For youth with type 2 diabetes, to facilitate changes in eating and physical activity habits that reduce insulin resistance and improve metabolic status.
- For pregnant and lactating women, to provide adequate energy and nutrients needed for optimal outcomes.
- For older adults, to provide for the nutritional and psychosocial needs of an aging individual.
- For individuals treated with insulin or insulin secretagogues, to provide self-management education for treatment (and prevention) of hypoglycemia, acute illnesses, and exercise-related blood glucose problems.
- For individuals at risk for diabetes, to decrease risk by

encouraging physical activity and promoting food choices that facilitate moderate weight loss or at least prevent weight gain.

This chapter provides information on theories and facts about diabetes. The effects of specific nutrients, sweeteners, alcohol, and exercise on blood glucose levels are described. Methods and means of managing diabetes through glucose monitoring, insulin regimens, and dietary intervention are reviewed. Adherence to diabetic eating patterns is covered in a section describing research in this area. Also included are eating behaviors that are inappropriate for optimum adherence to diabetic eating patterns. For step 1, assessment, methods to determine eating patterns prior to instruction on a diabetic dietary recommendation are described. As a part of step 3 intervention, the chapter discusses theories and treatment strategies for lack of knowledge related to general dietary modifications that affect blood glucose levels and lack of knowledge regarding fat intake and weight gain. Strategies designed to deal with lack of planning and lack of commitment provide the nutrition counselor with tools to increase the likelihood of adherence to eating patterns that allow for normalization of blood glucose levels.

Theories and Facts about Nutrition and Type 2 Diabetes

The person with type 2 diabetes is usually overweight and has peripheral resistance to insulin. The treatment of choice is lifestyle change with reduced energy intake by decreasing dietary fat and increasing energy expenditure by adding tailored exercise habits to normal daily schedules.[7-10]

These changes in energy balance will allow for decreased insulin resistance and reduced and normalized blood glucose levels. The single most important goal in managing a person with obesity and type 2 diabetes is to achieve and maintain desirable body weight by reducing total energy intake to levels below energy expenditure. With the loss of weight, blood glucose levels normalize.

For weight reduction, the diet should be adequate in nutrients but restricted in calories. Diets very low in calories and suboptimal in micronutrients may require the addition of a vitamin and mineral supplement. For persons who cannot adhere to a weight-loss diet, insulin or oral agents may be necessary to lower blood glucose levels. Three oral agents are commonly used in treatment of type 2 diabetes: sulfonylureas, the biguanide metformin, the alpha-glucosidase inhibitor acarbose, and the thiazolidinedione troglitazone. Each reduces blood glucose in a different way. Sulfonylureas act to reduce the release of glucose from the pancreas. Metformin works to reduce the liver's production of glucose. Acarbose blocks the digestion of complex carbohydrates, resulting in the reduction of glucose absorption. Finally, thiazolidinedione increases the insulin sensitivity of skeletal muscle, adipose tissue, and liver cells. While insulin therapy is the last resort in treatment of type 2 diabetes, it is becoming a common method of treating this chronic disease.[11]

The presence of hepatic or renal disease may exclude the use of oral agents. Although effective in type 2 diabetes, these drugs are absolutely contraindicated in persons with type 1 diabetes because they are only effective in patients who are able to produce endogenous insulin. Irregular exercise and eating patterns for persons taking oral agents can lead to periods of severe hypoglycemia. Weight loss is the key to achieving control in type 2 diabetes.

Several current studies are designed to determine the treatment options to delay or prevent type 2 diabetes. These studies show that it is possible to achieve a risk reduction that can delay type 2 diabetes, if not prevent it.[12-18] Three of these studies showed a decreased incidence of type 2 diabetes with the following reductions in risk: in the Diabetes Prevention Program (DPP), metformin lowered risk by 31%[12]; in the STOP-IDDM trial, acarbose lowered risk by 32%[15]; and troglitazone lowered risk by 56% in the TRIPOD study.[14] In the DPP, changes in diet, exercise, and lifestyle were nearly twice as effective in delaying the onset of diabetes overall as was metformin.[12]

Theories and Facts about Nutrition and Type 1 Diabetes

Insulin-dependent persons have complete beta cell failure, cannot produce insulin, are prone to ketoacidosis, and require exogenous insulin. Therapy revolves around insulin, diet, and exercise.

Effective insulin treatment to avoid extremely high and low blood glucose levels requires a standardized daily dietary regimen. The insulin regimen is closely tied to dietary intake, and the entire lifestyle of the client is important in tailoring a meal plan. Several factors in dietary control are important: (1) timing of meals, (2) dietary composition, (3) caloric intake, and (4) level and regularity of physical activity. With new, fast-acting insulin, timing of meals is less important because it is not necessary to allow 30 minutes between insulin injection and meals; however, with regular insulin, it is still important to allow 30 minutes between an insulin injection and the meal. At present, few clients are on regular insulin.

In the Diabetes Control and Complications Trial (DCCT), when study participants in the intensive intervention reported that they were adhering to their individualized meal plan and adjusting their insulin to meet changes in their carbohydrate intake 90% of the time, their HbA1c levels were reduced by 0.9 of a point (11% lower) compared to those who reported following their meal plan less than 45% of the time. A second dietary behavior that resulted in achievement of a normal HbA1c target without hypoglycemia or weight gain was responding to hyperglycemia with less carbohydrate/food or more insulin. This behavior resulted in 0.5 points lower (5% lower) HbA1c than observed in those who used these behaviors less than half the time. A third behavior was adjusting the dose of insulin to match meal size and content. Results showed that those who used this behavior 90% of the time reduced their HbA1c by 0.5 points (7% lower) compared to those who never used this behavior. A fourth behavior which often resulted in problematic blood glucose levels when not used was the appropriate treatment of low blood glucose levels. When hypoglycemia symptoms occur, the client will often over-treat without waiting 15 minutes for the initial glucose dose to begin working in an effort to immediately reduce negative symptoms. For those clients who appropriately treated hypoglycemia, their HbA1c was 0.5 points lower (7% lower) than those who almost always over-treated their low blood glucose levels. A fifth behavior that often resulted in elevated blood glucose levels was nighttime snacking. HbA1c was lower in those who ate bedtime snacks in a consistent fashion. Additionally, those who ate extra snack foods less than once per week had 4% lower HbA1c levels than those who reported eating extra snacks more than three times in a week.[19]

In summary, the DCCT results showed that there are three important outcomes that should be a focus when counseling clients with type 1 diabetes: HbA1c levels (as discussed above), hypoglycemia, and weight gain. Delahanty provides a list of items that nutrition counselors should focus on when facilitating behavior change in clients. For hypoglycemic episodes, the following areas are important:

- Provide the client with information on appropriate ways to treat elevated blood glucose levels. In the DCCT, quick-acting glucose tablets were the treatment of choice for hypoglycemia. Clients kept these tablets in their cars, office desks, purses or pockets, and numerous places in their homes. Another method of treating hypoglycemia was to try 10 to 15 grams of fast-acting carbohydrate sources on various levels of blood sugar. Adjustments in the number of grams could then be made to accommodate a variety of situations.
- Emphasize the concept that inconsistent carbohydrate intake is a key culprit in erratic blood glucose levels. Often the reason for symptoms that accompany elevated glucose levels—feeling tired, for example—are a result of eating patterns that vary in content and amount. Wide swings in blood glucose levels often result in problematic symptoms.
- Tailor insulin levels to activities in the client's life.[20]

Because weight gain was a problem in the DCCT, nutrition counselors should focus on facilitating behaviors in clients that minimize this outcome. Methods to accomplish this are below:

- For those with a family history of overweight or obesity, discuss the potential for gaining weight as blood glucose control increases.
- Indicate the need to reduce calories by 250–300 per day when beginning intensive therapy.
- Caution against over treating a hypoglycemic reaction because of the increase in caloric intake that may result.
- Adjust insulin rather than increasing dietary intake to accommodate physical activity.
- If patterns of hypoglycemia are noted, decrease insulin rather than increasing dietary intake with meal size and/or snacking.
- Discuss making reduced fat intake a priority. Keeping carbohydrate intake consistent will minimize hypoglycemia and reduce the calories associated with treating it.[20]

The DCCT showed that tailored dietary patterns and lifestyle change were important to achieving dietary and exercise goals. Several meal-planning strategies were used: simple and advanced carbohydrate counting, the Exchange system, Healthy Food Choices, and Total Available Glucose.[21,22]

An extended follow-up study to the DCCT, Epidemiology of Diabetes Interventions and Complications study (EDIC), shows that the benefits of intensive therapy remain after 10 years beyond the 6.5-year intensive intervention of the DCCT. Results from this follow-up study showed that the intensive intervention group compared to the usual care group not only maintained a difference, but also increased that difference in incidence of nephropathy, retinopathy and hypertension. The group that previously received intensive intervention also experienced less cardiovascular disease and slower progression of vascular intima-media thickness.[23-26]

Controversy exists with regard to the best nutrient distribution for dietary prescription. The American Dietetic Association and American Diabetes Association recommend the following nutrient distribution:

1. Individuals should limit protein intake with no more than the adult Recommended Dietary Allowance (RDA) (0.8 g/kg/day) with evidence of nephropathy; and protein intake adjusted for very young children, pregnant and lactating women, and some elderly persons.
2. The goal for dietary fat intake in individuals with type 1 and 2 diabetes is the same as that for persons who have a history of cardiovascular disease. The most recent guidelines from the National Cholesterol Education Program are 25–35% of total calories from fat and saturated fat at 7% of total calories.[27] Intake of trans fat should be minimized.[6]
3. It is important to individualize the percentage of daily calories from carbohydrate based on the patient's eating habits. The percentage of daily calories from carbohydrate can be devised after the protein and fat goals have been met. The percentage and distribution will vary with insulin regimens and treatment goals.[6,28] For the average person without diabetes, the National Academy of Science recommends that intake of carbohydrate represent from 45–65% of total calories.[29] These recommendations are general, flexible requirements. The major goal should be to normalize blood sugars with glycosylated hemoglobin (HbA1c) in the normal range. (See Table 6–1 and "Blood Glucose Monitoring" on page 249 for a detailed discussion of HbA1c.)

Table 6–1   Glycemic Control for People with Diabetes

Biochemical Index	Nondiabetic	Goal	Action Suggested
Preprandial glucose (mg/dL)	< 115	80–120	< 80, > 140
Bedtime glucose (mg/dL)	< 120	100–140	< 100, > 160
Hemoglobin A1c (%)	< 6	< 7	> 8

Notes: Values are for nonpregnant individuals. "Action suggested" depends on individual patient circumstances. Hemoglobin A1c is referenced to a nondiabetic range of 4.0–6.0% (mean 5.0%; standard deviation 0.5%). *In the Diabetes Control and Complications Trial, the experimental group had glycosylated hemoglobins of approximately 7.0% and the standard group 9.0%.[†]

*American Diabetes Association Position Statement: Standards of Medical Care for Patients with Diabetes Mellitus. *Diabetes Care* 1994;17:616–624.
[†]The Diabetes Control and Complications Research Group, "The effect of intensive treatment of diabetes on the development and progression of long-term complications in insulin-dependent diabetes mellitus," *N Engl J Med* 1993;329:977–986.

4. Lifestyle change is the primary goal for achieving weight loss with decreases in intake and increases in physical activity. Caloric intake should be decreased by 500–1000 kcal/day with a resulting weight loss of 1–2 pounds per week.[6]
5. The optimal macronutrient mix for adults in general, not those with diabetes, based on the Dietary Reference Intakes (DRIs) is 45–65% of total energy from carbohydrate, 20–35% from fat and 10–35% from protein.[29]

It is unlikely that there is a perfect combination of macronutrients and that tailoring of these combinations of macronutrients would seem to be best for persons with diabetes.[6]

Effects of Specific Nutrients, Sweeteners, Alcohol, and Exercise on Blood Glucose Levels

Carbohydrates

Traditionally, dietary recommendations focused on use of complex carbohydrate and minimization of simple carbohydrate, assuming that the latter was absorbed rapidly and thus produced swings in blood glucose.[30,31] Subsequent studies demonstrated that when sucrose is substituted for other carbohydrate, it does not increase blood glucose to a greater extent than isocaloric amounts of starch.[32–34]

Following is a discussion on the types of carbohydrate that are digestible. It should be kept in mind that affects on blood glucose are dependent on the facts discussed above.

Digestible Carbohydrate

Digestible dietary carbohydrate has traditionally been classified as simple (monosaccharides, disaccharides, and oligosaccharides) or complex (polysaccharides). Most foods do not fall into just one category, but are in a combination of categories. In human nutrition, the monosaccharides of greatest importance are the six-carbon sugars—glucose, fructose, and galactose. Glucose, also known as dextrose or corn sugar, is present in sweet fruits such as berries, grapes, pears, and oranges, and in certain vegetables, notably corn and carrots. Relatively large amounts occur in honey as well. Dextrose from corn syrup is often used commercially as a sweetener in prepared foods. Fructose, also called levulose or fruit sugar, is also found in most fruits and vegetables. Galactose is not found free in foods, although it is a major constituent of the principal carbohydrate in milk, lactose.

Disaccharides are formed when two monosaccharides are chemically bonded together. When glucose and fructose are bonded, sucrose, or table sugar, results. It is found in most fruits and vegetables and is a major component of brown sugar, maple sugar, and molasses. Many processed foods are sweetened with sucrose. When glucose and galactose are bonded, the disaccharide lactose results. Lactose, the only significant carbohydrate of animal origin, is found in milk and milk products. Maltose is another important disaccharide that results when two identical glucose units bond. Maltose is found in germinating seeds, some breakfast cereals, and fermented products, such as beer.

Oligosaccharides are next in complexity, containing between three and ten monosaccharide units. The oligosaccharides, stachyose and raffinose, occur in small amounts in legumes such as kidney beans and lentils and, although believed to be inert metabolically, they are acted on by bacteria in the lower small intestine and colon and may cause increased flatus production.

The term polysaccharide denotes the combination of a number of monosaccharides. Polysaccharides of plant origin are commonly known as starches, of which there are several types. Different carbohydrate-containing foods (for example, corn, wheat, and apples) have different starches, each genetically determined. For example, amylose is a plant starch in which hundreds of glucose units are combined to form one long, straight chain. Amylopectin is another plant starch, also composed solely of glucose units, but arranged in branched chains. Various plants contain both amylose and amylopectin, although in different proportions.

The most abundant polysaccharide (and probably the most common organic molecule on earth) is cellulose, a component of plant cell walls. The body cannot digest cellulose because the human digestive system does not have the capacity to break the cellulose linkage structure. However, the amylose structure is readily digested. In summary, small structural distinctions make the difference in how each molecule behaves and is used.

The one animal polysaccharide, glycogen, is not present in the food supply to an appreciable extent. Although it is stored as an energy source in some animal tissue (muscle and liver), it disappears with the death of the animal, leaving only negligible amounts in foods such as liver and fresh shellfish. The significance of glycogen for humans is its manufacture by the body during the course of glucose metabolism.[35]

During digestion, even large molecules of carbohydrate, such as starch, are eventually hydrolyzed to monosaccharides. Through enzymatic activity and chemical activity involving gastric acid, dietary carbohydrate is converted to the three monosaccharides (Figure 6-1).

In diabetes management, one of the most controversial topics is the type of dietary carbohydrate consumed. In the past, a commonly accepted belief was that because sugars are smaller molecules, they are more rapidly digested and absorbed than complex carbohydrates. Researchers believed that the larger molecules of complex carbohydrate took longer to be absorbed, resulting in a slower and more moderate rise in blood glucose levels. Patients were advised to avoid simple carbohydrate and encouraged to increase their intake of complex carbohydrate. In the 1970s and 1980s, researchers began to challenge this dietary dogma, asserting that glycemic changes were not related solely to the molecular structure of the carbohydrate consumed.[30,36,37]

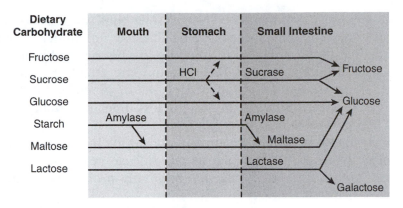

FIGURE 6-1   Schematic Diagram of Carbohydrate Digestion.
Source: Reprinted by permission from Kreutler PA, *Nutrition in Perspective,*
2nd ed. Copyright © 1987 by Allyn and Bacon.

Several investigators have conducted research in people with diabetes indicating that glycemic response is not related solely to the molecular structure of the carbohydrate consumed. As indicated previously, Bantle and his coworkers found no differences in metabolism of glucose between diets containing predominantly starch or simple sugar in patients with type 1 or type 2 diabetes.[32,38,39] Additional research shows no adverse effects of sucrose on glycemia.[40–46]

Although much research is still necessary to explain fully how carbohydrates affect diabetic control, past research has provided some very interesting clues.[47] Over the years, studies point to the following factors in the relationship of complex carbohydrates and their effect on blood glucose values:

- nature of the starch
- protein-starch interaction
- antinutrients other than fiber
- physical form
    1. cooking method
    2. particle size (blending, grinding, etc.)

Crapo and coworkers studied the glycemic and insulin responses to a group of carbohydrate-containing foods, including bread, rice, potato, and corn, of normal and glucose-intolerant volunteers. Their findings indicated that the differences in responses to these foods are related to differences in the digestibility of starches.[30,37,48,49] Studies have also shown that, because of its chemical structure, amylopectin can be digested more quickly than amylase. The glucose chains of amylose are bound by hydrogen bonds, making them less available for amylitic attack than amylopectin, which has many branched chains of glucose.[50] Indeed, raw legume starch (high in amylose) is less digestible than cornstarch in rats.[51]

An interaction between the protein and starch in food may also influence the digestibility and blood glucose response to the starch.[52] Anderson et al. found that removing protein from flour increased its digestibility.[53]

In addition to the starch and protein components of foods, antinutrients (natural enzyme inhibitors, lectins, phytates, and tannins) may affect starch digestibility and the blood glucose response. Enzyme inhibitors, lectins, and phytates were shown to produce hypoglycemia and decreased growth in rats.[54-58] Furthermore, antinutrients may inhibit starch digestion in the gastrointestinal tract.[57,59-61]

The physical form of complex carbohydrates also affects blood glucose responses. A greater rise in blood glucose was reported after consumption of cooked as opposed to raw starches. Researchers found that raw plant foods produced lower blood glucose responses than did cooked plant foods.[62-64] Researchers have looked at moist and dry heat methods of cooking. Jenkins found that drying cooked red lentils in a warm oven for 12 hours resulted in significantly enhanced glycemic response and rate of in vitro digestion as compared with lentils boiled 20 minutes.[65]

The size of the starch particle is also important in starch digestibility. Digestibility increased when beans were ground first and then cooked as opposed to when they were cooked first and then ground.[65] O'Dea and others found that the blood glucose response to whole apples increased when apples were blended to a puree or when the juice was extracted.[63,66,67]

Indigestible Carbohydrate

Fiber is carbohydrate that is not hydrolyzed by human digestive enzymes. It consists of plant cell walls composed mostly of three polysaccharides—cellulose, pectic substances, and hemicellulose—as well as noncarbohydrate lignin. Fiber is a component of plant foods only; it is not found in foods of animal origin.

It is important to draw a clear distinction between the effects of purified fiber added to a diet and fiber naturally present in food. In general, the viscous, water-soluble fibers, such as guar and pectin (purified fiber), have been most effective in flattening postprandial glycemia in normal and diabetic volunteers and reducing urinary glucose loss in diabetic subjects. Part of this action may stem from the ability of these fibers to slow gastric emptying and reduce the rate of small intestinal absorption, possibly by increasing the thickness of the unstirred water layer immediately adjacent to the small intestinal absorptive surface.

Fiber that occurs naturally in foods may reduce the rate of small intestinal digestion by changing the degree to which digestive enzymes penetrate foods. Viscous forms of fiber may also have this same effect impeding the penetration of the food by digestive enzymes, as may viscous forms of fiber. However, disruption of the normal relationship of starch and fiber, as in the milling of wheat products, may greatly reduce any effect the fiber might have on postprandial glycemia.

Concerns have been raised about the vitamin and mineral status of people who change from a habitually low-fiber diet to a diet of higher fiber content. Studies of vitamin and mineral status in adult subjects on high-fiber diets have not found evidence of deficiency.[68-70] Two populations at greatest risk, children[71-73] and pregnant women,[74,75] also have shown no harmful effects of fiber. Another population at risk is the elderly. Studies have not been done to evaluate mineral malabsorption in this age group. Use of high-fiber diets in this group should be approached with caution.[68] Use of high-fiber diets in persons with gastroparesis is contraindicated.[76]

Many natural food fiber/diabetes studies report improvement in glucose control.[77-79] One limiting factor in these studies is the difficulty in knowing what caused this improvement—the fiber component of the diet or other simultaneous changes in macronutrient content. Anderson indicates that most of the reduction in insulin requirements for lean diabetic patients eating high-carbohydrate and fiber diets may be related to the 70% carbohydrate and 12% fat content, with only a small role assigned to fiber content.[80] Studies that have included the soluble-fiber supplements guar and pectin have demonstrated improved glucose control.[78,79] By contrast, insoluble-fiber supplements such as wheat bran and cellulose have usually produced no significant change.[81,82]

Lafrance showed no beneficial glycemic effect of 56 grams of fiber ingested by persons with type 1 diabetes.[83] Giacco also studied persons with type 1 diabetes and showed positive effects of 50 gram fiber diets on blood glucose but not lipids.[84] Hollenbeck chose to study persons with type 2 diabetes using fiber from 11–27 grams per 1000 kcal.[85] Findings showed that glycemia, insulinemia and lipids did not improve. Another study conducted by Chandalia and coworkers compared 24 with 50 grams of fiber and found decreased blood glucose, reduced hyperinsulinemia, and decreased lipids in the 50 gram arm.[86]

The amounts of dietary fiber were high in studies showing improved glycemic control. These high amounts (more than 50 grams per day) would be difficult to achieve for most persons in the Western world. The 1994 recommendations for persons with diabetes do not suggest high-fiber diets for one reason: because the levels necessary to improve glycemic control would be difficult to obtain from foods.[82,87]

In summary, studies have shown that even with a variety of starches and sugars in the diet, the blood glucose response is the same if the amount of carbohydrate remains the same.[88]

Classifying Carbohydrates Using the Glycemic Index

As stated earlier, researchers have found variations in blood sugars when specific foods within the categories of simple and complex carbohydrate were tested for post-ingestion blood glucose excursions. Wolever and colleagues provided one method of classifying foods according to their effect on blood glucose levels.[89]

In theory, the higher the glycemic index value, the higher the blood glucose values would be expected to rise after the ingestion of the food. Results of early glycemic index research proved contrary to previous beliefs about the effect of carbohydrate on blood glucose levels. For example, researchers were surprised to find that instant potatoes had a higher glycemic index (120) than ice cream (69) (Table 6-2). As a class, legumes are the foods that produce the flattest glycemic response, which is thought to be due to the slow release of carbohydrate during digestion rather than to slowed carbohydrate absorption.[90,91]

Table 6–2 Glycemic Index of Selected Foods

Food	Glycemic Index	Food	Glycemic Index
Breads		Legumes	
White	100	Kidney beans, canned	74
Whole meal	100	Lentils, green, canned	74
Pumpernickel	68	Baked beans, canned	70
Pasta		Kidney beans, dried	43
Spaghetti, white,		Lentils, green, dried	36
boiled 15 min	67	Soybeans, canned	22
Spaghetti, brown,		Soybeans, dried	20
boiled 15 min	61	Fruit	
Spaghetti, white,		Banana	84
boiled 5 min	45	Orange juice	71
Cereal Grains		Orange	59
Millet	103	Apple	52
Rice, brown	81	Apple juice	45
Rice, instant, boiled 1 min	65	Sugars	
Barley, pearled	36	Maltose	152
Breakfast Cereals		Glucose	138
Cornflakes	121	Sucrose	83
Puffed wheat	110	Lactose	57
Shredded wheat	97	Fructose	26
Porridge oats	89	Dairy Products	
"All Bran"	74	Ice cream	69
Root Vegetables		Yogurt	52
Potato, instant	120	Skim milk	46
Potato, mashed	98	Whole milk	44
Potato, new/white, boiled	80	Snack Foods	
Potato, sweet	70	Corn chips	99
Vegetables		Potato chips	77
Carrots, cooked	92		
Peas, frozen	74		

Source: Data from Wolever TM, *World Review of Nutrition Dietetics,* Vol. 62, pp. 120–185, copyright © 1990.

The glycemic index (GI) is defined as:

$$GI = 100 \times F/R$$
$$F = \text{test food}$$
$$R = \text{reference food (bread)}$$

Franz has reported that blood glucose levels in persons with both type 1 and 2 diabetes did not improve with low glycemic diets.[92] Currently, the American Diabetes Association states that there is not enough evidence to recommend diets that have a low glycemic index as a primary strategy in planning meals when assisting patients who have diabetes.[88] Franz suggests that there may be a place for use of the glycemic index in fine-tuning postprandial blood glucose levels. Use of the glycemic index should only occur after emphasis on total carbohydrate.[93] A more recent concept is the glycemic load, which includes both the number of grams of carbohydrate in a usual food serving or meal and the glycemic index. This value has no evidence-based intervention research behind it and therefore is not recommended at this time. In summary, any change in the diet creates counterchange; therefore, counselors must always consider the total diet and its appropriateness for an individual.

Fat

The fat content of the diet is important for individuals with diabetes. Persons with diabetes have a two to three times greater incidence of atherosclerosis and risk of death from cardiovascular disease than do persons who do not have diabetes, with an expected reduction in lifespan of five to seven years.[94] Lower saturated fat, cholesterol, and total fat intake may help avoid coronary complications. The American Diabetes Association states that persons with diabetes have risk factors similar to those who have had a history of cardiovascular disease. Therefore, the recommendations are the same for individuals with diabetes and for those with a past CVD history, as previously discussed.[6]

Although fat has been associated with decreased gastric emptying, the addition of fat to a carbohydrate load does not necessarily alter its effect on blood glucose levels. Studies on the effect of fat on blood glucose levels showed varying responses.[95] Two showed that fat, regardless of type, has no impact on digestion rates or blood glucose responses.[96,97] Parillo found that diets enriched with monounsaturated fats may reduce insulin resistance.[98] Others found reduced postprandial blood glucose responses when a saturated fat (butter) was eaten with carbohydrate. There was no associated decrease in insulin response.[99,100] One study showed no significant changes in acute postprandial glucose responses and insulin levels when subjects ate amounts of fat smaller than those described in the studies above. However, the subjects demonstrated a large impairment of carbohydrate tolerance following a standard meal eaten four hours after the high-fat breakfast.[101] The exact mechanism behind this effect is unclear. Studies show that energy intake plays a role in determining the effects of a high-carbohydrate versus a high monounsaturated fat eating pattern.[102,103]

For persons who need to reduce weight, a lower energy and low-fat, moderate-carbohydrate eating pattern is recommended. Persons at normal body weight would have improved triglycerides and postprandial glycemia if a high-monounsaturated fat dietary approach were followed.[88]

Brackenridge stresses that food combinations can alter rates of carbohydrate digestion and absorption, modifying the pattern of glucose rise after a meal.[104] When this occurs, although the total amount of glucose released into the bloodstream may be unchanged, the postprandial glucose rise can be delayed or blunted. This reaction will change insulin demand and availability. Exhibit 6-1 shows two meals with identical carbohydrate content, but very different fat and fiber content. These two meals may produce significantly different 2-hour postprandial glucose levels. Post-meal glucose testing will provide data to determine the optimal size and timing of the pre-meal insulin bolus for specific meals.

Protein

Protein is also important in the diabetic person's diet. Approximately 58% of animal protein intake may eventually be converted to glucose, but at a much slower rate than carbohydrate.[105-107] High-protein diets have been recommended for the treatment of diabetes and may be associated with beneficial effects in some people with diabetes, but these diets have not yet been investigated scientifically. Concern about high-protein diets seems to center on the increased fat and cholesterol content that accompanies such diets unless food choices are made carefully. High-protein diets are

Exhibit 6-1   Isocarbohydrate Meals

Item		CHO (g)	Fat (g)	Fiber (g)
Meal 1:	8 oz orange juice	27	0	< 1
	2 slices white bread	26	2	2
	2 oz part-skim cheese	2	8	< 1
	1 oz puffed rice cereal	13	0	< 1
	4 oz skim milk	6	0	< 1
	Black coffee	0	0	0
	Total	74	10	~ 4
Meal 2:	1 apple (3/lb)	18	1	3
	2 slices bran bread	26	4	6
	2 tsp soft margarine	1	10	< 1
	1/2 cup 100% Bran	23	2	13
	4 oz low-fat milk	6	3	< 1
	Total	74	~ 20	~ 22

Source: Reprinted from Brackenridge B, Carbohydrate counting for diabetes therapy, in *Handbook of Diabetes Medical Nutrition Therapy*, M.A. Powers, ed., p. 262. Copyright © 1996, Aspen Publishers, Inc.

contraindicated in diabetic patients with renal disease in predialysis states.

Calories

The caloric content of the diet is very important, as the majority of persons with type 1 diabetes initially lose a significant amount of weight. A diet must be adequate in calories for normal growth and development in pediatric age groups and for desirable body weight in adults. In the pregnant diabetic individual, caloric intake must be adjusted for normal growth and development of the fetus. Excess weight can lead to insulin resistance. Chapter 4 discusses strategies to aid in decreasing calories.

Sweeteners

Many alternatives are open to diabetic persons who want to use nonglucose-containing sweeteners. Four low-calorie sweeteners currently approved for use in the United States are acesulfame potassium, aspartame, saccharin, and sucralose. Low-calorie sweeteners with approval or reapproval pending include alitame and cyclamate.

Acesulfame Potassium

Acesulfame potassium is 200 times sweeter than sucrose, is heat stable, and blends well with other nutritive and nonnutritive sweeteners. Studies using both humans and animals have shown that acesulfame potassium is not metabolized, nor does it accumulate in the body. Because it is not metabolized, it has no caloric value. It has no effect on blood glucose, cholesterol, total glycerol, or free glycerol levels.[108] In terms of safety, no adverse effects were documented even at administered doses of 1,000 times higher than anticipated maximum dietary intake by humans. It has been deemed safe for all segments of the population.[87,109] In one packet of sweetener, equivalent to the sweetness of two teaspoons of sugar, there are only 10 milligrams of potassium (1 medium-sized banana = 440 milligrams potassium).

Aspartame

Aspartame has a slow onset of a sweet taste that is sustained over time. It is stable in dry foods but decomposes on prolonged exposure to high temperatures or in liquid form. Aspartame is metabolized in the gastrointestinal tract to aspartic acid, phenylalanine, and methanol. The aspartic acid is primarily used for energy through conversion to CO_2 in the Krebs cycle. The phenylalanine is primarily incorporated into body protein, either unchanged or as tyrosine. The methyl group is hydrolyzed by intestinal esterases to methanol. The metabolism of aspartame is the same as that of its equivalent natural components. The individual components are rapidly metabolized and do not accumulate at recommended intakes.[110] It would be extremely difficult to consume amounts large enough to accumulate to toxic levels because the body continuously clears the byproducts from the system.[111,112] Aspartame in the amount of 2.7 grams per day does not affect blood glucose control.[111] The Food and Drug Administration (FDA) has found aspartame to be a safe sweetener for the general population, in-cluding pregnant women and children. One qualifier is that persons who do not tolerate phenylalanine should avoid aspartame-containing products.[113]

Saccharin

Saccharin is a white, crystalline powder synthesized from toluene. It is approximately 300 times sweeter than sucrose. Despite many claims that saccharin has a bitter aftertaste, it continues to be a popular tabletop sweetener. Saccharin is only slightly soluble in water and is stable under many conditions. The continued use of saccharin is due at least in part to its long shelf life, low price, and heat stability. Saccharin is not metabolized and is excreted unchanged, primarily by the kidneys in the urine.[114] Researchers have found that "as a group, users of artificial sweeteners (saccharin and cyclamates) have little or no excess risk of cancer of the lower urinary tract."[115] The American Medical Association reviewed experimental data and reaffirmed its stand that saccharin should continue to be available as a food additive.[116] Both the American Dietetic Association and the American Diabetes Association have stated that saccharin poses no health hazard.[87,117]

Sucralose

Sucralose is 600 times sweeter than sucrose. It is made from sugar by selectively substituting three chlorine atoms for three hydroxyl groups on the sugar molecule. It has a similar taste profile to sugar with no unpleasant aftertaste, and it has no calories. It is stable in solutions and at varying pH levels and temperatures. It can be used in cooking and baking. Sucralose is essentially nonmetabolized. It passes rapidly through the body without being broken down. It is not digested in the gastrointestinal tract and only a small amount (about 15% of that ingested) is absorbed through the small intestine. The remainder passes through the digestive system unchanged and is excreted in the feces. Sucralose does not accumulate in any tissues and is not actively transported across the blood–brain barrier to the central nervous system, across the placental barrier, or from the mammary gland into breast milk.[118] Studies indicate that sucralose can be used safely by everyone, including pregnant and lactating women, children, and persons with type 1 and type 2 diabetes.[119] Also, sucralose does not promote tooth decay.[120] The FDA has approved the use of sucralose in 15 food and beverage categories.[121]

The American Dietetic Association states that all FDA-approved nonnutritive sweeteners can be used by persons with diabetes, including pregnant women.[88]

Sweeteners Pending FDA Approval

Alitame

Alitame is a dipeptide-based amide formed from L-aspartic acid and D-alanine. It is 2,000 times sweeter than sucrose. It is stable at high temperatures and over a broad pH range and less stable in lower ranges (acids). It can be used in sodas, fruit drinks, baked goods, confections, and tabletop sweeteners.[122] Alitame is metabolized to its two proteins and other components. The amino acids are metabolized and the remainder excreted unchanged.

Cyclamate

Cyclamate, a derivative of cyclohexylsulfamic acid, is 30 times sweeter than sucrose. It enhances the sweetness of other sweeteners, is heat stable, mitigates the bitter aftertaste of saccharin when saccharin is the second sweetener, increases the product's stability or shelf life, and usually reduces product cost.[122] Cyclamate is metabolized in the digestive tract, and its byproducts are secreted by the kidneys. Its primary metabolite is cyclohexylamine, which some scientists believe may be more toxic than cyclamate. Cyclohexylamine is formed from the nonabsorbed cyclamate by bacteria in the gastrointestinal tract. Not all persons are able to metabolize cyclamate, and those who do only metabolize a portion of what is consumed.[123] It has been shown that cyclamate has no significant effect on blood glucose.[122] The FDA continues to review data for other safety issues in addition to carcinogenicity (such as genetic damage and testicular atrophy).[124] However, the safety of cyclamate for human use has been supported.[125]

Alcohol

Alcohol intake may cause hypoglycemia because the enzyme most common in alcohol metabolism, alcohol dehydrogenase (ADH), inhibits gluconeogenesis in the liver. In a fasting person with diabetes, 2 ounces of distilled liquor may result in hypoglycemia. In a non-fasting person with well-controlled diabetes, moderate alcohol intake of either 8 ounces of regular beer, 4 ounces of dry wine, or 2 ounces of distilled liquor along with a meal does not seem to affect the blood glucose level dramatically.[126,127]

Individuals with well-controlled diabetes who have eaten minimal amounts of food may experience hypoglycemia within 6 to 36 hours after alcohol ingestion.[128] Self-monitoring blood glucose levels before and after alcohol intake and a meal enables the person to predict potential hypoglycemia and prevent it from occurring.

Alcohol has been shown to cause hyperglycemia in a non-fasting person who has diabetes due to glycogenolysis in the liver and peripheral insulin resistance.[129] The rise in blood glucose depends on the quantity of alcohol consumed and the amount of liver glycogen stores available.[130]

Intoxication can result in decreased competence in administering insulin or other hypoglycemic agents or lack of ability to time and plan meals appropriately. In addition, alcohol intoxication can mask the symptoms of hypoglycemia and impede appropriate treatment. Another potential metabolic consequence of alcohol ingestion is elevated plasma triglyceride levels. Because diabetes is associated with an increased incidence of hypertriglyceridemia, nutrition counselors should consider the effect of alcohol on plasma triglyceride levels in the dietary therapy of any diabetic client. It would seem prudent to curtail alcohol ingestion significantly in clients with preexisting elevations of plasma triglyceride. The caloric content of the alcohol must be considered and included in the diabetic meal plan. Finally, because alcohol intake may cause hypoglycemia, clients should be warned about and given strategies to deal with this potential problem.[131]

In summary, persons with diabetes should avoid alcohol abuse. Counselors can explain the specific risks for people with diabetes. Moderate ingestion of alcohol is the key for diabetic individuals, with caution regarding its effect on caloric balance, control of plasma triglyceride levels, and reduced reaction time.

Exercise

Exercise can modulate the body's sensitivity to insulin and increase peripheral glucose use, resulting in improved metabolic control for those with diabetes. In type 1 diabetes, the effect of exercise can vary depending on blood glucose control. Those individuals who are poorly controlled may experience elevated blood glucose levels. For those in good blood glucose control, the opposite may result, with the symptoms of hypoglycemia. For those with type 2 diabetes, blood glucose control will improve with an exercise regimen. The reason for this improvement lies in decreased insulin resistance and increased insulin sensitivity, with resulting increased peripheral use of glucose both during and after activity.[93,132]

The goals of an exercise program for individuals with diabetes are:

1. to maintain or improve cardiovascular fitness to prevent or minimize the long-term cardiovascular complications of diabetes
2. to improve flexibility, which is impaired as muscle collagen becomes glycated
3. to improve muscle tone and bulk, which may deteriorate as a result of neuropathy and which uses glucose as fuel
4. to ensure that persons with type 1 diabetes can participate safely in and enjoy physical or sports activities
5. to assist in glucose management and weight control in people with type 2 diabetes
6. to allow individuals with diabetes to experience the same benefits and enjoyment that people without diabetes gain from a regular exercise program.[133,134]

Management of Diabetes

To manage diabetes, counselors must understand blood glucose testing, insulin types and their effect on blood glucose levels, and management schemes.

Blood Glucose Monitoring

Methods are available for accurate and convenient self-measurement of blood glucose. In one, a small drop of blood is obtained from the finger with a device called an autolet and placed on a strip (Chemstrip or Dextrostick). An enzymatic reaction takes place to cause the strip to change color, indicating the amount of glucose in the blood. The stick is read through comparison with a color chart or by a machine, the glucometer. Thorough instruction in monitoring is crucial and should be given by trained medical personnel. Home blood glucose monitoring that is completed incorrectly may not reflect actual blood glucose levels.

Monitoring blood glucose levels requires measurement up to eight times a day, including before each meal (breakfast, lunch and dinner), during the night, or one to two hours after meals. The postprandial blood glucose values indicate how well insulin matches the foods eaten at meals. The goal is to prevent hyperglycemia and hypoglycemia after a meal. Nighttime blood glucose levels are important because they can provide a reason for high levels of glycosylated hemoglobin (HbA1c) when no other rationale may be available. When multiple injections of regular insulin are given, it is preferable to measure blood glucose levels before each meal (preprandially) (15–30 minutes before a meal at approximately the time of an injection or a bolus) rather than two hours after a meal. For clients who are willing, measurement 15–30 minutes before and 2 hours after a meal may give information that helps in normalizing blood glucose levels. Changes in insulin regimens are based on these blood glucose determinations, looking at a pattern over a period of three days.

In persons with type 2 diabetes, daily self-monitoring of blood glucose should occur one to four times a day, often before breakfast. Additional monitoring should be done three to four times a week before and 2 hours after the largest meal.[93]

In addition to blood glucose monitoring, the measurement of glycosylated hemoglobin indicates the degree of long-term control of diabetes. Glucose in the blood reacts with free amino groups in proteins in a stable and irreversible nonenzymatic process called glycosylation. Thus glucose is attached to the protein for the life of the protein. Hemoglobin, one of several proteins exhibiting glycosylation, has a lifespan of 100 to 120 days. The percentage of glycosylated hemoglobin in the blood reflects the time-averaged blood glucose levels from the preceding two to three months.[135–138] Table 6-1 (page 234) indicates optimum levels for glycosylated hemoglobin.

In persons with type 1 diabetes, it is important to document ketones in the urine. When blood glucose levels are out of control or when clients are acutely ill, ketone bodies can be important early warning signs of impending diabetic ketoacidosis. On sick days, it is important for clients to take insulin, test their blood glucose frequently, test their urine for ketones, and try to eat their usual amount of carbohydrate, divided into smaller meals and snacks. If blood glucose levels rise above 240 mg/dL, the entire amount of usual carbohydrate grams is not necessary. Frequent non-caloric fluid intake is also recommended.

Types of Insulin

Diet and insulin must be matched closely to achieve normalized blood glucose levels. The insulin preparations available today fall into four categories:

1. Rapid short-acting insulin (insulin analogs named lispro and aspart): onset of action in 15 minutes, peaks in $1/2$ to $1^1/2$ hours, and the effective duration is 2–4 hours.
2. Short-acting insulin: onset of action in 30–60 minutes, peaks in 2–3 hours, and the effective duration is 3–6 hours. Included in this category is regular insulin.
3. Intermediate-acting insulin: onset of action is 2–4 hours, peaks in 6–12 hours after injection, and the effective duration is 10–18 hours. NPH (Neutral Protamine Hagedorn) and lente are intermediate-acting insulins.
4. Long-acting insulin: onset of action is 6–10 hours, peaks in 10–16 hours, and the effective duration is 18 to 20 hours. Ultralente and glargine are long-acting insulins. Unlike ultralente, glargine has a slow dissolution at the site of injection resulting in a constant and peakless delivery over 24 hours.[93,139]

The newest of the four insulins described above are lispro and aspart. They allow persons with diabetes to inject a dose and eat immediately. This eliminates the need for injecting regular insulin 30 minutes prior to a meal. Without this time lag, patients have increased flexibility in food choices and a spontaneity that they are not afforded with regular insulin on injection regimens.

Insulin manufacturers have developed premixed ratios of NPH

and regular insulin. The most commonly prescribed premixed insulin is 70/30 (70% NPH and 30% regular, a standard based on the two-thirds to one-third guideline). Also available is 50/50 insulin, which can reduce postprandial hyperglycemia and the risk of subsequent hypoglycemia.

Other premixed insulins include the addition of neutral protamine to lispro, creating an intermediate-acting insulin that has been used in 75/25 combinations with lispro. Another premixed insulin includes the addition of neutral protamine to aspart, creating an immediate-acting insulin with 75% neutral protamine aspart and 30% aspart.

Multiple daily injection (MDI) therapy and the constant subcutaneous infusion insulin (CSII) pump provide the dietitian with a wealth of flexibility in dietary recommendations. Timing of meals, dietary composition, caloric content of the diet, and physical activity are immensely important to the successful use of MDI or CSII. Teamwork among physician, nurse, and dietitian is crucial to success. During the DCCT, subjects in the experimental study group (following an intensive management protocol) had the option of using either MDI therapy consisting of three or more injections per day or the CSII pump.

Insulin pump therapy involves administration of regular insulin subcutaneously via a CSII pump attached to the abdomen with a needle. From a syringe attached to the pump, insulin flows through tubing to the needle injection site. The pump is a kind of computer that, when programmed, allows insulin to enter the body to maintain a constant insulin level throughout the day, much as the pancreas does when functioning properly. The pump also allows the client to increase the amount of insulin in a bolus at each meal, which also mimics the normally functioning pancreas. A basal dose of insulin is programmed into the computer-like pump to provide a constant, small dose of regular insulin at all times. Meals are covered by bolusing or pushing a button on the pump with the appropriate number (shown in a window) that coincides with the correct units of regular insulin to match a meal.

MDI therapy is similar to the pump concept in that regular insulin is injected via syringe to cover each meal. Basal needs are usually met with NPH, frequently given at supper or bedtime for overnight control, or with one to two injections of ultralente insulin given before breakfast or before both breakfast and supper.

Dietary Intervention

Both CSII and MDI therapy require the use of a dietary exchange pattern, which should be based upon individual needs and preferences (for example, for cardiovascular problems, The American Heart Association's recommendations as discussed in Chapter 5 may be necessary). The exchange list shown in Adherence Tool 6-6 in the Treatment Strategies section includes only items preferred by one particular client. Each food is placed in a category with items that have approximately equivalent carbohydrate, protein, and fat contents. For persons on the pump or MDI, an additional step that allows more flexibility without sacrificing accuracy is carbohydrate counting or counting total available glucose.

The major rationale for using carbohydrate counting is that dietary carbohydrate is the main determinant of meal-related insulin demand. Although the absolute glucose excursion and rate of glucose appearance differ among individual carbohydrate foods,[90] it is estimated that 90–100% of digestible dietary carbohydrate enters the bloodstream as glucose in the first few hours after a meal.[140] This system recognizes that only a portion of fat and protein are metabolized to glucose and that overall these nutrients yield much less glucose than does an equal amount of carbohydrate.[140] When fat and protein intake are relatively consistent from day to day, the basal or intermediate-acting insulin present between meals is adjusted to handle the glucose released by their metabolism. A precise estimate of the insulin demand created by a particular meal or snack can therefore be derived by simply counting the grams of carbohydrate it contains.

The basic meal plan for a patient who uses carbohydrate counting is composed of gram totals of carbohydrate to be eaten at each planned meal and snack. There are two ways to develop such a plan.[104] The preferred method for patients with type 1 diabetes is to base the plan on the client's current eating habits. An average or usual meal pattern can be identified using several days of food records provided by the client. This pattern can then be translated into the carbohydrate gram equivalent that is consumed at each meal or snack. This approach can also be used for patients with type 2 diabetes, with adjustments to the usual intake negotiated to match intake with available insulin (endogenous or exogenous) as needed. Any desirable changes to improve overall nutritional intake or to address specific risk factors are negotiated on a staged basis as education progresses.

Alternatively, a carbohydrate plan can be derived from an estimated or calculated calorie prescription by multiplying the desired caloric intake by the desired proportion of carbohydrate and dividing the resulting value by 4. For example, a client is estimated to require 2,000 calories for weight maintenance, and the goal is for the client to consume 50% of calories as carbohydrate. Multiply 2,000 calories by 0.5 and divide the resulting value (1,000) by 4 calories/gram of carbohydrate. The total daily carbohydrate allowance would be 250 grams. This total allowance is then distributed among the day's meals and snacks with attention to the client's preferences for meal size and composition, and subsequently fine-tuned on the basis of blood glucose results.

The next step is to calculate pre-meal doses of regular insulin using the insulin-to-carbohydrate ratio. For persons with diabetes, there is an identifiable ratio between grams of carbohydrate eaten and the number of units of insulin required. This ratio can be used to calculate the appropriate pre-meal dose of insulin (bolus) for any meal or snack of known carbohydrate content. The ratio varies significantly from client to client: from as little as 5 grams of carbohydrate per unit of insulin up to 20 grams. The 150-pound jogger with type 1 diabetes may require only one unit of insulin for each 20 grams of carbohydrate, while the 200-pound woman with type 2 diabetes may require one unit of insulin for each 10 grams of carbohydrate. In the DCCT, persons with type 1 diabetes usually required one unit of pre-meal bolus of regular insulin for each 10 to 15 grams of carbohydrate. In general, the lower the total daily insulin dose, the greater the number of grams of carbohydrate covered by a single unit of insulin. The precise ratio for each person should be individually determined.

The total available glucose (TAG) system[107] is based on research described by Munro and Allison in their classic text, *Mammalian Protein Metabolism, Volume 1*, in which these authors discuss the gluconeogenic properties of certain proteins.[105] The amino acids that are definitely gluconeogenic are those that rapidly degrade to intermediates of glycolysis during the tricarboxylic acid cycle. Amino acids that give irregular results when administered in a large, single dose degrade relatively slowly, either because of the low activity of the enzymes of intermediary metabolism or because of the slow absorption. The high yield of glucose on feeding proteins in dogs indicates that the conversion of protein to carbohydrate can be maximal. Munro and Allison identify amino acids as rapidly gluconeogenic, variably gluconeogenic, and nongluconeogenic.

Lusk reported in 1928 that meat protein yields 58 grams of glucose per 100 grams of protein metabolized.[141] He also studied the gluconeogenic effects of casein, whose amino acid composition is similar to that of mixed meat protein. The calculated maximum yield of casein is 57 grams of glucose per 100 grams of protein. This idea has resulted in the use of a fixed number (TAG) for each meal as a way of controlling blood sugars. The number is derived from calculations with exact figures of carbohydrate and animal protein, found in *Bowes and Church's Food Values of Portions Commonly Used*.[142] For example, cooked beef cubed steak weighs 3.5 ounces (100 grams), contains 0.0 grams of carbohydrate, 28.6 grams of animal protein, and 14.4 grams of fat.

To calculate TAG, the following formula is used:

0.0 grams of carbohydrate + (28.6 grams of animal protein × 0.58) = TAG.

The conversion factor for animal protein is the value discovered in Lusk's animal studies. TAG is a value that approximates the amount of ingested glucose that will be available for cell use. Lusk also found that about 10% of fat is converted to carbohydrate. Some nutritionists add in this value for a total TAG calculation.[107] In an attempt to simplify calculations, this value, usually low if diets include 30–35% of calories from fat, is not used here. By giving each meal a total figure for TAG, individuals can vary intake of fat without going over the recommended grams of TAG. TAG for each exchange is as follows:

- 1 fruit exchange = 15 grams of TAG
- 1 meat exchange = 4 grams of TAG
- 1 vegetable exchange = 5 grams of TAG
- 1 bread exchange = 15 grams of TAG
- 1 milk exchange = 17 grams of TAG

Table 6-3 shows calories, carbohydrate, protein, and fat values for each exchange. At the end of the chapter, Exchange List 6-A and Exchange List 6-B show exchange groups with amounts of

Table 6–3   Summary of the 1995 Exchange Lists

List	Carbohydrate (g)	Protein (g)	Fat (g)	Calories
Carbohydrates				
Starch	15	3	1 or less	80
Fruit	15	—	—	60
Milk				
Skim	12	8	0–3	90
Low-fat	12	8	5	120
Whole	12	8	8	150
Other carbohydrates	15	Varies	Varies	Varies
Vegetables	5	2	—	25
Meat/meat substitutes				
Very lean	—	7	1	35
Lean	—	7	3	55
Medium fat	—	7	5	75
High fat	—	7	8	100
Fat	—	—	5	45

Source: Data from Exchange Lists for Meal Planning, copyright © 1995, The American Dietetic Association and the American Diabetes Association.

food equivalent to one exchange. Exhibit 6-2 provides a sample bolus calculation.

There are several guidelines to follow to cover intake (TAG) with insulin. One unit of regular insulin covers approximately 10 to 15 grams of TAG, depending upon the individual. For one person, one unit of insulin may cover 11 grams of TAG, with normal blood glucose values resulting; for a second person, one unit of regular insulin may cover 9 grams of TAG. For each person, the ratio of TAG to insulin depends on the time of day and physical activity. The ratio may be different at breakfast than at lunch or supper. As a general rule of thumb, a person with diabetes should wait 30 minutes before eating a meal after bolusing or injecting regular insulin (Table 6-4). Exhibit 6-3 contains tips to adjust insulin.

There are several cautions in using TAG and carbohydrate counting. These values do not take into consideration the fat or vegetable protein calories for TAG or fat and total protein for car-bohydrate counting. Clients may consume a diet very high in calo-

Exhibit 6–2 Sample Bolus Calculation by Different Methods

Patient: 37-year-old woman, 112 lb
Estimated Ratio: 15 g carbohydrate (CHO) per unit insulin or
      1 interchange per unit of insulin

	Method of Carbohydrate Counting		
Sample Meal	Gram Counting	Exchanges	TAG
1 ham sandwich	36 g CHO	2 starch = 30 g	36 g CHO + 12.6 g CHO (21 g protein × 0.6)
4 oz serving bean soup	11 g CHO	½ starch = 8 g	11 g CHO + 1.8 g CHO (3 g protein × 0.6)
Green salad	5 g CHO	Free	5 g CHO
8 oz low-fat milk	12 g CHO	1 milk = 12 g	12 g CHO + 4.8 g CHO (8 g protein × 0.6)
3 fresh apricots	12 g CHO	1 fruit = 15 g	12 g CHO
Total carbohydrate	76 g	65 g	95.2 g
Calculated pre-meal dose of short-acting insulin or bolus	5.1 U[a]	4.3 U[a]	6.3 U[a,b]

[a]Doses containing fractional units can be given by pump; for injections with syringe or pen, round dose to nearest whole unit.
[b]In patients using systems such as total available glucose (TAG) that account for dietary protein in the bolus insulin dose calculation, total daily insulin doses will not be different, as compared with the same patient using simply carbohydrate counting. However, different basal insulin rates or insulin-to-carbohydrate ratios may be derived under the TAG approach because of the different way in which pre-meal doses are being determined.

Source: Reprinted from Brackenridge B, Carbohydrate counting for diabetes therapy, in *Handbook of Diabetes Medical Nutrition Therapy*, M.A. Powers, ed., p. 259. Copyright © 1996, Aspen Publishers, Inc.

Table 6–4 Timing Boluses Using Regular Insulin To Cover Snacks or Meals That Are Very High in Fiber, Fat, or Simple Sugars as Compared with Usual Snacks or Meals

Time of Bolus	Usual Meal	High in Fiber	High in Fat	High in Simple Sugars
15 Minutes		X	X	
30 Minutes	X			
45 Minutes				X

ries but have normal blood glucose levels. Even though the TAG system and carbohydrate counting allow for flexibility, a low-fat diet that emphasizes nutrient adequacy is very important. One last qualifying statement is important: Munro and Allison stated that, while it is possible to determine whether an amino acid can cause a net increase in total carbohyrate, it cannot be predicted whether this gluconeogenic effect is significant.[105] TAG, in combination with a standard exchange system, can result in good blood glucose control in compliant persons.

Facilitating control in the client with type 1 diabetes mellitus requires understanding the time-action curves of all insulin preparations. The DCCT used 38 different insulin regimens, including the combinations such as ultralente with NPH or NPH three times daily, to achieve specified blood glucose targets.[4] Figure 6-2 visually depicts the time-action curves of various combination insulin regimens. Information on these time-action curves is essential to ensure appropriate meal planning. The goal is to match foods and their specific amounts to be eaten at the best times in order to prevent glycemic excursions. The dietitian must be involved as a strategic member of the team to maximize blood glucose control. Problem solving for common blood glucose patterns is summarized in Table 6-5, providing a generic basis for alterations in meal composition, amounts, and timing.

The constant subcutaneous infusion insulin pump's effect is schematically shown in Figure 6-3. The amount of insulin given to cover each meal varies for each individual. It requires blood glucose monitoring and constant supervision by a physician to find the right match of insulin for TAG to achieve normal blood glucose

Exhibit 6-3 Adjusting Insulin

Nutrition counselors should keep the following in mind as they help patients with diabetes to problem solve to reach target blood glucose values.

1. Make sure target blood glucose ranges have been set or negotiated with the patient. Otherwise, the patient has no idea what is to be accomplished. An old saying applies: "If you don't know where you're going, any road will get you there!"
2. Fix the fasting first. Because blood glucose levels will stay in about the same range or elevate throughout the day for those with NIDDM, getting the fasting blood glucose level normalized sets the tone for the rest of the day, provided the patient continues to eat appropriately.
3. Look to the previous medication dose when solving a problem time of day. For example, if there is a high midafternoon blood glucose pattern and the morning shot of NPH/regular insulin was the last administration, perhaps more NPH is required.
4. Do not be reactionary. Observe patterns of blood glucose levels versus responding to one or two isolated values. Practitioners may want to discard the lowest and highest values as outliers when perusing blood glucose logs. Allow a new regimen (an increase or decrease in food, medications, or activity) to be tried for at least three days before considering another change.
5. Do not automatically blame the diet. Just because you are a dietitian does not mean that diet is the only aspect of diabetes care you must consider. Timing of meals and medications, poor fluid intake, site selection and rotation for insulin administration, activity changes, acute stress, illness, or other medications can account for out-of-range blood glucose values.
6. Change only one or two things at a time when modifying the diet so that the effectiveness of each change can be documented separately. If too many components are altered at once, the cause cannot be determined because it is confounded by other variables.
7. Correct the basal rates first. For those on intensive therapy (MDI or CSII), boluses of regular insulin can only be accurately determined if basal insulin (Lente, NPH, Ultralente, or basal rate on an insulin pump) is correct. Similarly, insulin-to-carbohydrate ratios cannot be refined unless basal rates have been correctly adjusted. Basal rates are correct when the individual with diabetes can skip a meal and the blood glucose remains stable (hypoglycemia or hyperglycemia does not occur).

Source: Reprinted from Thom SL, Diabetes medications and delivery methods, in *Handbook of Diabetes Medical Nutrition Therapy*, ed. M.A. Powers, p. 102, © 1996, Aspen Publishers, Inc.

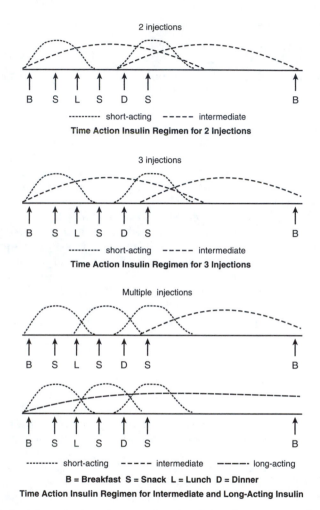

FIGURE 6–2 Time-Action Curves of Various Combination Insulin Regimens. *Source:* Reprinted with permission from *Physician's Guide to Insulin-Dependent (Type 1) Diabetes,* 1988. Copyright © 1994 by American Diabetes Association.

levels. For example, at breakfast three units of regular insulin may be given to cover 45 grams of TAG, equivalent to one unit of insulin for every 15 grams of TAG (45 grams TAG ÷ 3 units of regular insulin = 15 grams of TAG per unit of regular insulin). If this client were to plan an increase in food intake at this meal to 60 grams of TAG or an increase of 15 grams over the recommended TAG, one extra unit of insulin will be needed. At lunch, this client

Table 6–5 Common Problem Patterns Identified Using Blood Glucose Monitoring

Problem	Potential Cause*	Potential Solutions
High fasting glucose	Insulin resistance,[†] insufficient insulin available overnight, rebound hyperglycemia overnight (Somogyi effect), Dawn Phenomenon	Adjust P.M. intermediate- or long-term acting insulin dose or time Weight reduction to reduce insulin resistance
High glucose after breakfast	Inadequate insulin produced or injected to cover breakfast, peak insulin action not at anticipated time	Adjusted time or dose of short-acting A.M. insulin Decrease size of breakfast or adjust amount of breakfast carbohydrate or divide breakfast into two smaller morning meals
Insulin reactions (hypo-glycemia) before lunch	Insufficient breakfast for A.M. short-acting insulin or peak action later than anticipated time	Adjust time, type, or dose of A.M. short-acting insulin Add morning snack or increase breakfast
Insulin reactions (hypo-glycemia) in afternoon	Excessive A.M. intermediate-acting insulin, skipping, or inadequate lunch	Adjust time, type, or dose of A.M. intermediate-acting insulin Add afternoon snack or increase lunch
High glucose in afternoon	Inadequate insulin produced or intermediate-acting A.M. insulin is insufficient for need, or excessive snack or lunch	Adjust time or dose of P.M. insulin Add afternoon snack or increase lunch
High glucose at night after evening meal	Inadequate insulin produced or insufficient insulin to cover dinner, or evening meal too large	Adjust time or dose of P.M. insulin Reduce size of meal or alter meal composition (_ carbohydrate)
Insulin reactions (hypo-glycemia) at night	Excessive amount of insulin, or insufficient dinner meal or evening snack	Adjust time, type, or dose of evening or bedtime insulin Increase dinner and/or snack carbohydrate

*In addition to food and insulin, other factors may affect blood glucose (e.g., exercise, sick days, infection).

[†]Insulin resistance associated with obesity is likely to result in high glucose levels throughout the day.

Source: Adapted from Powers MA, Barr P, Franz M, Holler H, Wheeler ML, Wylie-Rosett J. *Nutrition Guide for Professionals: Diabetes Education and Meal Planning,* p. 6, copyright © 1989, American Dietetic Association/American Diabetes Association.

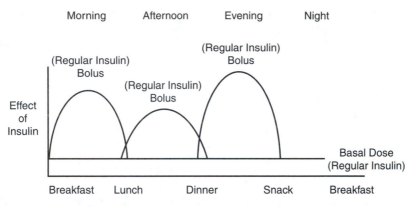

FIGURE 6–3   Schematic Representation of Mealtimes and Their Correspondence with Insulin Delivered by the Constant-Infusion Insulin Pump

boluses two units of regular insulin for every 66 grams of TAG, which equals one unit of insulin for every 33 grams of TAG (66 grams of TAG ÷ 2 units of regular insulin = 33 grams of TAG per unit of regular insulin). If the client planned to eat only 33 grams of TAG at lunch, a bolus of one unit of insulin would cover the decreased intake. At dinner, nine units of regular insulin are given to cover 81 grams of TAG, or one unit of insulin for every 9 grams of TAG (81 grams of TAG ÷ 9 units of regular insulin = 9 grams of TAG per unit of regular insulin). If 47 grams of TAG were planned for dinner, this client could bolus with 5.2 units of regular insulin (47 grams of TAG ÷ 9 grams of TAG per unit of regular insulin = 5.2 units of insulin).

Research on Adherence to Eating Patterns Controlled for Carbohydrate, Protein, and Fat

Adherence to a prescribed dietary plan is one of the most important aspects of diabetes management and perhaps the most difficult for clients to learn or with which to comply. Researchers have found that many clients do not understand or follow their diabetic diet regimens.[143] As a solution to this problem, clinicians are beginning to advocate highly individualized, flexible approaches to diet management that can accommodate individual eating habits and preferences.[4]

A number of studies have examined correlates of diabetic diet noncompliance, including knowledge, health values, and social and cultural factors.[144-146] None of these studies provides a clear, unified direction for diabetic nutrition education, but when reviewed in combination, they emphasize the need for comprehensive interventions that include social support, promotion of self-care and active participation, and emphasis on how (as well as why) to follow the dietary eating pattern.[147] Because of the complexity of the optimal educational approach, few studies have rigorously evaluated the effectiveness of strategies to improve dietary adherence among clients with diabetes.

Weinsier et al. achieved excellent compliance with an individualized diet prescription, frequent follow-up and feedback, and social support in a controlled trial of an experimental diabetic diet.[148] However, there have been few controlled educational experiments. One found that a group program was more effective than individual bedside teaching.[149] Another demonstrated that a programmed learning unit that reduced the amount of professional time needed resulted in knowledge increases comparable to those achieved after a longer individual counseling session.[150] Dunn et al. found that a comprehensive program resulted in knowledge gains.[151] The Webb et al. study of a multimethod group program demonstrated the program's effects in improving adherence to the carbohydrate and fat composition of the diet, as well as glycemic control.[152] Because of the generally accepted comprehensive approach to diabetes education, along with the complex self-care regimens prescribed for clients with diabetes, it is unlikely that research can tell nutritionists exactly which educational strategies contribute the most to diet adherence. Self-monitoring of blood glucose is a technology that has been found acceptable to clients and effective for improving glycemic control.[4,153-155] Unfortunately, the investigators of this strategy did not collect dietary data to discern the behavioral effects of self-monitoring; nor did they employ a control group receiving similar management without glucose self-monitoring.

Several implications for practice emerge from the studies reviewed here and the published commentaries of clinicians. Most important, dietary adherence is best when the diet is tailored to the individual client. The education plan should also be tailored, as seen in Slowie's case studies.[156] Comprehensive educational diagnosis tools have been developed, and validated knowledge tests toward this end are available.[157] Computerized dietary analysis with simple recommendations as part of a printout can provide both assessment and feedback.[152]

Social support from family members as well as other clients with diabetes is important in facilitating lifestyle changes.[158] Schwartz et al. found a higher percentage of abnormal blood glucose control measures (fasting blood glucose values and HbA1c) in individuals with many recent life events. These researchers felt that social support may decrease the individual's isolation and help deal with life events, with resulting improved control.[159] Frequent follow-up, feedback (including glucose self-monitoring), and behavioral methods such as contingency contracting and self-reinforcement can improve outcomes.[160-162] A large number of print and audiovisual instructional aids are available through health agencies, the American Diabetes Association, and commercial sources. Educational materials must be appropriate for the comprehension level of program participants; a mismatch can impede understanding of the regimen.[163]

Researchers who studied compliance with accuracy in describing food portions found that men with diabetes underestimated chicken portions (i.e., ate portions that were larger than estimated) by an average of 30–40% and underestimated rice portions (i.e., ate portions that were smaller than estimated) by an average of 25–35%.[164] In another study, clients with diabetes (24 with type 1 diabetes and 184 with type 2 diabetes) were asked what factors contributed to nonadherence to their diabetic regimens. Standardized questions revealed few differences between type 1 and type 2 participants on the level of reported adherence or reasons for nonadherence. Subjects reported adhering least well to dietary and physical activity components of the regimen. Open-ended questions revealed that the most common reasons for dietary nonadherence were the situational factors of eating out at restaurants and inappropriate food offers from others. These researchers suggested that diabetes education programs should inform clients of high-risk situations and provide training in covert modeling and behavioral rehearsal to enhance assertive skills.[165,166]

Inappropriate Eating Behaviors

Most persons with type 1 diabetes complain about the lack of spontaneity in their new eating patterns. The joy of eating seems to rely partially on the element of surprise, but one very important way to normalize blood sugars is to keep the eating pattern consistent from day to day. This is one of the most difficult dilemmas facing the client with type 1 diabetes. Without consistency in the eating pattern, changes in insulin levels are difficult to adjust and dangerous.

A second common problem involves social eating. The major problem is knowing how to count foods with unknown ingredients. Secondary, but also important, is the ability to avoid large quantities of foods that elevate blood glucose levels. As do many clients on new eating patterns, the insulin-dependent person initially finds the diet new and exciting. Adherence to diet and control of blood glucose levels are excellent. With time, the newness of the diet diminishes and the desire to be "like everyone else" can overcome the desire to achieve good control or normalized blood glucose levels.

Assessment of Eating Behaviors

A thorough initial assessment is crucial to future dietary success. Assessing the client's prior experience with dieting and diabetic eating patterns is very important. Many persons with type 1 diabetes have followed weight-loss diets in the past, even though one of the initial symptoms of diabetes is weight loss. Some younger diabetic persons may have never followed a diet. If this is the case, setting the stage for successful adherence to diet is crucial.

Carefully assessing daily eating patterns is important. Time may not allow for food record collection, but a thorough diet history or quantified food frequency may provide some useful information on past eating habits. Counselors should attend to variations in eating patterns. For example, a clue to potential problems with weekend blood glucose levels is dietary patterns that are very different from weekday patterns.

The diet history can also give the counselor an impression of nutrient intake. Many persons, particularly teenagers, may be eating diets low in calcium, iron, or vitamin A and C. Fat intake may be high, with a large portion coming from saturated fat. In addition to a quantified food frequency or diet history, the Client Eating Questionnaire for Low-Calorie Eating Patterns in Treating Obesity, Adherence Tool 4–1 in Chapter 4, may be useful in identifying past and present weight loss and resulting dietary behaviors. Once the client begins the new eating pattern, food records can be very helpful. The food record in Adherence Tool 6-1 might be used in assessing adherence to the new eating pattern.

Throughout the initial assessment phase, family support is crucial to eventual success. For adolescents, positive support without overbearing dictation of rules is important. For older clients, positive support from spouse or significant others should be assessed.

Prior knowledge about foods is also important. Some persons who are newly diagnosed may have a variety of misconceptions about a diabetic eating pattern. "I can no longer eat carbohydrates," is one common fallacy. Counselors should determine whether the client has followed a previous diet with an exchange pattern that might conflict with the new diabetic exchange pattern. Some concepts learned in Weight Watchers may no longer apply. Some clients may begin using only commercial foods labeled "dietetic." Counselors should assess each client's understanding of what is eliminated in "dietetic" products. Frequently fat, not carbohydrate, is reduced, leaving a product that may be high in carbohydrate.

Once a client is instructed on the new eating pattern, frequent and consistent assessment of adherence to the pattern is important. This may involve diet records, 24-hour recalls on the phone (if possible, for three days with one weekend day), or short diet records requiring simple check-off systems, such as Adherence Tool 6-2. This tool can be used to help clients monitor and avoid snacking if it is not a part of the recommended regimen. Tracking eating behaviors with a graph may be helpful. If the recommendation for TAG is 40 at breakfast, 40 at lunch, and 60 at dinner, graphing intake over one month's time may be helpful. Adherence Tool 6-3 shows an example of a graph in which TAG for breakfast is represented by a line. One heavy horizontal line represents the desired TAG for this meal.

Dietary nonadherence will be reflected in biochemical data such as blood glucose and glycosylated hemoglobin levels. Graphing these two parameters can illustrate trends. For example, drawing a graph of weekly blood sugar and glycosylated hemoglobin levels once every three months will show difficult weeks and "in-control" weeks (see Adherence Tool 6-4). Adherence Tool 6-5 allows the client to make a check mark when boluses are administered an appropriate number of minutes prior to a meal. Assessing what might have happened to cause changes in blood sugars may be the first step to changes in adherence.

Treatment Strategies

Problems with following diabetic eating patterns fall into three categories: lack of knowledge, lack of planning, and lack of commitment. This section provides suggestions for strategies to deal with lack of knowledge and cueing devices to help increase meal planning. Lack of commitment, the most difficult problem to solve, is obvious from repeated highs and lows in blood sugars, elevated glycosylated hemoglobins, or both, in spite of information given to help correct the situation.

Strategies Dealing with Lack of Knowledge

Lack of Knowledge Related to General Dietary Modifications That Affect Blood Glucose

To begin a nutrition counseling session appropriately, counselors must provide the client with adequate information. The counselor might provide a skeleton of an instructional plan to provide information on a diabetic eating pattern, including one week of intensive dietary counseling, possibly a three-day hospital stay, while the client is beginning the new diet pattern. Additional information is given in subsequent visits one month apart. Information should be given in small amounts, with practice time included in each session to allow the client to complete exercises with the nutrition counselor. This valuable practice is a way of setting the stage for behaviors that will be required in daily life.

Tailoring is once again very important to diet adherence (see Adherence Tool 6-6). Ideally each client should receive a diet pattern that fits the individual's lifestyle. An electronic program might be used to create an individual exchange list and dietary pattern.

For the person with diabetes, this type of tailoring makes for less work in learning the carbohydrate content of many food items, provides greater detail, and can stimulate learning because it creates a feeling of ownership.

In teaching the concept of TAG, counselors should use concrete and tailored examples (see Exhibit 6-4). Adherence Tools 6-7 and 6-8 provide practice and tips on using TAG. Adherence Tools 6-9 to 6-11 help the client practice calculating TAG and exchanges in recipes. In applying TAG, clients need a basic understanding of weighing and measuring (see Adherence Tool 6-12). For clients

---

Exhibit 6-4   Teaching TAG

1. Give an example:

Exchange	TAG
2 Fruit	= 30
1 Bread	= 15
1 Meat	= 4
1 Fat	= 0
	49 = TAG at breakfast

2. Describe clearly what the client can eat:

   Breakfast — **Breakfast TAG**
   Carbohydrate (grams) +
   Animal Protein (grams) × 0.58

Breakfast	Carbohydrate	Animal Protein
1 large apple	30.0	—
(197 grams)	—	
1 slice of bread	11.7	—
1 teaspoon margarine	—	—
1 ounce Canadian bacon	—	+ (5.6 grams × 0.58 = 3.3)
	41.7	+ 3.3 = 45.0 grams of TAG

The same example can be used with exchanges only:

Breakfast	Breakfast Exchanges
1 large apple	2 Fruit
1 slice of bread	1 Bread
1 teaspoon margarine	1 Fat
1 ounce Canadian bacon	1 Meat

who want to take home information about TAG, Adherence Tools 6-13 and 6-14 are helpful. Similar tools could be used for carbohydrate counting. Written as well as verbal advice is important.

Meal planning is also extremely important. Adherence Tool 6-15 provides practice in planning a menu using a new eating pattern.

Counselors should emphasize the importance of knowing the contents of commercial products. Adherence Tool 6-16 provides practice in reading labels.

If clients frequently eat in restaurants, counselors should select the menus from a few favorite places, calculate TAG or carbohydrate for a meal, ask the client to bolus with insulin, and actually visit the restaurant with the client. If problems arise, the counselor can guide the client through the meal.

After presenting crucial information in a way that tailors the eating pattern to each person, counselors must stage changes in eating habits to coincide with recommendations. Clients can find it difficult to follow all dietary restrictions immediately. Focus on the least difficult problem first, while asking clients to continue to follow all restrictions to the greatest degree possible. In addition, work closely with clients and let them decide which problem is the least difficult. An example of this type of staging with information follows:

Client: "I think learning the specific amounts of foods in each of these exchange categories will be difficult. I am not sure that I can do this. It seems to be more than I can handle."

Nutrition counselor: "Let's begin slowly, taking each category one week at a time. Continue to look up amounts for the categories you must follow, but learn amounts of your favorite foods in one category by reviewing them daily over a one-week period." (Initial/Brief Nutrition Education)

Client: "That sounds more manageable; I think I might be able to handle that."

Lack of Knowledge Related to Fat Intake and Weight Gain

Lack of knowledge about foods can make a crucial difference in weight gain for insulin-dependent persons. Many clients are upset by the initial and frequently steady weight gain that results when blood glucose levels normalize. Weight gain occurs because calories, no longer being lost in the urine, are used for energy and, eventually, weight gain results. Many clients misuse the idea that fat contributes little to elevations in blood glucose. They think that if fat is "free," it may be used to add to meals when a TAG or carbohydrate limit or exchange pattern is "used up" in a day.

Table 6-6 illustrates the case of one client whose blood glucose levels were normal on the average but whose fat intake was causing significant climbs in weight based on monthly determinations. The diet was checked very carefully to determine where caloric intake might be contributing to weight gain. This client was doing

Table 6–6 Recommended and Actual Fat Consumption before Instruction

RECOMMENDED BREAKFAST PATTERN

	Carbohydrate	Protein	Fat	
Breakfast	(g)	(g)	(g)	TAG
1 Meat	—	7	5	4
2 Bread	30	4	—	30
3 Fat	—	—	15	—
2 Fruit	30	—	—	30
	60	11	20	64

464 kilocalories
3.86 g saturated fat
5.19 g polyunsaturated fat

ACTUAL HIGH-FAT BREAKFAST

	Carbohydrate	Protein	Fat	
Breakfast	(g)	(g)	(g)	TAG
1 ounce sausage (28 g)	0.5	4.0	8.1	2.8
2 muffins (40 g)	32.0	6.2	8.0	32.0
4 teaspoons margarine	—	—	16.4	—
1 large apple (197 g)	30.0	0.4	0.7	30.0
	62.5	10.6	33.2	64.8

591 kilocalories
14.40 g saturated fat
2.68 g polyunsaturated fat

Source: Reprinted with permission from Pennington JA, Douglass JS. *Bowes and Church's Food Values of Portions Commonly Used,* Eighteenth Edition. Philadelphia: Lippincott Williams & Wilkins, 2005.

everything requested in terms of following exchanges and TAG for breakfast. Blood glucose levels were normal, but unfortunately weight and blood cholesterol levels increased because the breakfast eaten contained 127 more calories than the recommended meal. Blood low-density lipoprotein cholesterol levels were up, mainly because of the extremely high intake of saturated fat (the recommended amount of saturated fat is 3.86 grams; actual consumption was up to 14.40 grams).

Following in-depth dietary instruction on the fat and saturated fat content of certain foods, this client can alter intake to reduce weight and blood cholesterol levels. Table 6-7 indicates recommended intake and actual intake after instruction. The figures show that TAG is actually a bit low in the low-fat meal. A suggestion might be to add 4.6 grams of carbohydrate, or approximately 5 grams ($^1/_3$ fruit exchange). Table 6-8 compares nutrient intake for the recommended high- and low-fat diets. It clearly illustrates how careful instruction on fat content of foods can minimize eventual problems with weight gain and increases in low-density lipoprotein cholesterol.

Figure 6-4 shows two weight graphs for a client. One indicates an increase in weight following high fat intake. The second shows how weight comes down with a change in the fat content of the diet. Clear instructions on monitoring blood glucose levels are essential. A client who is not monitoring appropriately or who is guessing at blood glucose levels can be counseled to increase or decrease insulin and dietary intake inappropriately.

For persons on the constant subcutaneous infusion insulin (CSII) pump, eating three meals a day is very important. Snacking can lead to problems, as Exhibit 6-5 shows. This example illustrates several rules. First, clients on the CSII pump must limit meals to three a day or at least keep three hours between meals. Second, timing boluses is extremely important. In most cases, clients should give an injection or punch in a bolus on the pump 30 minutes before eating. The blood glucose of 60 at 5:00 PM indicates a timing problem: insufficient time (five minutes) between bolus and snack. The candy bar caused a rise in blood glucose before the regular insulin could have an effect. By the time the insulin peaked, the effect of the candy bar was gone, resulting in low blood glucose. Third, it is important to cover snacks with adequate amounts of regular insulin. Exhibit 6-5 shows insufficient amounts of in-

Table 6–7   Recommended and Actual Fat Consumption after Instruction

RECOMMENDED BREAKFAST PATTERN				
	Carbohydrate	Protein	Fat	
Breakfast	(g)	(g)	(g)	TAG
1 Meat	—	7	5	4
2 Bread	30	4	—	30
3 Fat	—	—	15	—
2 Fruit	30	—	—	30
Total	60	11	20	64
464 kilocalories				
3.86 grams saturated fat				
5.19 grams polyunsaturated fat				
ACTUAL LOW-FAT BREAKFAST				
	Carbohydrate	Protein	Fat	
Breakfast	(g)	(g)	(g)	TAG
1 ounce Canadian bacon (28 g)	—	5.6	2.00	3.2
1 English muffin (57 g)	26.2	4.5	1.10	26.2
4 teaspoons margarine	—	—	11.34	—
1 large apple (197 g)	30.0	0.4	0.70	30.0
Total	56.2	10.5	15.14	59.4
403 kilocalories				
2.67 grams saturated fat				
5.14 grams polyunsaturated fat				

Source: Reprinted with permission from Pennington JAT, Church HN. *Bowes and Church's Food Values of Portions Commonly Used,* copyright © 1995, Lippincott-Raven Publishers.

sulin given to cover both snacks. In this case, assume that one unit of insulin covers 10 grams of TAG. (Remember, in reality the ratio of insulin to TAG varies for different times of day and different persons.) The bedtime snack was very high in fat and fiber. Timing was changed to allow for high fat and fiber intake, but the bolus for the bedtime snack did not sufficiently cover TAG (assuming one unit of insulin for every 10 grams of TAG, one unit of insulin will not cover 64 grams of TAG). Some clients may not need to cover bed-

Table 6–8 Comparison of Recommended versus High- and Low-Fat Diet

Nutrients (g)	Recommended Diet	High-Fat Diet	Low-Fat Diet
Carbohydrate	60.00	62.5	56.2
Protein	11.00	10.60	10.50
Fat	20.00	33.20	15.14
Saturated Fat	3.86	14.40	2.67
Polyunsaturated Fat	5.19	2.68	5.14
Kilocalories	464.00	591.00	403.00

Baseline:
Ideal Body Weight = 85 kg
Average Blood Sugar for Week = 100
Blood Sugar Range for Week = 80–120

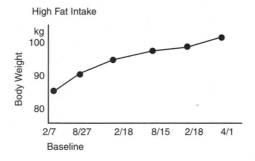

High Fat Intake

Ideal Body Weight = 85 kg
Average Blood Sugar for Week = 100
Blood Sugar Range for Week = 80–120

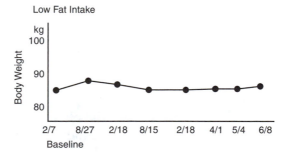

Low Fat Intake

Average Blood Sugar for Week = 100
Blood Sugar Range for Week = 80–120

FIGURE 6–4 Weight Graphs

Exhibit 6–5   Meal, Blood Glucose, and Insulin Diary, #1

Blood Glucose Levels	**Actual Intake**
	Breakfast (10:30 AM) Nothing Eaten
Pre-Lunch (10:30 AM) Blood Glucose = 100 mg/dL Recommended Insulin Given	
	Lunch (11:00 AM) Recommended Pattern Followed
Pre-Afternoon Snack (2:55 PM) No Blood Glucose Taken Insulin Given = 2 Units Regular Insulin	

Afternoon Snack (3:00 PM)
2-ounce Snicker's Candy Bar

Carbohydrate	Protein	Fat	Kilocalories
33.0	6.0	13.0	270

Pre-Dinner (5:00 PM) Blood Glucose = 60 mg/dL Took glucose tablet	
	Dinner (5:30 PM) Recommended Dietary Pattern Followed
Pre-Bedtime Snack (9:45 PM) No Blood Glucose Taken Insulin Given = 1 Unit Regular Insulin	

Bedtime Snack (10:00 PM)
Popped Corn (6 cups) +
5 tablespoons margarine

Carbohydrate	Protein	Fat	Kilocalories
64.2	10.8	34.2	607.8

time snacks with regular insulin, but the client in Exhibit 6-5 has very high nighttime blood sugars if regular insulin is not used to cover the snack.

Table 6-4 provides a rough guide for timing boluses on the CSII pump. These times are helpful when covering a snack (if necessary) that is very different in fat and/or fiber content from the usual snack. Changing the timing of a bolus may help to allow for increased digestion time such as 15 minutes instead of 30 minutes for popped corn with a large amount of fat. In addition, allowing three hours between meals can prevent one bolus of regular insulin from affecting the bolus that follows. Exhibit 6-6 illustrates this idea. In this example the regular insulin bolus for breakfast peaks too close to the peak of the lunch bolus, resulting in a reaction at 12:30 PM. The pre-lunch blood glucose is actually postprandial breakfast glucose. Because the pre-lunch blood glucose is high, extra insulin is given to adjust for it, which brings blood glucose levels down. With extra insulin for lunch and less than three hours between breakfast and lunch, the regular insulin peaks are too close, resulting in hypoglycemia.

In summary, many of the difficulties encountered by clients with type 1 diabetes can be eliminated through monitoring (via diary) and thus identifying problems contributing to poor adherence. Basic early instruction on diet is crucial. Tailoring the regimen helps eliminate certain problems with later backsliding. For example, although fat intake may be of minor significance in alter-

---

Exhibit 6–6 Meal, Blood Glucose, and Insulin Diary, #2

Blood Glucose Levels	**Actual Intake**
Breakfast (9:30 AM) Blood Glucose = 100 Recommended Insulin Given	
	Breakfast (10:00 AM) Recommended Pattern Followed
Prelunch (11:00 AM) Blood Glucose = 285 Extra Dose of Regular Insulin Given	
	Lunch (11:30 AM) Recommended Pattern Followed
Postlunch (12:30 PM) Blood Glucose = 45 (REACTION) Treated with Glucose Tablets	

ing blood glucose values, it is important to eventual weight gain. Information about fat is important. Three basic rules for clients on the CSII pump or MDI are also important:

1. Limit meals to three a day and/or allow three hours between meals.
2. Bolus or inject insulin 30 minutes prior to eating (or 5 minutes for Lispro).
3. Cover diet intake with adequate amounts of insulin.

Strategies Dealing with Lack of Planning

Cueing devices can help persons with type 1 diabetes remember to bolus or inject insulin on time. Reminders on the refrigerator to give insulin 30 minutes before eating are important. If a morning or evening dose is a problem, signs on the mirror in the bathroom can cue clients.

A simple calendar requiring check marks can help the client who constantly forgets to bolus or inject insulin 30 minutes (or 5 minutes for Lispro) before a meal. Adherence Tool 6-5 is an example of a monthly monitoring device that, if placed in a visible area and used as a daily recording device, could serve as a cue. The same calendar might serve as a reminder of problems for clients who eat in restaurants frequently. A star might remind clients to plan for a restaurant meal by calling the restaurant to find out what is on the menu and ask questions to determine what is in a recipe. By planning ahead, clients can select food appropriately with little effort while in the restaurant. Most people can save favorite restaurant menus and calculate exchange, TAG or carbohydrate values for favorite selections. Extra care and effort initially can make eating in restaurants more enjoyable.

Strategies Dealing with Lack of Commitment

Most insulin-dependent persons enter periods of low commitment to keeping blood glucose levels normal. This can be evidenced in a variety of ways. One is "bouncing" blood glucose levels that have a roller coaster appearance when graphed. Another is relatively good blood glucose levels with high glycosylated hemoglobin levels. This may indicate problems with high blood sugars at night, but it can also signal fabricated glucose values. A third clue to lack of commitment is the client who comes in saying, "I just want to have one day where I don't have to worry about blood glucose levels, fingersticks, diet, and exercise."

The extracted text that follows illustrates the thoughts that are familiar to many persons with diabetes. This monologue was written by a person with diabetes and illustrates the dilemma that occurs in trying to lead a normal life and be in good diabetes control at all times.

> "So you begin on the perfection side. Your whole world revolves around your diabetes. You weigh and measure and time everything. You learn to eat when you're not hungry. You learn not to eat when you are hungry. You do everything right, and you have reactions anyway. There is never a break. There is never a vacation from your diabetes.
>
> Even one slight deviation from perfection causes you to panic. You just know something horrible is going to happen. You're going to go into a coma and die like everyone keeps telling you. But then you realize nothing really bad happened. You don't even feel bad physically. So you ease up just a little on the strictness of the requirements. You allow yourself a little more freedom. You realize you're not even having as many reactions. You're not quite as uptight about doing things perfectly. But you do begin to feel a little guilty, especially when people tell you about people with diabetes who were on the imperfect side and they died. But really you're doing fine. You begin to experiment—see how far you can push your limits. You find you feel awful here, and you have more reactions. So you find a very comfortable place somewhere in the middle. You still structure things, and you don't just eat anything you want to. But your world allows other things besides diabetes now. And then it happens: PROBLEMS, accompanied by GUILT compounded by FEAR of more PROBLEMS. You're told that there never was a middle ground. Either you are all the way over on the perfection side, or you are totally on the imperfection side. And your problems are evidence that you are as far over on the imperfection side as you can possibly be. So everyone tells you that you could avoid more problems IF you will just switch back to the perfection side. So you

switch back. But you are human. There are other things to think about besides diabetes. You make choices. Now what? You know you're really on the imperfection side. But you must try to convince everyone that you're on the perfection side, because you find out that family and friends will nag you if they find out that you are imperfect. And your doctors don't really want to know you're not perfect. They only want to hear how perfectly their regimen is working. So you live a normal life. You learn to take tests only when you know they're going to be perfect; or if you take a test that isn't perfect you simply don't record it. MORE GUILT!

You eat only what's on your diet when you're with others. But when you're by yourself, you find the only thing you can think about eating is anything that's forbidden. You "pig out."

You make sure your random blood sugars are in the perfect range when you visit the doctor. You learn to be so good at deception that you begin to wonder just where you really are in your control. You realize you've even been deceiving yourself. How good has your control really been? You feel fine. Your A1c's are good. You've had very few reactions, and the tests that you take for your own knowledge are mostly good. And then it happens: MORE PROBLEMS.

Now everyone knows that you really weren't perfect. So they remind you that it's your own fault. If you had just been perfect, the problems would never have happened. So now what? You just learn to live with not only the physical pain, but the GUILT that comes with it for the rest of your life. Or until someone comes along who is not afraid that your humanness will make her a failure. She listens. She hears you. Then she speaks the magic words: "IT'S NOT YOUR FAULT!" It takes a while for the words to sink in. The layers of guilt have been building for years. But then it hits you. You can let go of all the guilt. It's honestly okay to be HUMAN. But best of all you know that someone understands you and accepts you just the way you are. And because she cares, you know you don't have to face your problems alone. Then the pain isn't so hard to live with."[167] (Theory: Cognitive-Behavioral Theory; Strategy: Cognitive Restructuring)

A problem with lack of commitment is not solved with recipes, information on the nutrient content of a commercial product, or more telephone contact without appropriate intervention. The following dialogue illustrates one possible initial approach to dealing with lack of commitment. Strategies include open questions to identify the problem, paraphrasing, empathy, and contracting.

Client: "I just want to have one day without diabetes, without fingersticks, and without dietary calculations. Living with diabetes is not like other tasks in life. You can't say, 'I worked hard and now I am finished. I did a good job.' Diabetes is forever!" (Theory: Transtheoretical Model, Precontemplator/Contemplator)

Nutrition counselor: "You have thought about this for a long time. Describe why you feel this way now and initially you seemed to be more enthusiastic." (Open Question)

Client: "When you first start treating your diabetes, it's fun and exciting. You feel better for the first time in a long while. You feel in control. You are given responsibility for diet and fingersticks and exercise."

Nutrition counselor: "You're sort of in a honeymoon phase." (Paraphrase)

Client: "Yes, exactly. But things change. Your friends get tired of hearing about how well you are doing. They don't give you as much positive reinforcement for your labor. In fact they seem to get tired of hearing you talk about your disease and how well you are doing. Without this support, you get tired of doing everything well." (Contemplator's negative thoughts)

Nutrition counselor: "So you need to have some kind of reward for your efforts, but your friends don't always come through." (Reflection)

Client: "Yes."

Nutrition counselor: "Let's try to list a few ways that you can provide positive reinforcement for yourself. What things in your life really make you feel good?"

Client: "Well, I like to read. I love to watch MTV. I like eating pizzas."

Nutrition counselor: "Great, let's set up a contract. Whenever you have blood sugars on three consecutive pre-prandial sticks between 100 and 130 in a day, you can reward yourself with one of these fun things. We will even figure out how to count pizza. I can help by calling the restaurant. Let's write the contract." (See Exhibit 6-7.) (Theory: Behavior Modification; Strategy: Contingency Management)

As with other diets, lack of commitment may be a direct result of a change in life events. Clients who go through a divorce may blame their preoccupation with diabetes care, resulting in changes in the care taken to follow a dietary regimen.

Significant family changes such as marriage or remarriage, birth of a child, or death of a close relative can have devastating effects on blood sugars. In one family the husband, Mr. X, was on an insulin pump. His father died of complications of the disease. Following her father-in-law's death, the client's wife began looking at the disease differently. She felt that she should not have married someone with a disease so devastating and was concerned about her children eventually being diagnosed with diabetes. For several months, Mr. X's blood glucose values were uncontrolled and his attitude toward his care was very casual. His wife finally sought psychiatric care, and Mr. X's dietary adherence began to improve.

Exhibit 6–7   Contract

I will reward myself each day for preprandial blood sugars between 100 and 130 on three consecutive occasions in a day. The following things will be used as rewards:

1. Going to the library for a good novel
2. Watching MTV
3. Eating three slices of a Pizza Hut Canadian Bacon Pizza containing approximately 63 grams of TAG.

If my blood sugars are not between 100 and 130 preprandially, I will not receive any of the above three rewards.

(*Nutrition counselor*) will call me each Friday at 10:00 AM at work to check on my progress.

Patient _____

Nutrition Counselor _____

Job-related changes can also affect blood glucose values. The loss of a job and beginning of a new one can cause schedule changes that make lunch hours less predictable or stimulate snacking. One woman who began babysitting in her home snacked every time the children ate. Her blood glucose values were very high and occasionally low from insulin boluses taken too close together. Another woman moved from a secretarial position to a job in a bakery. Everyone snacked on doughnut holes at 10:00 AM, and she joined the group. Loss of a job can make matters other than diabetes care a higher priority.

The insulin-dependent person who is diagnosed with another disease, such as heart disease, may become very discouraged. One man stated, "I am too young to have to worry about both diabetes and heart disease." Frequently, another illness may require added dietary restrictions that complicate the regimen and make it more difficult to follow, adding stress to an already complicated life situation.

One of the positive aspects of good adherence and normalized blood glucose levels is fewer symptoms. When a client can connect diet with positive, healthful feelings, he or she has a great deal of incentive to work hard for good dietary adherence. Reminding clients how well they felt while they were strictly following the new eating pattern may be enough to change lack of commitment to enthusiasm. In some cases, planning a one-week menu may help the client cut back on dietary calculations and worry just before a meal. After planning the menu with the nutrition counselor on several occasions, clients may begin planning on their own, allowing for more spontaneity and fewer calculations for the rest of the week.

Counselors can involve family members in helping with diet by asking them to reinforce good dietary behaviors. They might even participate in signing a contract. With the client, the counselor can make a list of stressful events that take place in one week and ask the family to assist in making certain times of the day less stressful. The children might help with laundry or pack a sack lunch.

In some cases, constructive confrontation may be beneficial to increasing dietary commitment. For example:

Nutrition counselor: "I really thought we were doing well in working together on dietary problems. (Personal Relationship Statement) I see your glycosylated hemoglobin has gone up one whole point. Your diet records also show an increase in snacking." (Description of Behavior—Theory: Behavior Modification)

Client: "I know I just don't have any motivation. I really want to do well."

Nutrition counselor: "You seem to be saying two things: (1) you want to do well, and (2) you just don't care. (Description of Feelings and Interpretation of Client's Situation—Theory = Cognitive-Behavioral) Am I right?"

Client: "Yes." (Understanding Response)

Nutrition counselor: "How do you feel about what I am saying?" (Perception Check)

Client: "I'm trying to do two things, and I feel like a failure all the time. Sometimes I just say I might as well give up, and I do. I don't check my blood sugars or I check them at times when I know they are good and write those numbers down. Then I just throw my hands up in despair and say what's the use and start snacking."

Nutrition counselor: "Good, you seem to be able to talk about exactly what you are feeling and that's pretty low sometimes. (Interpretive Response and Constructive Feedback) Would you be willing to do a diary of your thoughts?"

Client: "What's that?"

Nutrition counselor: "It's not difficult. Just record what you think in a few sentences every time you eat. Use this form (Appendix G). We will talk about your thought diary when you come to the next visit."

Client: "I will try to record before and after each meal, but may miss on weekends."

Nutrition counselor: "Record as often as you can. This is to help you. I do not want it to become a burden."

At the next visit, the discussion could revolve around how to replace negative thoughts with positive thoughts, such as "I only ate one small cracker. I won't eat any more. I'm doing great today."

The transtheoretical model is useful when facilitating changes in behavior in persons who are not ready to change. The example below is one in which the transtheoretical model is used with a person who is in the precontemplation stage after many years of dealing with diabetes. While symptom relief can occur with controlled blood glucose, many persons with diabetes wish for a vacation. In the example below, the client is dealing with the day-to-day monotony of managing her diabetes. While she thoroughly understands what is required to achieve normal blood glucose control, her ability to make dietary adherence a priority has recently dropped, leaving her blood glucose levels erratic and her HbA1c high.

Counselor: "Hi, how are things going?"

Client: "Well, I just want a vacation from my diabetes. I know what to do but just want to be like all of my friends." (Precontemplation)

Counselor: "So sometimes living with diabetes makes you different from your friends, and you just want to be like everyone else." (Reflection)

Client: "Yes! I know that I can't take a vacation."

Counselor: "Maybe it would help to list some of the reasons you want to stop adhering to your diet."

Client: "Oh this will be easy. When I go to a party, I will stuff myself and not worry about drinking alcohol or pigging out on all those delicious things everyone else is eating."

Counselor: "Anything else?"

Client: "It is a great vacation from diabetes to just not care about my diet."

Counselor: "Is that all?"

Client: "One more thing. I would not feel different any more."

Counselor: "What are some positive things about following your dietary pattern?"

Client: "One is that I would be taking better care of my health overall and avoid complications."

Counselor: "Others . . ."

Client: "I would have more energy."

Counselor: "Anything else?"

Client: "I love being with my grandchildren. I would have enough energy to do things with them. My grandchildren mean the world to me. This is a very important part of my life."

Counselor: "OK, so you have several reasons for not changing your eating habits. One is that you could go to a party and do what everyone else is doing. You could also just relax and not worry about following an eating pattern. And you would not have to feel different from everyone else. On the other hand, some of the positives are that you would be taking better care of your health and would have more energy. Finally and very importantly, you want to spend quality time with your grandchildren. So where do you stand now with this decision regarding following your diet?"

Client: "Well, my grandchildren must come first. This is what tips the scales in favor of trying my best to follow my diet. I just must find a way to be sure that I keep them in mind."

Strategies to deal with lack of commitment are very important to a client's long-term success with a diabetic regimen. Identifying changes in life events can signal eventual problems. Many strategies to deal with these changes are included in this chapter and focus on identifying positive support persons and appropriate use of constructive confrontation. Also, a person in precontemplation can be helped to reappraise values and find new reasons to follow a dietary pattern.

Review of Chapter 6

1. List three factors that are commonly associated with eating patterns designed to control blood glucose levels and lead to inappropriate eating behaviors:

    a. _____

    b. _____

    c. _____

2. List two nutrients to emphasize in collecting baseline information on eating patterns for persons with diabetes.

    a. _____

    b. _____

3. Identify four strategies to help combat inappropriate eating behaviors when working with clients on new diabetic eating patterns:

    a. _____

    b. _____

c. _____

d. _____

4. The following describes a problem situation with a client who has been instructed on a diabetic diet. Identify a theory and strategies that might help solve this client's problem and explain your reason for selecting it.

   Mr. J. has been placed on an eating pattern to control diabetes by his physician. During nutrition assessment you found that he has most difficulty with afternoon snacks. At his company during break, everyone eats frosted cupcakes, candy bars, or jellybeans. (a) What further questions would you ask to elicit more information? (b) What strategies would you use to help alleviate the problem? (c) Why did you choose these strategies?

   a. _____

   b. _____

   c. _____

References

1. American Diabetes Association. *All About Diabetes, Diabetes Statistics, National Diabetes Fact Sheet, 2005.* Available at: http//www .diabetes.org. Accessed April 18, 2007.
2. McBean AM, Li S, Gilbertson DT, Collins AJ. Differences in diabetes prevalence, incidence, and mortality among the elderly of four racial/ethnic groups: whites, blacks, Hispanics, and Asians. *Diabetes Care* 2004;27(10):2317–2324.
3. Narayan KM, Boyle JP, Thompson TJ, Sorensen SW, Williamson DF. Lifetime risk for diabetes mellitus in the United States. *JAMA* 2003;290(14):1884–1890.
4. The effect of intensive treatment of diabetes on the development and progression of long-term complications in insulin-dependent diabetes mellitus. The Diabetes Control and Complications Trial Research Group. *N Engl J Med* 1993;329(14):977–986.
5. Franz MJ, Bantle JP, Beebe CA, et al. Nutrition principles and recommendations in diabetes. *Diabetes Care* 2004;27(Suppl 1):S36–S46.
6. Standards of medical care in diabetes–2006. *Diabetes Care* 2006;29(Suppl 1):S4–S42.
7. Wing RR, Blair EH, Bononi P, Marcus MD, Watanabe R, Bergman RN. Caloric restriction per se is a significant factor in improvements in

glycemic control and insulin sensitivity during weight loss in obese NIDDM patients. *Diabetes Care* 1994;17(1):30–36.

8. Kelley DE, Wing R, Buonocore C, Sturis J, Polonsky K, Fitzsimmons M. Relative effects of calorie restriction and weight loss in noninsulin-dependent diabetes mellitus. *J Clin Endocrinol Metab* 1993;77(5):1287–1293.

9. Markovic TP, Jenkins AB, Campbell LV, Furler SM, Kraegen EW, Chisholm DJ. The determinants of glycemic responses to diet restriction and weight loss in obesity and NIDDM. *Diabetes Care* 1998;21(5):687–694.

10. Albright A, Franz M, Hornsby G, et al. American College of Sports Medicine position stand. Exercise and type 2 diabetes. *Med Sci Sports Exerc* 2000;32(7):1345–1360.

11. Lipkin E. New strategies for the treatment of type 2 diabetes. *J Am Diet Assoc* 1999;99(3):329–334.

12. Knowler WC, Barrett-Connor E, Fowler SE, et al. Reduction in the incidence of type 2 diabetes with lifestyle intervention or metformin. *N Engl J Med* 2002;346(6):393–403.

13. Tuomilehto J, Lindstrom J, Eriksson JG, et al. Prevention of type 2 diabetes mellitus by changes in lifestyle among subjects with impaired glucose tolerance. *N Engl J Med* 2001;344(18):1343–1350.

14. Buchanan TA, Xiang AH, Peters RK, et al. Preservation of pancreatic beta-cell function and prevention of type 2 diabetes by pharmacological treatment of insulin resistance in high-risk Hispanic women. *Diabetes* 2002;51(9):2796–2803.

15. Chiasson JL, Josse RG, Gomis R, Hanefeld M, Karasik A, Laakso M. Acarbose for prevention of type 2 diabetes mellitus: the STOP-NIDDM randomised trial. *Lancet* 2002;359(9323):2072–2077.

16. Knowler WC, Hamman RF, Edelstein SL, et al. Prevention of type 2 diabetes with troglitazone in the Diabetes Prevention Program. *Diabetes* 2005;54(4):1150–1156.

17. Torgerson JS, Hauptman J, Boldrin MN, Sjostrom L. XENical in the prevention of diabetes in obese subjects (XENDOS) study: a randomized study of orlistat as an adjunct to lifestyle changes for the prevention of type 2 diabetes in obese patients. *Diabetes Care* 2004;27(1): 155–161.

18. Yusuf S, Gerstein H, Hoogwerf B, et al. Ramipril and the development of diabetes. *JAMA* 2001;286(15):1882–1885.

19. Delahanty LM, Halford BN. The role of diet behaviors in achieving improved glycemic control in intensively treated patients in the Diabetes Control and Complications Trial. *Diabetes Care* 1993;16(11): 1453–1458.

20. Delahanty LM, Nathan DM. Research navigating the course of clinical practice in diabetes. *J Am Diet Assoc* 2004;104(12):1846–1853.

21. Anderson EJ, Richardson M, Castle G, et al. Nutrition interventions for intensive therapy in the Diabetes Control and Complications Trial. The DCCT Research Group. *J Am Diet Assoc* 1993;93(7):768–772.

22. Wolever TM, Hamad S, Chiasson JL, et al. Day-to-day consistency in amount and source of carbohydrate associated with improved blood glucose control in type 1 diabetes. *J Am Coll Nutr* 1999;18(3):242–247.

23. Retinopathy and nephropathy in patients with type 1 diabetes four years after a trial of intensive therapy. The Diabetes Control and Complications Trial/Epidemiology of Diabetes Interventions and Complications Research Group. *N Engl J Med* 2000;342(6):381–389.

24. Effect of intensive therapy on the microvascular complications of type 1 diabetes mellitus. *JAMA* 2002;287(19):2563–2569.

25. Sustained effect of intensive treatment of type 1 diabetes mellitus on development and progression of diabetic nephropathy: the Epidemiology of Diabetes Interventions and Complications (EDIC) study. *JAMA* 2003;290(16):2159–2167.

26. Nathan DM, Lachin J, Cleary P, et al. Intensive diabetes therapy and carotid intima-media thickness in type 1 diabetes mellitus. *N Engl J Med* 2003;348(23):2294–2303.

27. Executive Summary of the Third Report of the National Cholesterol Education Program (NCEP) Expert Panel on Detection, Evaluation, and Treatment of High Blood Cholesterol in Adults (Adult Treatment Panel III). *JAMA* 2001;285(19):2486–2497.

28. Nutrition recommendations and principles for people with diabetes mellitus. *Diabetes Care* 2000;23(Suppl 1):S43–46.

29. Institute of Medicine. *Dietary Reference Intakes: Energy, Carbohydrate, Fiber, Fat, Fatty Acids, Cholesterol, Protein and Amino Acids.* Washington, D.C.: National Academies Press, 2002.

30. Crapo PA, Reaven G, Olefsky J. Plasma glucose and insulin responses to orally administered simple and complex carbohydrates. *Diabetes* 1976;25(9):741–747.

31. Anderson JW, Ward K. Long-term effects of high-carbohydrate, high-fiber diets on glucose and lipid metabolism: a preliminary report on patients with diabetes. *Diabetes Care* 1978;1(2):77–82.

32. Bantle JP, Swanson JE, Thomas W, Laine DC. Metabolic effects of dietary sucrose in type 2 diabetic subjects. *Diabetes Care* 1993;16(9):1301–1305.

33. Peterson DB, Lambert J, Gerring S, et al. Sucrose in the diet of diabetic patients—just another carbohydrate? *Diabetologia* 1986;29(4):216–220.

34. Rickard KA, Loghmani ES, Cleveland JL, Fineberg NS, Freidenberg GR. Lower glycemic response to sucrose in the diets of children with type 1 diabetes. *J Pediatr* 1998;133(3):429–434.

35. Thom SL. Diabetes medications and delivery methods. In: Powers MA, ed. *Handbook of Diabetes Medical Nutrition Therapy.* Gaithersburg, MD: Aspen Publishers, Inc., 1996:95.

36. Crapo PA, Reaven G, Olefsky J. Postprandial plasma-glucose and -insulin responses to different complex carbohydrates. *Diabetes* 1977;26(12):1178–1183.

37. Crapo PA, Kolterman OG, Waldeck N, Reaven GM, Olefsky JM. Post-

prandial hormonal responses to different types of complex carbohydrate in individuals with impaired glucose tolerance. *Am J Clin Nutr* 1980;33(8):1723–1728.

38. Bantle JP, Laine DC, Castle GW, Thomas JW, Hoogwerf BJ, Goetz FC. Postprandial glucose and insulin responses to meals containing different carbohydrates in normal and diabetic subjects. *N Engl J Med* 1983;309(1):7–12.

39. Bantle JP, Laine DC, Thomas JW. Metabolic effects of dietary fructose and sucrose in types 1 and 2 diabetic subjects. *JAMA* 1986;256(23):3241–3246.

40. Slama G, Haardt MJ, Jean-Joseph P, et al. Sucrose taken during mixed meal has no additional hyperglycaemic action over isocaloric amounts of starch in well-controlled diabetics. *Lancet* 1984;2(8395):122–125.

41. Bornet F, Haardt MJ, Costagliola D, Blayo A, Slama G. Sucrose or honey at breakfast have no additional acute hyperglycaemic effect over an isoglucidic amount of bread in type 2 diabetic patients. *Diabetologia* 1985;28(4):213–217.

42. Abraira C, Derler J. Large variations of sucrose in constant carbohydrate diets in type 2 diabetes. *Am J Med* 1988;84(2):193–200.

43. Forlani G, Galuppi V, Santacroce G, et al. Hyperglycemic effect of sucrose ingestion in IDDM patients controlled by artificial pancreas. *Diabetes Care* 1989;12(4):296–298.

44. Wise JE, Keim KS, Huisinga JL, Willmann PA. Effect of sucrose-containing snacks on blood glucose control. *Diabetes Care* 1989;12(6):423–426.

45. Peters AL, Davidson MB, Eisenberg K. Effect of isocaloric substitution of chocolate cake for potato in type I diabetic patients. *Diabetes Care* 1990;13(8):888–892.

46. Loghmani E, Rickard K, Washburne L, Vandagriff J, Fineberg N, Golden M. Glycemic response to sucrose-containing mixed meals in diets of children with insulin-dependent diabetes mellitus. *J Pediatr* 1991;119(4):531–537.

47. Wolever TM, Josse RG. The role of carbohydrate in the diabetes diet. *Med Exercise Nutr Health* 1993;2:84–99.

48. Coulston A, Greenfield M, Kraemer F, Tobey T, Reaven G. Effect of source of dietary carbohydrate on plasma glucose and insulin responses to test meals in normal subjects. *Am J Clin Nutr* 1980;33(6):1279–1282.

49. Coulston A, Greenfield MS, Kraemer FB, Tobey TA, Reaven GM. Effect of differences in source of dietary carbohydrate on plasma glucose and insulin responses to meals in patients with impaired carbohydrate tolerance. *Am J Clin Nutr* 1981;34(12):2716–2720.

50. Sandstedt RM, Strahan D, Ueda S, Abbot RC. The digestibility of high amylose corn starches. The apparent effect of the ae gene on susceptibility to amylose action. *Cereal Chem* 1962;39:123–131.

51. Geervani P, Theophilus R. Influence of legume starches on protein nutrition and availability of lysine and methionine to albino rats. *J Food Sci* 1981;46:817–828.

52. Nuttall FQ, Mooradian AD, Gannon MC, Billington C, Krezowski P. Effect of protein ingestion on the glucose and insulin response to a standardized oral glucose load. *Diabetes Care* 1984;7(5): 465–470.

53. Anderson IH, Levine AS, Levitt MD. Incomplete absorption of the carbohydrate in all-purpose wheat flour. *N Engl J Med* 1981;304(15): 891–892.

54. Bowman DE. Amylase inhibitor of navy beans. *Science* 1945;102: 358–359.

55. Rea RL, Thompson LU, Jenkins DJA. Lectins in foods and their relation to starch digestibility. *Nutr Res* 1985;5(9):919–929.

56. Hintz HF, Hogue DE, Krook L. Toxicity of red kidney beans (*Phaseolus vulgaris*) in the rat. *J Nutr* 1967;93(1):77–86.

57. Yoon JH, Thompson LU, Jenkins DJ. The effect of phytic acid on in vitro rate of starch digestibility and blood glucose response. *Am J Clin Nutr* 1983;38(6):835–842.

58. Kakade ML, Evans RJ. Growth inhibition of rats fed raw navy beans (*Phaseolus vulgaris*). *J Nutr* 1966;90(2):191–198.

59. Puls W, Keup U. Influence of an amylase inhibitor (BAY d 7791) on blood glucose, serum insulin and NEFA in starch loading tests in rats, dogs and man. *Diabetologia* 1973;9(2):97–101.

60. Hillebrand I, Boehme K, Frank G, Fink H, Berchtold P. The effects of the alpha-glucosidase inhibitor BAY g 5421 (Acarbose) on meal-stimulated elevations of circulating glucose, insulin, and triglyceride levels in man. *Res Exp Med (Berl)* 1979;175(1):81–86.

61. Snow P, O'Dea K. Factors affecting the rate of hydrolysis of starch in food. *Am J Clin Nutr* 1981;34(12):2721–2727.

62. Collings P, Williams C, MacDonald I. Effects of cooking on serum glucose and insulin responses to starch. *Br Med J (Clin Res)*1981;282(6269):1032.

63. Wolever TM, Jenkins DJ, Kalmusky J, et al. Glycemic response to pasta: effect of surface area, degree of cooking, and protein enrichment. *Diabetes Care* 1986;9(4):401–404.

64. Wolever TM, Jenkins DJ, Kalmusky J, et al. Comparison of regular and parboiled rices: explanation of discrepancies between reported glycemic responses to rice. *Nutr Res* 1986;6:349–357.

65. Jenkins DJ, Thorne MJ, Camelon K, et al. Effect of processing on digestibility and the blood glucose response: a study of lentils. *Am J Clin Nutr* 1982;36(6):1093–1101.

66. O'Dea K, Nestel PJ, Antonoff L. Physical factors influencing postprandial glucose and insulin responses to starch. *Am J Clin Nutr* 1980;33(4):760–765.

67. Collier G, O'Dea K. Effect of physical form of carbohydrate on the postprandial glucose, insulin, and gastric inhibitory polypeptide responses in type 2 diabetes. *Am J Clin Nutr* 1982;36(1):10–14.

68. James WP, Branch WJ, Southgate DA. Calcium binding by dietary fibre. *Lancet* 1978;1(8065):638–639.

69. Jenkins DJ, Wolever TM, Taylor RH, Reynolds D, Nineham R, Hocka-

day TD. Diabetic glucose control, lipids, and trace elements on long-term guar. *Br Med J* 1980;280(6228):1353–1354.

70. Anderson JW, Ferguson SK, Karounos D, O'Malley L, Sieling B, Chen WJ. Mineral and vitamin status on high-fiber diets: long-term studies of diabetic patients. *Diabetes Care* 1980;3(1):38–40.

71. Lindsay AN, Hardy S, Jarrett L, Rallison ML. High-carbohydrate, high-fiber diet in children with type 1 diabetes mellitus. *Diabetes Care* 1984;7(1):63–67.

72. Baumer JH, Drakeford JA, Wadsworth J, Savage DC. Effects of dietary fibre and exercise on mid-morning diabetic control—a controlled trial. *Arch Dis Child* 1982;57(12):905–909.

73. Kinmonth AL, Angus RM, Jenkins PA, Smith MA, Baum JD. Whole foods and increased dietary fibre improve blood glucose control in diabetic children. *Arch Dis Child* 1982;57(3):187–194.

74. Kuhl C, Molsted-Pedersen L, Hornnes PJ. Guar gum and glycemic control of pregnant insulin-dependent diabetic patients. *Diabetes Care* 1983;6(2):152–154.

75. Ney D, Hollingsworth DR, Cousins L. Decreased insulin requirement and improved control of diabetes in pregnant women given a high-carbohydrate, high-fiber, low-fat diet. *Diabetes Care* 1982;5(5):529–533.

76. Canivet B, Creisson G, Freychet P, Dageville X. Fibre, diabetes, and risk of bezoar. *Lancet* 1980;2(8199):862.

77. Story L, Anderson JW, Chen WJ, Karounos D, Jefferson B. Adherence to high-carbohydrate, high-fiber diets: long-term studies of non-obese diabetic men. *J Am Diet Assoc* 1985;85(9):1105–1110.

78. Jenkins DJ, Goff DV, Leeds AR, et al. Unabsorbable carbohydrates and diabetes: Decreased post-prandial hyperglycaemia. *Lancet* 1976;2(7978):172–174.

79. Vuorinen-Markkola H, Sinisalo M, Koivisto VA. Guar gum in insulin-dependent diabetes: effects on glycemic control and serum lipoproteins. *Am J Clin Nutr* 1992;56(6):1056–1060.

80. Anderson JW. The role of dietary carbohydrate and fiber in the control of diabetes. *Adv Intern Med* 1980;26:67–96.

81. Jenkins DJ, Wolever TM, Jenkins AL, Lee R, Wong GS, Josse R. Glycemic response to wheat products: reduced response to pasta but no effect of fiber. *Diabetes Care* 1983;6(2):155–159.

82. Tinker L, Wheeler M. Fiber metabolism and use in diabetes therapy. In: Powers MA, ed. *Handbook of Diabetes Medical Nutrition Therapy.* Gaithersburg, MD: Aspen Publishers, Inc., 1996:405.

83. Lafrance L, Rabasa-Lhoret R, Poisson D, Ducros F, Chiasson JL. Effects of different glycaemic index foods and dietary fibre intake on glycaemic control in type 1 diabetic patients on intensive insulin therapy. *Diabet Med* 98;15(11):972–978.

84. Giacco R, Parillo M, Rivellese AA, et al. Long-term dietary treatment with increased amounts of fiber-rich low-glycemic index natural foods improves blood glucose control and reduces the number of

hypoglycemic events in type 1 diabetic patients. *Diabetes Care* 2000;23(10):1461–1466.

85. Hollenbeck CB, Coulston AM, Reaven GM. To what extent does increased dietary fiber improve glucose and lipid metabolism in patients with noninsulin-dependent diabetes mellitus (NIDDM)? *Am J Clin Nutr* 86;43(1):16–24.

86. Chandalia M, Garg A, Lutjohann D, von Bergmann K, Grundy SM, Brinkley LJ. Beneficial effects of high dietary fiber intake in patients with type 2 diabetes mellitus. *N Engl J Med* 2000;342(19):1392–1398.

87. Nutrition recommendations and principles for people with diabetes mellitus. *Diabetes Care* 1994;17(5):519–522.

88. Evidence-based nutrition principles and recommendations for the treatment and prevention of diabetes and related complications. *Diabetes Care* 2002;25(1):202–212.

89. Wolever TM, Jenkins DJ. The use of the glycemic index in predicting the blood glucose response to mixed meals. *Am J Clin Nutr* 1986;43(1):167–172.

90. Jenkins DJ, Wolever TM, Taylor RH, et al. Glycemic index of foods: a physiological basis for carbohydrate exchange. *Am J Clin Nutr* 1981;34(3):362–366.

91. Jenkins DJ, Wolever TM, Taylor RH, Barker HM, Fielden H. Exceptionally low blood glucose response to dried beans: comparison with other carbohydrate foods. *Br Med J* 1980;281(6240):578–580.

92. Franz MJ. Carbohydrate and diabetes: is the source or the amount of more importance? *Curr Diab Rep* 2001;1(2):177–186.

93. Franz M. Medical nutrition therapy for diabetes mellitus and hypoglycemia of nondiabetic origin. In: Mahan L, Escott-Stump S, eds. *Krause's Food, Nutrition, and Diet Therapy*, 2004:804–814.

94. Summary of the Second Report of the National Cholesterol Education Program (NCEP) Expert Panel on Detection, Evaluation, and Treatment of High Blood Cholesterol in Adults (Adult Treatment Panel II). *JAMA* 1993;269(23):3015–3023.

95. Jenkins DJ, Wolever TM, Bacon S, et al. Diabetic diets: high carbohydrate combined with high fiber. *Am J Clin Nutr* 1980;33(8):1729–1733.

96. Wong S, Traianedes K, O'Dea K. Factors affecting the rate of hydrolysis of starch in legumes. *Am J Clin Nutr* 1985;42(1):38–43.

97. Lovejoy J, DiGirolamo M. Habitual dietary intake and insulin sensitivity in lean and obese adults. *Am J Clin Nutr* 1992;55(6):1174–1179.

98. Parillo M, Rivellese AA, Ciardullo AV, et al. A high-monounsaturated-fat/low-carbohydrate diet improves peripheral insulin sensitivity in non-insulin-dependent diabetic patients. *Metabolism* 1992;41(12):1373–1378.

99. Collier G, O'Dea K. The effect of coingestion of fat on the glucose, insulin, and gastric inhibitory polypeptide responses to carbohydrate and protein. *Am J Clin Nutr* 1983;37(6):941–944.

100. Collier G, McLean A, O'Dea K. Effect of co-ingestion of fat on the

metabolic responses to slowly and rapidly absorbed carbohydrates. *Diabetologia* 84;26(1):50–54.

101. Collier GR, Wolever TM, Jenkins DJ. Concurrent ingestion of fat and reduction in starch content impairs carbohydrate tolerance to subsequent meals. *Am J Clin Nutr* 1987;45(5):963–969.

102. Garg A, Bantle JP, Henry RR, et al. Effects of varying carbohydrate content of diet in patients with non-insulin-dependent diabetes mellitus. *JAMA* 1994;271(18):1421–1428.

103. Heilbronn LK, Noakes M, Clifton PM. Effect of energy restriction, weight loss, and diet composition on plasma lipids and glucose in patients with type 2 diabetes. *Diabetes Care* 1999;22(6):889–895.

104. Brackenridge B. Carbohydrate counting for diabetes therapy. In: Powers MA, ed. *Handbook of Diabetes Medical Nutrition Therapy.* Gaithersburg, MD: Aspen Publishers, 1996:262–263.

105. Munro H, Allison J. *Mammalian Protein Metabolism, Volume 1.* New York: Academic Press, 1964.

106. Nuttall FQ, Gannon MC. Plasma glucose and insulin response to macronutrients in nondiabetic and NIDDM subjects. *Diabetes Care* 1991;14(9):824–838.

107. Oexmann MJ. *Total Available Glucose Diabetic Food System.* Charleston, SC: Medical University of South Carolina Printing Service, 1987.

108. Evaluation of certain food additives and contaminants. Thirty-seventh report of the Joint FAO/WHO Expert Committee on Food Additives. *WHO Tech Rep Ser* 1991;806:1–52.

109. American Dietetic Association. Position statement: use of nutritive and non-nutritive sweeteners. *J Am Diet Assoc* 1993;93(7): 816–820.

110. Stegink LD. Aspartame metabolism in humans: acute dosing studies. In: Stegink LD, Filer LJJ, eds. *Aspartame: Physiology and Biochemistry.* New York: Marcel Dekker, 1984:509–554.

111. Nehrling JK, Kobe P, McLane MP, Olson RE, Kamath S, Horwitz DL. Aspartame use by persons with diabetes. *Diabetes Care* Sep-1985;8(5):415–417.

112. Monte WC. Aspartame: Methanol and the public health. *J Appl Nutr* 1984;36:42–54.

113. Aspartame: Commissioner's Final Decision. *Federal Register* 1981;46: 38283.

114. Saccharin and Its Salts. *Federal Register* 1977;42:62209.

115. Morrison AS, Buring JE. Artificial sweeteners and cancer of the lower urinary tract. *N Engl J Med* 1980;302(10):537–541.

116. Saccharin. Review of safety issues. Council on Scientific Affairs. *JAMA* 1985;254(18):2622–2624.

117. American Dietetic Association. Position statement on nutritive and nonnutritive sweeteners. *Nutr Res Newsl* 1998.

118. McNeil Specialty Products Company. *Sucralose: An Introduction to a New Low-Calorie Sweetener.* New Brunswick, NJ: McNeil Specialty Products Company, 1994.

119. Mezitis N, Koch P, Maggio C, Quoddoos A, Pi-Sunyer FX. Glycemic response to sucralose, a novel sweetener, in subjects with diabetes mellitus. *Diabetes* 1994;43(5):S261A.

120. Bowen WH, Young DA, Pearson SK. The effects of sucralose on coronal and root-surface caries. *J Dent Res* 1990;69(8):1485–1487.

121. Warshaw HS. Alternative sweeteners–past, present and potential. *Diabetes Spectr* 1990;3(5):335.

122. Bopp BA, Price P. Cyclamate. In: O'Brien L, Gelardi RC, eds. *Alternative Sweeteners*. New York: Marcel Dekker, Inc., 1991.

123. Bopp BA, Sonders RC, Kesterson JW. Toxicological aspects of cyclamate and cyclohexylamine. *Crit Rev Toxicol* 1986;16(3):213–306.

124. Newsome R. Sugar substitutes. In: Altschul AM, ed. *Low-Calorie Foods Handbook*. New York: Marcel Dekker, Inc., 1993:139–170.

125. O'Brien L, Miller WT. Cyclamate–a toxicological review. *Toxicology* 1989;3(4):307.

126. Walsh CH, O'Sullivan DJ. Effect of moderate alcohol intake on control of diabetes. *Diabetes* 1974;23(5):440–442.

127. Koivisto VA, Tulokas S, Toivonen M, Haapa E, Pelkonen R. Alcohol with a meal has no adverse effects on postprandial glucose homeostasis in diabetic patients. *Diabetes Care* 1993;16(12):1612–1614.

128. Franz MJ. Diabetes mellitus: considerations in the development of guidelines for the occasional use of alcohol. *J Am Diet Assoc* 1983;83(2):147–152.

129. Menze R. Effect of moderate ethanol ingestion on overnight diabetes control and hormone secretion in type 1 diabetic patients. *Diabetologia* 1991;34:A188.

130. American Diabetes Association. Technical review: nutrition principles for the management of diabetes and related complications. *Diabetes Care* 1994;17(5):490.

131. Kulkarni KD. *Adjusting Nutrition Therapy for Special Situations. Handbook of Diabetes Medical Nutrition Therapy*. Gaithersburg, MD: Aspen Publishers, Inc, 1996:437–442.

132. Wasserman DH, Zinman B. Exercise in individuals with IDDM. *Diabetes Care* 1994;17(8):924–937.

133. Franz M. Exercise benefits and guidelines for persons with diabetes. In: Powers MA, ed. *Handbook of Diabetes Medical Nutrition Therapy*. Gaithersburg, MD: Aspen Publishers, Inc., 1996:107–129.

134. American Diabetes Association. Diabetes mellitus and exercise. *Diabetes Care* 2002;25(Suppl 1):S64.

135. Jovanovic L, Peterson CM. The clinical utility of glycosylated hemoglobin. *Am J Med* 1981;70(2):331–338.

136. Bunn HF. Nonenzymatic glycosylation of protein: relevance to diabetes. *Am J Med* 1981;70(2):325–330.

137. Jovanovic L, Peterson CM. Hemoglobin A1c–the key to diabetic control. *Lab Med Practic Phys* 1978;Jul–Aug:11.

138. Peterson CM, Jones RL. Glycosylation reactions and reversible sequelae of diabetes mellitus. In: Peterson CM, ed. *Diabetes Management in the Eighties*. New York: Praeger Publishers, 1982:12–25.

139. Franz M, Reader D, Monk D. *Implementing Group and Individual Medical Nutrition Therapy for Diabetes.* Alexandria, VA: American Diabetes Association, 2002.
140. Choppin J, Jovanovic L, Peterson CM. Matching food with insulin. *Diabetes Prof* 1991;Spring:1–14.
141. Lusk G. *The Elements of the Science of Nutrition.* Philadelphia: W. B. Saunders Co., 1928.
142. Pennington JA, Douglass JS. *Bowes and Church's Food Values of Portions Commonly Used*, Eighteenth Edition. Philadelphia: Lippincott Williams & Wilkins, 2005.
143. West KM. Diet therapy of diabetes: an analysis of failure. *Ann Intern Med* 1973;79(3):425–434.
144. Watkins JD, Williams TF, Martin DA, Hogan MD, Anderson E. A study of diabetic patients at home. *Am J Public Health Nations Health* 1967;57(3):452–459.
145. Broussard BA, Bass MA, Jackson MY. Reasons for diabetic diet noncompliance among Cherokee Indians. *J Nutr Educ* 1982;14:56–57.
146. Schlenk EA, Hart LK. Relationship between health locus of control, health value, and social support and compliance of persons with diabetes mellitus. *Diabetes Care* 1984;7(6):566–574.
147. Eckerling L, Kohrs MB. Research on compliance with diabetic regimens: applications to practice. *J Am Diet Assoc* 1984;84(7):805–809.
148. Weinsier RL, Seeman A, Herrera MG, Simmons JJ, Collins ME. Diet therapy of diabetes. Description of a successful methodologic approach to gaining diet adherence. *Diabetes* 1974;23(8):669–673.
149. Hassell J, Medved E. Group/audiovisual instruction for patients with diabetes. Learning achievements and time economics. *J Am Diet Assoc* 1975;66(5):465–470.
150. Tani GS, Hankin JH. A self-learning unit for patients with diabetes. *J Am Diet Assoc* 1971;58(4):331–335.
151. Dunn SM, Bryson JM, Hoskins PL, Alford JB, Handelsman DJ, Turtle JR. Development of the diabetes knowledge (DKN) scales: forms DKNA, DKNB, and DKNC. *Diabetes Care* 1984;7(1):36–41.
152. Webb KL, Dobson AJ, O'Connell DL, et al. Dietary compliance among insulin-dependent diabetics. *J Chronic Dis* 1984;37(8):633–643.
153. Sonksen PH, Judd SL, Lowy C. Home monitoring of blood–glucose. Method for improving diabetic control. *Lancet* 1978;1(8067):729–732.
154. Walford S, Gale EA, Allison SP, Tattersall RB. Self-monitoring of blood-glucose. Improvement of diabetic control. *Lancet* 1978;1(8067):732–735.
155. Cohen M, Zimmet P. Self-monitoring of blood glucose levels in non-insulin-dependent diabetes mellitus. *Med J Aust* 1983;2(8):377–380.
156. Slowie LA. Patient learning—segments from case histories. *J Am Diet Assoc* 1971;59(6):563–567.
157. Boutaugh ML, Hull AL, Davis WK. An examination of diabetes educational assessment forms. *Diabetes Educ* Winter 1982;7(4):29–34.
158. Shenkel RJ, Rogers JP, Perfetto G, Levin RA. Importance of "signifi-

cant others" in predicting cooperation with diabetic regimen. *Int J Psychiatry Med* 1985;15(2):149–155.

159. Schwartz LS, Springer J, Flaherty JA, Kiani R. The role of recent life events and social support in the control of diabetes mellitus. A pilot study. *Gen Hosp Psychiatry* 1986;8(3):212–216.

160. Bush MA. Compliance, education, and diabetes control. *Mt Sinai J Med* 1987;54(3):221–227.

161. Wing RR, Epstein LH, Nowalk MP, Lamparski DM. Behavioral self-regulation in the treatment of patients with diabetes mellitus. *Psychol Bull* 86;99(1):78–89.

162. McCulloch DK, Mitchell RD, Ambler J, Tattersall RB. Influence of imaginative teaching of diet on compliance and metabolic control in insulin dependent diabetes. *Br Med J (Clin Res Ed)* 1983;287(6408):1858–1861.

163. McNeal B, Salisbury Z, Baumgardner P, Wheeler FC. Comprehension assessment of diabetes education program participants. *Diabetes Care* 1984;7(3):232–235.

164. Rapp SR, Dubbert PM, Burkett PA, Buttross Y. Food portion size estimation by men with type II diabetes. *J Am Diet Assoc* 1986;86(2):249–251.

165. Ary DV, Toobert D, Wilson W, Glasgow RE. Patient perspective on factors contributing to nonadherence to diabetes regimen. *Diabetes Care* 1986;9(2):168–172.

166. Glanz K. Nutrition education for risk factor reduction and patient education: a review. *Prev Med* 1985;14(6):721–752.

167. Martinez B. Perfection/imperfection. *Diabetes Spectr* 1995;8:304–307.

Exchange List 6-A   Exchange Lists for Meal Planning

STARCH LIST

Cereals, grains, pasta, breads, crackers, snacks, starchy vegetables, and cooked dried beans, peas, and lentils are starches. In general, one starch is:

- $^1/_2$ cup of cereal, grain, pasta, or starchy vegetable
- 1 ounce of a bread product, such as 1 slice of bread
- $^3/_4$ to 1 ounce of most snack foods (Some snack foods may also have added fat.)

Nutrition Tips
1. Most starch choices are good sources of B vitamins.
2. Foods made from whole grains are good sources of fiber.
3. Dried beans and peas are a good source of protein and fiber.

Selection Tips
1. Choose starches made with little fat as often as you can.
2. Starchy vegetables prepared with fat count as one starch and one fat.
3. Bagels or muffins can be 2, 3, or 4 ounces in size, and can, therefore, count as 2, 3, or 4 starch choices. Check the size you eat.
4. Dried beans, peas, and lentils are also found on the Meat and Meat Substitutes list.
5. Regular potato chips and tortilla chips are found on the Other Carbohydrates list.
6. Most of the serving sizes are measured after cooking.
7. Always check Nutrition Facts on the food label.

One starch exchange equals 15 grams carbohydrate,
3 grams protein, 0–1 grams fat, and 80 calories.

Bread

Bagel. . . . . $^1/_2$ (1 oz)

Bread, reduced-calorie . . . . 2 slices (1$^1/_2$ oz)

Bread, white, whole-wheat, pumpernickel, rye . . . . 1 slice (1 oz)

Bread sticks, crisp, 4 in long × $^1/_2$ in . . . . 2 ($^2/_3$ oz)

English muffin . . . . $^1/_2$
Hot dog or hamburger bun . . . . $^1/_2$ (1 oz)
Pita, 6 in across . . . . $^1/_2$
Roll, plain, small. . . . . 1 (1 oz)
Raisin bread, unfrosted . . . . 1 slice (1 oz)
Tortilla, corn, 6 in across 1
Tortilla, flour, 7–8 in across 1
Waffle, 4$^1/_2$-in square, reduced-fat 1

Cereals and Grains
Bran cereals . . . . $^1/_2$ cup
Bulgur . . . . $^1/_2$ cup
Cereals . . . . $^1/_2$ cup
Cereals, unsweetened, ready-to-eat . . . . $^3/_4$ cup
Cornmeal (dry) . . . . 3 Tbsp
Couscous . . . . $^1/_3$ cup
Flour (dry) . . . . 3 Tbsp
Granola, low-fat. . . . . $^1/_4$ cup
Grape-nuts. . . . . $^1/_4$ cup
Grits. . . . . $^1/_2$ cup
Kasha. . . . . $^1/_2$ cup
Millet . . . . $^1/_4$ cup
Muesli . . . . $^1/_4$ cup
Oats . . . . $^1/_2$ cup
Pasta . . . . $^1/_2$ cup
Puffed cereal. . . . . 1$^1/_2$ cups
Rice milk . . . . $^1/_2$ cup
Rice, white or brown . . . . $^1/_3$ cup
Shredded wheat . . . . $^1/_2$ cup
Sugar-frosted cereal. . . . . $^1/_2$ cup
Wheat germ . . . . 3 Tbsp

Starchy Vegetables
Baked beans. . . . . $^1/_3$ cup
Corn. . . . . $^1/_2$ cup
Corn on cob, medium . . . . 1 (5 oz)
Mixed vegetables with corn, peas, or pasta . . . . 1 cup
Peas, green. . . . . $^1/_2$ cup
Plaintain . . . . $^1/_2$ cup
Potato, baked or boiled . . . . 1 small (3 oz)
Potato, mashed. . . . . $^1/_2$ cup
Squash, winter (acorn, butternut). . . . . 1 cup
Yam, sweet potato, plain . . . . $^1/_2$ cup

Crackers and Snacks

Animal crackers 8
Graham crackers, $2^1/2$-in square 3
Matzoh . . . . $^3/_4$ oz
Melba toast . . . . 4 slices
Oyster crackers 24
Popcorn (popped, no fat added or low-fat microwave) . . . . 3 cups
Pretzels . . . . $^3/_4$ oz
Rice cakes, 4 in across 2
Saltine-type crackers 6
Snack chips, fat-free (tortilla, potato). . . . . 15–20 ($^3/_4$ oz)
Whole-wheat crackers, no fat added . . . . 2–5 ($^3/_4$ oz)

Dried Beans, Peas, and Lentils (Count as 1 starch
   exchange, plus 1 very lean meat exchange.)
Beans and peas (garbanzo, pinto, kidney, white, split, black-eyed) . $^1/_2$ cup
Lima beans. . . . . $^2/_3$ cup
Lentils . . . . $^1/_2$ cup
Miso* . . . . 3 Tbsp

Starchy Foods Prepared with Fat (Count as 1 starch
   exchange, plus 1 fat exchange)
Biscuit, $2^1/2$ in across 1
Chow mein noodles . . . . $^1/_2$ cup
Corn bread, 2-in cube . . . . 1 (2 oz)
Crackers, round butter type. 6
Croutons . . . . 1 cup
French-fried potatoes . . . . 16–25 (3 oz)
Granola . . . . $^1/_4$ cup
Muffin, small. . . . . 1 ($1^1/2$ oz)
Pancake, 4 in across 2
Popcorn, microwave. . . . . 3 cups
Sandwich crackers, cheese or peanut butter filling 3
Stuffing, bread (prepared). . . . . $^1/_3$ cup
Taco shell, 6 in across. 2
Waffle, $4^1/2$-in square 1
Whole-wheat crackers, fat added. 4–6 (1 oz)

Some food you buy uncooked will weigh less after you cook it. Starches
will often swell in cooking, so a small amount of uncooked starch will
become a much larger amount of cooked food. The following table shows
some of the changes.

*400 mg or more sodium per exchange.

Food (Starch Group)	Uncooked	Cooked
Oatmeal	3 Tbsp	$1/2$ cup
Cream of Wheat	2 Tbsp	$1/2$ cup
Grits	3 Tbsp	$1/2$ cup
Rice	2 Tbsp	$1/3$ cup
Spaghetti	$1/4$ cup	$1/2$ cup
Noodles	$1/3$ cup	$1/2$ cup
Macaroni	$1/4$ cup	$1/2$ cup
Dried beans	$1/4$ cup	$1/2$ cup
Dried peas	$1/4$ cup	$1/2$ cup
Lentils	3 Tbsp	$1/2$ cup

Common Measurements

3 tsp = 1 Tbsp   4 ounces = $1/2$ cup
4 Tbsp = $1/4$ cup   8 ounces = 1 cup
$5 1/3$ Tbsp = $1/3$ cup   1 cup = $1/2$ pint

FRUIT LIST

Fresh, frozen, canned, and dried fruits and fruit juices are on this list. In general, one fruit exchange is:

- 1 small to medium fresh fruit
- $1/2$ cup of canned or fresh fruit or fruit juice
- $1/4$ cup dried fruit

Nutrition Tips

1. Fresh, frozen, and dried fruits have about 2 grams of fiber per choice. Fruit juices contain very little fiber.
2. Citrus fruits, berries, and melons are good sources of vitamin C.

Selection Tips

1. Count $1/2$ cup cranberries or rhubarb sweetened with sugar substitutes as free foods.
2. Read the Nutrition Facts on the food label. If one serving has more than 15 grams of carbohydrate, you will need to adjust the size of the serving you eat or drink.
3. Portion sizes for canned fruits are for the fruit and a small amount of juice.
4. Whole fruit is more filling than fruit juice and may be a better choice.
5. Food labels for fruits may contain the words "no sugar added" or "unsweetened." This means that no sucrose (table sugar) has been added.
6. Generally, fruit canned in extra light syrup has the same amount of carbohydrate per serving as the "no sugar added" or the juice pack. All

canned fruits on the fruit list are based on one of these three types of pack.

One fruit exchange equals 15 grams carbohydrate and 60 calories. The weight includes skin, core, seeds, and rind.

Fruit

Apple, unpeeled, small	1 (4 oz)
Applesauce, unsweetened	$^1/_2$ cup
Apples, dried	4 rings
Apricots, fresh	4 whole (5$^1/_2$ oz)
Apricots, dried	8 halves
Apricots, canned	$^1/_2$ cup
Banana, small	1 (4 oz)
Blackberries	$^3/_4$ cup
Blueberries	$^3/_4$ cup
Cantaloupe, small	$^1/_3$ melon (11 oz) or 1 cup cubes
Cherries, sweet, canned	$^1/_2$ cup
Dates	3
Figs, fresh	1$^1/_2$ large or 2 medium (3$^1/_2$ oz)
Figs, dried	1$^1/_2$
Fruit cocktail	$^1/_2$ cup
Grapefruit, large	$^1/_2$ (11 oz)
Grapefruit sections, canned	$^3/_4$ cup
Grapes, small	17 (3 oz)
Honeydew melon	1 slice (10 oz) or 1 cup cubes
Kiwi	1 (3$^1/_2$ oz)
Mandarin oranges, canned	$^3/_4$ cup
Mango, small	$^1/_2$ fruit (5$^1/_2$ oz) or $^1/_2$ cup
Nectarine, small	1 (5 oz)
Orange, small	1 (6$^1/_2$ oz)
Papaya	$^1/_2$ fruit (8 oz) or 1 cup cubes
Peach, medium, fresh	1 (6 oz)
Peaches, canned	$^1/_2$ cup
Pear, large, fresh	$^1/_2$ (4 oz)
Pears, canned	$^1/_2$ cup
Pineapple, fresh	$^3/_4$ cup
Pineapple, canned	$^1/_2$ cup
Plums, small	2 (5 oz)
Plums, canned	$^1/_2$ cup
Prunes, dried	3
Raisins	2 Tbsp
Raspberries	1 cup
Strawberries	1$^1/_4$ cup whole berries

Tangerines, small . . . . 2 (8 oz)
Watermelon . . . . 1 slice (13^1/$_2$ oz) or 1^1/$_4$ cup cubes

Fruit Juice
Apple juice/cider . . . . ^{1}/$_2$ cup
Cranberry juice cocktail . . . . ^{1}/$_3$ cup
Cranberry juice cocktail, reduced-calorie . . . . 1 cup
Fruit juice blends, 100% juice . . . . ^{1}/$_3$ cup
Grape juice . . . . ^{1}/$_3$ cup
Grapefruit juice . . . . ^{1}/$_2$ cup
Orange juice . . . . ^{1}/$_2$ cup
Pineapple juice . . . . ^{1}/$_2$ cup
Prune juice . . . . ^{1}/$_3$ cup

MILK LIST

Different types of milk and milk products are on this list. Cheeses are on the Meat list and cream and other dairy fats are on the Fat list. Based on the amount of fat they contain, milks are divided into skim/very low-fat milk, low-fat milk, and whole milk. One choice of these includes:

	Carbohydrate (g)	Protein (g)	Fat (g)	Calories
Skim/very low-fat	12	8	0–3	90
Low-fat	12	8	5	120
Whole	12	8	8	150

Nutrition Tips
1. Milk and yogurt are good sources of calcium and protein. Check the food label.
2. The higher the fat content of milk and yogurt, the greater the amount of saturated fat and cholesterol. Choose lower-fat varieties.
3. For those who are lactose intolerant, look for lactose-reduced or lactose-free varieties of milk.

Selection Tips
1. One cup equals 8 fluid ounces or ^{1}/$_2$ pint.
2. Look for chocolate milk, frozen yogurt, and ice cream on the Other Carbohydrates list.
3. Nondairy creamers are on the Free Foods list.
4. Look for rice milk on the Starch list.
5. Look for soy milk on the Medium-Fat Meat list.

**One milk exchange equals 12 grams carbohydrate
and 8 grams protein.**

Skim and Very Low-Fat Milk (0–3 grams fat per serving)
Skim milk . . . . 1 cup
$^1/_2$% milk . . . . 1 cup
1% milk. . . . . 1 cup
Nonfat or low-fat buttermilk . . . . 1 cup
Evaporated skim milk . . . . $^1/_2$ milk
Nonfat dry milk . . . . $^1/_3$ cup dry
Plain nonfat yogurt . . . . $^3/_4$ cup
Nonfat or low-fat fruit-flavored yogurt sweetened
  with aspartame or with nonnutritive sweetener . . . . 1 cup

Low-Fat Milk (5 grams fat per serving)
2% milk. . . . . 1 cup
Plain low-fat yogurt. . . . . $^3/_4$ cup
Sweet acidophilus milk . . . . 1 cup

Whole Milk (8 grams fat per serving)
Whole milk . . . . 1 cup
Evaporated whole milk. . . . . $^1/_2$ cup
Goat's milk . . . . 1 cup
Kefir . . . . 1 cup

OTHER CARBOHYDRATES LIST
You can substitute food choices from this list for a starch, fruit, or milk choice on your meal plan. Some choices will also count as one or more fat choices.

Nutrition Tips
1. These foods can be substituted in your meal plan, even though they contain added sugars or fat. However, they do not contain as many important vitamins and minerals as the choices on the Starch, Fruit, or Milk list.
2. When planning to include these foods in your meal, be sure to include foods from all the lists to eat a balanced meal.

Selection Tips
1. Because many of these foods are concentrated sources of carbohydrate and fat, the portion sizes are often very small.
2. Always check Nutrition Facts on the label. It will be your most accurate source of information.
3. Many fat-free or reduced-fat products made with fat replacers contain carbohydrate. When eaten in large amounts, they may need to be counted. Talk with your dietitian to determine how to count these in your meal plan.
4. Look for fat-free salad dressings in smaller amounts on the Free Foods list.

**One exchange equals 15 grams carbohydrate,
or 1 starch, or 1 fruit, or 1 milk.**

Food	Serving Size	Exchanges per Serving
Angel food cake, unfrosted	$1/12$ cake	2 carbohydrates
Brownie, small unfrosted	2-in square	1 carbohydrate, 1 fat
Cake, unfrosted	2-in square	1 carbohydrate, 1 fat
Cake frosted	2-in square	2 carbohydrates, 1 fat
Cookie, fat-free	2 small	1 carbohydrate
Cookie or sandwich cookie with creme filling	2 small	1 carbohydrate, 1 fat
Cupcake, frosted	1 small	2 carbohydrates, 1 fat
Cranberry sauce, jellied	$1/4$ cup	2 carbohydrates
Doughnut, plain cake	1 medium ($1^1/2$ oz)	$1^1/2$ carbohydrates, 2 fats
Doughnut, glazed	$3^3/4$ in across (2 oz)	2 carbohydrates, 2 fats
Fruit juice bars, frozen, 100% juice	1 bar (3 oz)	1 carbohydrate
Fruit snacks, chewy (pureed fruit concentrate)	1 roll ($3/4$ oz)	1 carbohydrate
Fruit spreads, 100% fruit	1 Tbsp	1 carbohydrate
Gelatin, regular	$1/2$ cup	1 carbohydrate
Gingersnaps	3	1 carbohydrate
Granola bar	1 bar	1 carbohydrate, 1 fat
Granola bar, fat-free	1 bar	2 carbohydrates
Hummus	$1/3$ cup	1 carbohydrate, 1 fat
Ice cream	$1/2$ cup	1 carbohydrate, 2 fats
Ice cream, light	$1/2$ cup	1 carbohydrate, 1 fat
Ice cream, fat-free, no sugar added	$1/2$ cup	1 carbohydrate
Jam or jelly, regular	1 Tbsp	1 carbohydrate
Milk, chocolate, whole	1 cup	2 carbohydrates, 1 fat
Pie, fruit, 2 crusts	$1/6$ pie	3 carbohydrates, 2 fats
Pie, pumpkin or custard	$1/8$ pie	1 carbohydrate, 2 fats
Potato chips	12–18 (1 oz)	1 carbohydrate, 2 fats
Pudding, regular (made with low-fat milk)	$1/2$ cup	2 carbohydrates
Pudding, sugar-free (made with low-fat milk)	$1/2$ cup	1 carbohydrate
Salad dressing, fat-free*	$1/4$ cup	1 carbohydrate

*400 mg or more sodium per exchange.

Food	Serving Size	Exchanges per Serving
Sherbet, sorbet	$1/2$ cup	2 carbohydrates
Spaghetti or pasta sauce, canned*	$1/2$ cup	1 carbohydrate, 1 fat
Sweet roll or danish	1 ($2^1/2$ oz)	$2^1/2$ carbohydrates, 2 fats
Syrup, light	2 Tbsp	1 carbohydrate
Syrup, regular	1 Tbsp	1 carbohydrate
Syrup, regular	$1/4$ cup	4 carbohydrates
Tortilla chips	6–12 (1 oz)	1 carbohydrate, 2 fats
Yogurt, frozen, low-fat, fat-free	$1/3$ cup	1 carbohydrate, 0–1 fat
Yogurt, frozen, fat-free, no sugar added	$1/2$ cup	1 carbohydrate
Yogurt, low-fat with fruit	1 cup	3 carbohydrates, 0–1 fat
Vanilla wafers	5	1 carbohydrate, 1 fat

VEGETABLE LIST

Vegetables that contain small amounts of carbohydrates and calories are on this list. Vegetables contain important nutrients. Try to eat at least two or three vegetable choices each day. In general, one vegetable exchange is:

- $1/2$ cup of cooked vegetables or vegetable juice
- 1 cup of raw vegetables

If you eat one to two vegetable choices at a meal or snack, you do not have to count the calories or carbohydrates because they contain small amounts of these nutrients.

Nutrition Tips

1. Fresh and frozen vegetables have less added salt than canned vegetables. Drain and rinse canned vegetables if you want to remove some salt.

2. Choose more dark green and dark yellow vegetables, such as spinach, broccoli, romaine, carrots, chilies, and peppers.

3. Broccoli, brussels sprouts, cauliflower, greens, pepper, spinach, and tomatoes are good sources of vitamin C.

4. Vegetables contain 1 to 4 grams of fiber per serving.

*400 mg or more sodium per exchange.

Selection Tips

1. A 1-cup portion of broccoli is a portion about the size of a light bulb.
2. Tomato sauce is different from spaghetti sauce, which is on the Other Carbohydrates list.
3. Canned vegetables and juices are available without added salt.
4. If you eat more than 4 cups of raw vegetables or 2 cups of cooked vegetables at one meal, count them as 1 carbohydrate choice.
5. Starchy vegetables such as corn, peas, winter squash, and potatoes that contain larger amounts of calories and carbohydrates are on the Starch list.

**One vegetable exchange equals 5 grams carbohydrate,
2 grams protein, 0 grams fat, and 25 calories.**

Vegetables

Artichoke
Artichoke hearts
Asparagus
Beans (green, wax, Italian)
Bean sprouts
Beets
Broccoli
Brussels sprouts
Cabbage
Carrots
Cauliflower
Celery
Cucumber
Eggplant
Green onions or scallions
Greens (collard, kale, mustard, turnip)
Kohlrabi
Leeks
Mixed vegetables (without corn, peas, or pasta)

Mushrooms
Okra
Onions
Pea pods
Peppers (all varieties)
Radishes
Salad greens (endive, escarole, lettuce, romaine, spinach)
Sauerkraut*
Spinach
Summer squash
Tomato
Tomatoes, canned
Tomato sauce*
Tomato/vegetable juice*
Turnips
Water chestnuts
Watercress
Zucchini

MEAT AND MEAT SUBSTITUTES LIST

Meat and meat substitutes that contain both protein and fat are on this list. In general, one meat exchange is:

- 1 oz meat, fish, poultry, or cheese
- $1/2$ cup dried beans

*400 mg or more sodium per exchange.

Based on the amount of fat they contain, meats are divided into very lean, lean, medium-fat, and high-fat lists. This is done so you can see which ones contain the least amount of fat. One ounce (one exchange) of each of these includes:

	Carbohydrate (g)	Protein (g)	Fat (g)	Calories
Very Lean	0	7	0–1	35
Lean	0	7	3	35
Medium-fat	0	7	5	75
High-fat	0	7	8	100

Nutrition Tips

1. Choose very lean and lean meat choices whenever possible. Items from the high-fat group are high in saturated fat, cholesterol, and calories and can raise blood cholesterol levels.
2. Meats do not have any fiber.
3. Dried beans, peas, and lentils are good sources of fiber.
4. Some processed meats, seafood, and soy products may contain carbo-hydrate when consumed in large amounts. Check the Nutrition Facts on the label to see if the amount is close to 15 grams. If so, count it as a carbohydrate choice as well as a meat choice.

Selection Tips

1. Weigh meat after cooking and removing bones and fat. Four ounces of raw meat is equal to 3 ounces of cooked meat. Some examples of meat portions are:
   - 1 ounce cheese = 1 meat choice and is about the size of a 1-inch cube
   - 2 ounces meat = 2 meat choices, such as
     - 1 small chicken leg or thigh
     - $^1/_2$ cup cottage cheese or tuna
   - 3 ounces meat = 3 meat choices and is about the size of a deck of cards, such as
     - 1 medium pork chop
     - 1 small hamburger
     - $^1/_2$ of a whole chicken breast
     - 1 unbreaded fish fillet
2. Limit your choices from the high-fat group to three times per week or less.
3. Most grocery stores stock Select and Choice grades of meat. Select grades of meat are the leanest meats. Choice grades contain a moder-ate amount of fat, and Prime cuts of meat have the highest amount of fat. Restaurants usually serve Prime cuts of meat.

4. "Hamburger" may contain added seasoning and fat, but ground beef does not.
5. Read labels to find products that are low in fat and cholesterol (5 grams or less of fat per serving).
6. Dried beans, peas, and lentils are also found on the Starch list.
7. Peanut butter, in smaller amounts, is also found on the Fat list.
8. Bacon, in smaller amounts, is also found on the Fat list.

Meal Planning Tips
1. Bake, roast, broil, grill, poach, steam, or boil these foods rather than frying.
2. Place meat on a rack so the fat will drain off during cooking.
3. Use a nonstick spray and a nonstick pan to brown or fry foods.
4. Trim off visible fat before or after cooking.
5. If you add flour, bread crumbs, coating mixes, fat, or marinades when cooking, ask your dietitian how to count it in your meal plan.

Very Lean Meat and Substitutes List

One exchange equals 0 grams carbohydrate, 7 grams protein, 0–1 grams fat, and 35 calories.

One very lean meat exchange is equal to one of the following items:

Poultry: Chicken or turkey (white meat, no skin), Cornish hen
(no skin). . . . . 1 oz
Fish: Fresh or frozen cod, flounder, haddock, halibut,
trout; tuna (fresh or canned in water). . . . . 1 oz
Shellfish: Clams, crab, lobster, scallops, shrimp, imitation shellfish . . 1 oz
Game: Duck or pheasant (no skin), venison, buffalo, ostrich . . . . 1 oz
Cheese with 1 gram or less of fat per ounce:
   Nonfat or low-fat cottage cheese . . . . $^{1}/_{4}$ cup
   Fat-free cheese. . . . . 1 oz
Other: Processed sandwich meats with 1 gram or less fat
per ounce, such as deli thin, shaved meats, chipped beef,*
turkey ham. . . . . 1 oz
   Egg whites 2
   Egg substitutes, plain . . . . $^{1}/_{4}$ cup
   Hot dogs with 1 gram or less fat per ounce*. . . . . 1 oz
   Kidney (high in cholesterol) . . . . 1 oz
   Sausage with 1 gram or less fat per ounce . . . . 1 oz

Count as one very lean meat and one starch exchange:

Dried beans, peas, lentils (cooked) . . . . $^{1}/_{2}$ cup

*400 mg or more sodium per exchange.

Lean Meat and Substitutes List

> **One exchange equals 0 grams carbohydrate, 7 grams protein,**
> **3 grams fat, and 55 calories.**

One lean meat exchange is equal to any one of the following items:

Beef: USDA Select or Choice grades of lean beef trimmed of fat,
  such as round, sirloin, and flank steak; tenderloin; roast (rib,
  chuck, rump); steak (T-bone, porterhouse, cubed), ground round . . . 1 oz

Pork: Lean pork, such as fresh ham; canned, cured, or boiled ham;
  Canadian bacon*; tenderloin, center loin chop . . . . 1 oz

Lamb: Roast, chop, leg . . . . 1 oz

Veal: Lean chop, roast. . . . . 1 oz

Poultry: Chicken, turkey (dark meat, no skin), chicken white
  meat (with skin), domestic duck or goose (well-drained of fat,
  no skin) . . . . 1 oz

Fish:
  Herring (uncreamed or smoked) . . . . 1 oz
  Oysters . . . . 6 medium
  Salmon (fresh or canned), catfish . . . . 1 oz
  Sardines (canned) . . . . 2 medium
  Tuna (canned in oil, drained) . . . . 1 oz

Game: Goose (no skin), rabbit . . . . 1 oz

Cheese:
  4.5%-fat cottage cheese . . . . $^{1}/_{4}$ cup
  Grated Parmesan . . . . 2 Tbsp
  Cheeses with 3 grams or less fat per ounce. . . . . 1 oz

Other:
Hot dogs with 3 grams or less fat per ounce* . . . . $1^{1}/_{2}$ oz

Processed sandwich meat with 3 grams or less fat per ounce,
  such as turkey pastrami or kielbasa . . . . 1 oz

Liver, heart (high in cholesterol). . . . . 1 oz

Medium-Fat Meat and Substitutes List

> **One exchange equals 0 grams carbohydrate, 7 grams protein,**
> **5 grams fat, and 75 calories.**

One medium-fat meat exchange is equal to any one of the following
  items:

Beef: Most beef products fall into this category (ground beef,
  meatloaf, corned beef, short ribs, Prime grades of meat
  trimmed of fat, such as prime rib) . . . . 1 oz

*400 mg or more sodium per exchange.

Pork: Top loin, chop, Boston butt, cutlet . . . . 1 oz
Lamb: Rib roast, ground . . . . 1 oz
Veal: Cutlet (ground or cubed, unbreaded). 1 oz
Poultry: Chicken dark meat (with skin), ground turkey or ground
  chicken, fried chicken (with skin). . . . . 1 oz
Fish: Any fried fish product . . . . 1 oz
Cheese with 5 grams or less fat per ounce:
  Feta . . . . 1 oz
  Mozzarella . . . . 1 oz
  Ricotta . . . . $1/4$ cup (2 oz)
Other:
Egg (high in cholesterol, limit to 3 per week) 1
Sausage with 5 grams or less fat per ounce . . . . 1 oz
Soy milk . . . . 1 cup
Tempeh . . . . $1/4$ cup
Tofu . . . . 4 oz or $1/2$ cup

High-Fat Meat and Substitutes List

**One exchange equals 0 grams carbohydrate, 7 grams protein,
8 grams fat, and 100 calories.**

Remember these items are high in saturated fat, cholesterol, and calories
and may raise blood cholesterol levels if eaten on a regular basis. One
high-fat meat exchange is equal to any one of the following items:

Pork: Spareribs, ground pork, pork sausage. . . . . 1 oz
Cheese: All regular cheeses, such as American,* cheddar,
  Monterey Jack, Swiss. . . . . 1 oz
Other: Processed sandwich meats with 8 grams or less fat
  per ounce, such as bologna, pimento loaf, salami. . . . . 1 oz
Sausage, such as bratwurst, Italian, knockwurst, Polish, smoked . . . . 1 oz
Hot dog (turkey or chicken)* 1 (10/lb)
Bacon . . . . 3 slices (20 slices/lb)

Count as one high-fat meat plus one fat exchange:

Hot dog (beef, pork, or combination)* 1 (10/lb)
Peanut butter (contains unsaturated fat). 2 Tbsp

FAT LIST
Fats are divided into three groups, based on the main type of fat they
contain: monounsaturated, polyunsaturated, and saturated. Small
amounts of monounsaturated and polyunsaturated fats in the foods we

*400 mg or more sodium per exchange.

eat are linked with good health benefits. Saturated fats are linked with heart disease and cancer. In general, one fat exchange is:

- 1 teaspoon of regular margarine or vegetable oil
- 1 tablespoon of regular salad dressings

Nutrition Tips

1. All fats are high in calories. Limit serving sizes for good nutrition and health.
2. Nuts and seeds contain small amounts of fiber, protein, and magnesium.
3. If blood pressure is a concern, choose fats in the unsalted form to help lower sodium intake, such as unsalted peanuts.

Selection Tips

1. Check the Nutrition Facts on food labels for serving sizes. One fat exchange is based on a serving size containing 5 grams of fat.
2. When selecting regular margarine, choose those with liquid vegetable oil as the first ingredient. Soft margarines are not as saturated as stick margarines. Soft margarines are healthier choices. Avoid those listing hydrogenated or partially hydrogenated fat as the first ingredient.
3. When selecting low-fat margarines, look for liquid vegetable oil as the second ingredient. Water is usually the first ingredient.
4. When used in smaller amounts, bacon and peanut butter are counted as fat choices. When used in larger amounts, they are counted as high-fat meat choices.
5. Fat-free salad dressings are on the Other Carbohydrates list and the Free Foods list.
6. See the Free Foods list for nondairy coffee creamers, whipped topping, and fat-free products, such as margarines, salad dressings, mayonnaise, sour cream, cream cheese, and nonstick cooking spray.

Monounsaturated Fats List

One fat exchange equals 5 grams fat and 45 calories.

Avocado, medium . . . . $^{1}/_{8}$ (1 oz)
Oil (canola, olive, peanut) . . . . 1 tsp
Olives: ripe (black) . . . . 8 large
    green, stuffed* . . . . 10 large
Nuts:
    almonds, cashews . . . . 6 nuts
    mixed (50% peanuts) . . . . 6 nuts

*400 mg or more sodium per exchange.

peanuts . . . . 10 nuts
pecans . . . . 4 halves
Peanut butter, smooth or crunchy . . . . 2 tsp
Sesame seeds . . . . 1 Tbsp
Tahini paste . . . . 2 tsp

Polyunsaturated Fats List

One fat exchange equals 5 grams fat and 45 calories.

Margarine: stick, tub, or squeeze . . . . 1 tsp
  lower-fat (30% to 50% vegetable oil) . . . . 1 Tbsp
Mayonnaise: regular . . . . 1 tsp
  reduced-fat . . . . 1 Tbsp
Nuts: walnuts, English . . . . 4 halves
Oil (corn, safflower, soybean) . . . . 1 tsp
Salad dressing: regular* . . . . 1 Tbsp
  reduced-fat . . . . 2 Tbsp
Miracle Whip Salad Dressing®: regular . . . . 2 tsp
  reduced-fat . . . . 1 Tbsp
Seeds: pumpkin, sunflower . . . . 1 Tbsp

Saturated Fats List**

One fat exchange equals 5 grams fat and 45 calories.

Bacon, cooked . . . . 1 slice (20 slices/lb)
Bacon, grease . . . . 1 tsp
Butter: stick . . . . 1 tsp
  whipped . . . . 1 tsp
  reduced-fat . . . . 1 Tbsp
Chitterlings, boiled . . . . 2 Tbsp ($1/2$ oz)
Coconut, sweetened, shredded . . . . 2 Tbsp
Cream, half and half . . . . 2 Tbsp
Cream cheese: regular . . . . 1 Tbsp ($1/2$ oz)
  reduced-fat . . . . 2 Tbsp (1 oz)
Fatback or salt pork, see below†
Shortening or lard . . . . 1 tsp
Sour cream: regular . . . . 2 Tbsp
  reduced-fat . . . . 3 Tbsp

*400 mg or more sodium per exchange.
**Saturated fats can raise blood cholesterol levels.
†Use a piece 1 in × 1 in × $1/4$ in if you plan to eat fatback cooked with vegetables. Use a piece 2 in × 1 in × $1/2$ in when eating only the vegetables with the fatback removed.

FREE FOODS LIST

A free food is any food or drink that contains less than 20 calories or less than 5 grams of carbohydrate per serving. Foods with a serving size listed should be limited to three servings per day. Be sure to spread them out throughout the day. If you eat all three servings at one time, it could affect your blood glucose level. Foods listed without a serving size can be eaten as often as you like.

Fat-Free or Reduced-Fat Foods

Cream cheese, fat-free . . . . 1 Tbsp
Creamers, nondairy, liquid . . . . 1 Tbsp
Creamers, nondairy, powdered . . . . 2 tsp
Mayonnaise, fat-free . . . . 1 Tbsp
Mayonnaise, reduced-fat. . . . . 1 tsp
Margarine, fat-free. . . . . 4 Tbsp
Margarine, reduced-fat . . . . 1 tsp
Miracle Whip®, nonfat . . . . 1 Tbsp
Miracle Whip®, reduced-fat. . . . . 1 tsp
Nonstick cooking spray
Salad dressing, fat-free. . . . . 1 Tbsp
Salad dressing, fat-free, Italian. . . . . 2 Tbsp
Salsa . . . . ¼ cup
Sour cream, fat-free, reduced-fat . . . . 1 Tbsp
Whipped topping, regular or light . . . . 2 Tbsp
Sugar-Free or Low-Sugar Foods
Candy, hard, sugar-free . . . . 1 candy
Gelatin dessert, sugar-free
Gelatin, unflavored
Gum, sugar-free
Jam or jelly, low-sugar or light. . . . . 2 tsp
Sugar substitutes*
Syrup, sugar-free . . . . 2 Tbsp

Drinks

Bouillon, broth, consommé**
Bouillon or broth, low-sodium

*Sugar substitutes, alternatives, or replacements that are approved by the Food and Drug Administration (FDA) are safe to use. Common brand names include: Equal® (aspartame); Sprinkle® (saccharin); Sweet One® (acesulfame K); Sweet-10® (saccharin); Sugar Twin® (saccharin); Sweet 'n Low® (saccharin).

**400 mg or more sodium per exchange.

Carbonated or mineral water
Cocoa powder, unsweetened. . . . . 1 Tbsp
Coffee
Club soda
Diet soft drinks, sugar-free
Drink mixes, sugar-free
Tea
Tonic water, sugar-free

Condiments
Catsup . . . . 1 Tbsp
Horseradish
Lemon juice
Lime juice
Mustard
Pickles, dill* . . . . 1^1/$_2$ large
Soy sauce, regular or light*
Taco sauce . . . . 1 Tbsp
Vinegar

Seasonings
Be careful with seasonings that contain sodium or are salts, such as
garlic or celery salt, and lemon pepper.

Flavoring extracts
Garlic
Herbs, fresh or dried
Pimiento
Spices
Tabasco® or hot pepper sauce
Wine, used in cooking
Worcestershire sauce

COMBINATION FOODS LIST
Many of the foods we eat are mixed together in various combinations.
These combination foods do not fit into any one exchange list. Often it is
hard to tell what is in a casserole dish or prepared food item. This is a list
of exchanges for some typical combination foods. This list will help you
fit these foods into your meal plan. Ask your dietitian for information
about any other combination foods you would like to eat.

*400 mg or more sodium per choice.

Food Entrees	Serving Size	Exchanges per Serving
Tuna noodle casserole, lasagna, spaghetti with meatballs, chili with beans, macaroni and cheese*	1 cup (8 oz)	2 carbohydrates, 2 medium-fat meats
Chow mein (without noodles or rice)	2 cups (16 oz)	1 carbohydrate, 2 lean meats
Pizza, cheese, thin crust*	1/4 of 10 in (5 oz)	2 carbohydrates, 2 medium-fat meats, 1 fat
Pizza, meat topping, thin crust*	1/4 of 10 in (5 oz)	2 carbohydrates, 2 medium-fat meats, 2 fats
Pot pie**	1 (7 oz)	2 carbohydrates, 1 medium-fat meat, 4 fats
Frozen Entrees		
Salisbury steak with gravy, mashed potato**	1 (11 oz)	2 carbohydrates, 3 medium-fat meats, 3–4 fats
Turkey with gravy, mashed potato, dressing*	1 (11 oz)	2 carbohydrates, 2 medium-fat meats, 2 fats
Entree with less than 300 calories**	1 (8 oz)	2 carbohydrates, 3 lean meats
Soups		
Bean**	1 cup	1 carbohydrate, 1 very lean meat
Cream (made with water)**	1 cup (8 oz)	1 carbohydrate, 1 fat
Split pea (made with water)**	1/2 cup (4 oz)	1 carbohydrate
Tomato (made with water)**	1 cup (8 oz)	1 carbohydrate
Vegetable beef, chicken noodle, or other broth-type**	1 cup (8 oz)	1 carbohydrate

*400 mg or more of sodium per exchange.
**400 mg or more sodium per choice.

FAST FOODS LIST

Food	Serving Size	Exchanges per Serving
Burritos with beef*	2	4 carbohydrates, 2 medium-fat meats, 2 fats
Chicken nuggets*	6	1 carbohydrate, 2 medium-fat meats, 1 fat
Chicken breast and wing, breaded and fried*	1 each 1 each	1 carbohydrate, 4 medium-fat meats, 2 fats
Fish sandwich/tartar sauce*	1	3 carbohydrates, 1 medium-fat meat, 3 fats
French fries, thin	20–25	2 carbohydrates, 2 fats
Hamburger, regular	1	2 carbohydrates, 2 medium-fat meats
Hamburger, large*	1	2 carbohydrates, 3 medium-fat meats, 1 fat
Hot dog with bun*	1	1 carbohydrate, 1 high-fat meat, 1 fat
Individual pan pizza*	1	5 carbohydrates, 3 medium-fat meats, 3 fats
Soft-serve cone	1 medium	2 carbohydrates, 1 fat
Submarine sandwich*	1 sub (6 in.)	3 carbohydrates, 1 vegetable, 2 medium-fat meats, 1 fat
Taco, hard shell**	1 (6 oz)	2 carbohydrates, 2 medium-fat meats, 2 fats

*400 mg or more of sodium per exchange.
**400 mg or more sodium per choice.

Food	Serving Size	Exchanges per Serving
Taco, soft shell*	1 (3 oz)	1 carbohydrate, 1 medium-fat meat, 1 fat

*400 mg or more of sodium per exchange.

Note: Ask your fast-food restaurant for nutrition information about your favorite fast foods.

Exchange List 6-B	Ethnic Food Exchanges	
Food	*Serving Size*	*Food Exchange*
Mexican Foods		
Burrito, bean	1 small	2 starch
	1 large	1 medium-fat meat, 3 starch, 2 fat
Burrito, meat (beef)	1 small	1 starch, 1 medium-fat meat
	1 large	$2^1/_2$ starch, 3 medium-fat meat, 1 fat
Chili	1 cup	2 starch, 2 medium-fat meat, 1 fat
Chili sauce	2 tsp	$^1/_3$ fruit
Corn chips	1 oz (1 cup)	1 starch, 2 fat
Enchilada: meat or cheese	1 small (6" tortilla)	1 medium-fat meat
Refried beans	$^1/_2$ cup	1 starch, 1 medium-fat meat
Spanish rice	1 cup	2 starch, 1 fat
Spanish sauce	$^1/_2$ cup	$^1/_3$ fruit, 1 fat
Tamale with sauce	1	1 starch, 1 medium-fat meat
Tortilla/taco shell	6" diameter	1 starch
Taco (meat, cheese, lettuce, tomato)	1	1 starch, 2 medium fat meat
Tostada		
with refried beans	1 small	2 starch
with meat	1 small	1 starch, 1 high-fat meat
Chinese Foods		
Egg flower, soup	1 cup	$^1/_2$ medium-fat meat

Source: Data from *McCance and Widdowson's The Composition of Foods* by Paul AA, Southgate DA, Elsevier Science Publishing Company, Inc., © 1985 and Pennington JAT, Douglass JS. *Bowes and Church's Food Values of Portions Commonly Used*, Eighteenth Edition. Philadelphia: Lippincott Williams & Wilkins, 2005.

Food	Serving Size	Food Exchange
Fried rice (rice, meat, eggs, onions)	1 cup	$1^1/_2$ starch, $^1/_2$ medium-fat meat
Fortune cookies	1	$^1/_2$ starch or $^1/_2$ fruit
Egg roll	1	$^1/_2$ starch, 1 vegetable
Chow mein	1 cup	1 starch, 1 medium-fat meat, 1 vegetable
Sukiyaki	1 cup	3 medium-fat meat, 1 fat
Tofu	2 oz	$^1/_2$ medium-fat meat
Chop suey	1 cup	2 medium-fat meat, 1 vegetable
Pepper steak	1 cup	1 starch, 3 medium-fat meat, 1 vegetable
Chow mein noodles	$^1/_2$ cup	1 starch, 1 fat
Egg foo young	1	1 vegetable, 2 medium-fat meat, 2 fat
East Indian Foods		
Alu Mattar (curried potatoes and peas)	1 cup	1 vegetable, $1^1/_2$ starch, 3 fat
Alu Paratha (flat whole wheat bread with spiced potato filling)	6" diameter	$2^1/_2$ starch, 6 fat
Chana Dal (curried chick peas)	$^1/_2$ cup	2 medium-fat meat
Kheema do Pyaza (curied ground lamb) with onions	1 cup	2 vegetable, 3 lean meat, 3 fat
Kofta (approx. $1^1/_2$" diameter)	3 balls	3 high-fat meat, 4 fat
Machli aur tomatar (curried halibut)	3 oz fish	$^1/_2$ vegetable, 3 lean meat, $1^1/_2$ fat

Food	Serving Size	Food Exchange
Masala dosai (crepe-like pancake with spiced potato filling)	1	2 starch, 4 fat
Chicken curry	3 oz chicken	$1/2$ vegetable, 3 lean meat, 2 fat
Samosas (deep-fried filled pastries)		
(potato filling)	1 large or 3 small	1 starch, 2 fat
(lamb filling)	1 large or 3 small	1 starch, $1/2$ lean meat, $2^1/2$ fat
Italian Foods		
Vermicelli soup	1 cup	1 starch
Minestrone soup	1 cup	1 starch, 1 fat
Pasta, cooked	$1/2$ cup	1 medium-fat meat
Italian ham (Prosciutto)	1 oz	1 medium-fat meat
Meatballs	1 oz	1 medium-fat meat
Chicken cacciatore	3 oz chicken with sauce	3 lean meat, 1 vegetable, 1 fat
Eggplant parmesan	1 cup	2 medium-fat meat, 2 vegetable, 1 starch, $1^1/2$ fat
Veal parmesan	1 cutlet (4 oz)	1 starch, 4 medium-fat meat, 1 vegetable, 1 fat
Italian spaghetti	1 cup	2 starch, 2 vegetable, 2 medium-fat meat
Lasagna	1 (3" × 4") serving	1 starch, 1 vegetable, $2^1/2$ medium-fat meat
Manicotti	1 shell	$1^1/2$ starch, 1 vegetable, 3 medium-fat meat, 2 fat
Pizza with cheese, sausage, pepperoni	$1/4$ of 16 oz pizza	2 starch, 1 vegetable, 2 medium-fat meat, 1 fat

Food	Serving Size	Food Exchange
Ravioli		2 starch, 1 vegetable
with cheese	1 cup	1 medium-fat meat, 1 fat
with beef	1 cup	2 starch, 1 vegetable, 1 medium-fat meat, 1 fat
Jewish Foods		
Bagel	$1/2$	1 starch
Bialy	1	1 starch
Challah	1 slice	1 starch
Matzo, 6" diameter	1	1 starch
Matzo, crackers	7 ($1^1/2$" square each)	1 starch
Potato latkes (calculate the fat used in cooking)	$1/2$ cup	1 starch
Kippered herring	1 oz	1 lean meat
Pickled herring	1 oz	1 lean meat
Smoked salmon (lox)	1 oz	1 lean meat
Corned beef	1 oz	1 high-fat meat
Chopped liver	1 oz	1 high-fat meat

Adherence Tool 6-1   One-Day Food Record (Monitoring Device)

Name _____

		No. of Exchanges	Type of Foods and Amount
Breakfast	Bread		
	Fruit		
	Milk		
	Meat		
	Fat		
Midmorning	Bread		
	Fruit		
	Milk		
	Meat		
	Fat		
Lunch	Bread		
	Fruit		
	Veg. A		
	Veg. B		
	Milk		
	Meat		
	Fat		
Midafternoon	Bread		
	Fruit		
	Milk		
	Meat		
	Fat		
Dinner	Bread		
	Fruit		
	Veg. A		
	Veg. B		
	Milk		
	Meat		
	Fat		
Bedtime	Bread		
	Fruit		
	Milk		
	Meat		
	Fat		

Adherence Tool 6-2   One-Week Check-Off System to Identify Morning Snacking Problems (Monitoring Device)

Monday

Tuesday

Wednesday

Thursday

Friday

Saturday

Sunday

+ = Had a snack
* = Avoided a snack

Adherence Tool 6-3   Graph of Breakfast TAG Values Based on Diet Records Completed Between Visits (Monitoring Device)

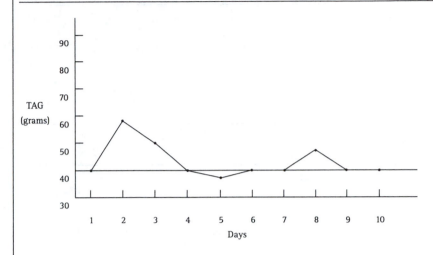

Adherence Tool 6-4   Graph of Blood Glucose and Glycosylated Hemoglobin Levels (Monitoring Device)

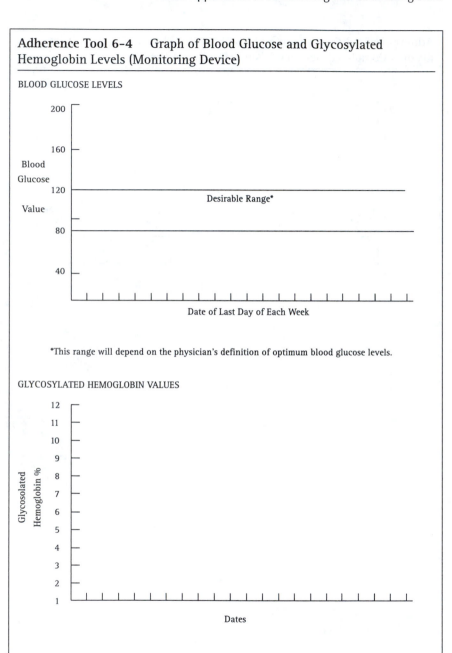

BLOOD GLUCOSE LEVELS

*This range will depend on the physician's definition of optimum blood glucose levels.

GLYCOSYLATED HEMOGLOBIN VALUES

Adherence Tool 6-5 Monthly Check-Off System for Pre-Meal Insulin Injections (Monitoring Device)

ONE–MONTH CALENDAR

Sun.	Mon.	Tues.	Wed.	Thur.	Fri.	Sat.

month of _____ 20_____. If you have any questions, please call: _____

Adherence Tool 6-6   Individualized Exchanges for Meal Planning (Informational Device)

Starch/Bread List
Cereals/grains and pasta, $1/2$ cup
   Grapenuts, $1/4$ cup
Starch vegetable
   Corn, $1/2$ cup
   Potato, baked, 1 small (3 ounces)
Bread
   Whole wheat bread, 1 slice
     (1 ounce)

Meat List
   Lean meats, 1 ounce
   Beef sirloin, 1 ounce
   Canned ham, 1 ounce
   Chicken, 1 ounce
   Tuna, 1 ounce
   Cottage cheese, $1/4$ cup

Vegetable List
   Cooked vegetables, $1/2$ cup
   Raw vegetables, 1 cup

Fruit List
   Apple, raw, 2 inches across, 1
   Banana (9 inches long), $1/2$
   Pear, large, $1/2$
   Raisins, 2 tablespoons
   Orange juice, $1/2$ cup

Milk List
   1% milk, 1 cup

Fat List
   Margarine, 1 teaspoon
   Reduced-calorie mayonnaise,
     1 tablespoon

Adherence Tool 6-7 Practice with Exchanges and Total Available
Glucose (TAG) (Informational Device)

Determine the exchanges and TAG for each of the following foods:

	Exchanges	TAG
Corn, $1/2$ cup		
Orange juice, 6 ounces		
Poached egg, 1		
Chicken, 3 ounces		
Pork chop, 2 ounces		
Tuna fish, $1/2$ cup		
Green beans, $3/4$ cup		
Saltine crackers, 6		
Party crackers (Triscuits), 5		
Graham crackers, 3		
Skim milk, 8 ounces		
Whole milk, 8 ounces		
Peanut butter, 2 tablespoons		
Italian dressing, 1 tablespoon		
Wheat bread, 2 slices		
Mayonnaise, 1 tablespoon		
Grape juice, $2/3$ cup		
Grapes, 15		
Watermelon, $1 1/4$ cup		
Small olives, 10		
Stick pretzels, $3/4$ ounces		
Dry nonfat milk, $1/3$ cup		
Baked beans, $1/2$ cup		
French fries, 10 ($3 1/2$ inches long)		
Muffin, 1, small plain		
Bacon, 2 slices		
American cheese, 1 ounce		
Bran Buds®, $1/2$ cup		
Oatmeal, 1 cup		
Plain nonfat yogurt, 1 cup		
Sour cream, $1/2$ cup		
Sherbet, $1/2$ cup		

continued

Adherence Tool 6-7 *continued*

List the amount of carbohydrate, protein, fat, and kilocalories in the following exchange groups:

Exchange	Carbohydrate (grams)	Protein (grams)	Fat (grams)	Kilo-calories (grams)	TAG
Bread					
Milk (skim)					
Fat					
Vegetable					
Meat					
Fruit					

Adherence Tool 6-8   Total Available Glucose (TAG) (Informational Device)

TAG = Carbohydrate (CHO) (g) + [Animal Protein (PRO) (g) 0.58]

	CHO	+ PRO (0.58)	= TAG
1 Fruit Exchange	= 15 g	+ 0	= 15
1 Meat Exchange	= 0	+ 7 g (0.58)	= 4
1 Milk Exchange	= 12 g	+ 8 g (0.58)	= 17
1 Bread Exchange	= 15 g	+ 0	= 15
1 Vegetable Exchange	= 5 g	+ 0	= 5

The number that results from this formula can be used to determine what each of your meals might include.

Counting total available glucose (TAG) is a way of ensuring consistency in diet from day to day. We count carbohydrate because we know it tends to raise blood sugars. Animal proteins also raise blood sugar levels because they are eventually converted to carbohydrate by our bodies. Fat does not raise blood sugar levels because very little of it is converted to carbohydrate. We do try to keep fat intake low enough to prevent increases in weight and also consider the type of fat you eat to prevent coronary heart disease.

Adherence Tool 6-9   Worksheet for Calculating Exchanges and Total Available Glucose (TAG) in a Recipe: Chocolate Cookies (Informational Device)

$1^1/_4$ cups flour	1 egg
$^1/_2$ teaspoon baking soda	$^1/_3$ cup buttermilk
$^1/_2$ teaspoon salt	1 teaspoon vanilla
$^1/_2$ cup butter or margarine	2 ounces melted unsweetened chocolate
1 cup white sugar	$^1/_2$ cup chopped walnuts

Ingredients	Fruit	Veg	Bread	Meat	Fat	Milk	TAG
$1^1/_4$ cups flour							
$^1/_2$ teaspoon baking soda							
$^1/_2$ teaspoon salt							
$^1/_2$ cup butter or margarine							
1 cup white sugar							
1 egg							
$^1/_3$ cup buttermilk							
1 teaspoon vanilla							
2 ounces melted chocolate							
$^1/_2$ cup walnuts							

Total Exchanges: Bread _____   Fruit _____
                    Meat _____   Vegetable _____
                    Fat _____   Milk _____
                    TAG _____
Exchanges per Serving _____
TAG per Serving   _____

Directions: Indicate what portion of an exchange each ingredient contains. Divide by the number of servings for each ingredient to obtain total exchanges and exchanges per serving. Use Pennington* to calculate TAG for each ingredient and per serving.

*Pennington JAT, Church HN, *Bowes and Church's Food Values of Portions Commonly Used,* copyright © 1995, Lippincott-Raven Publishers.

Adherence Tool 6-10   Worksheet for Calculating Exchanges and Total Available Glucose (TAG) in a Recipe: Chicken Soup (Informational Device)

12 ounces cooked chicken weigh after removing from bone	$1/4$ cup diced onion
	$1/2$ teaspoon salt
	$1/8$ teaspoon pepper
$1/3$ cup rice, uncooked	$1/2$ teaspoon celery salt
$1/2$ cup diced celery	4 cups water
$1/2$ cup carrots, chopped	

Ingredients	Fruit	Veg	Bread	Meat	Fat	Milk	TAG
12 ounces chicken							
$1/3$ cup rice, uncooked							
$1/2$ cup diced celery							
$1/2$ cup carrots, chopped							
$1/4$ cup diced onion							
$1/2$ teaspoon salt							
$1/8$ teaspoon pepper							
$1/2$ teaspoon celery salt							
4 cups water							

Total Exchanges: Bread _____   Fruit _____

Meat _____   Vegetable _____

Fat _____   Milk _____

TAG_____

Exchanges per Serving _____

TAG per Serving   _____

Adherence Tool 6-11   Worksheet for Calculating Exchanges and Total Available Glucose (TAG) in a Recipe: Chicken Almond Oriental (Informational Device) (4–6 Servings)

Ingredients	Fruit	Veg	Bread	Meat	Fat	Milk	TAG
1 pound chicken breast without bone and skin							
1¹/₂ cups broccoli cut into1" pieces							
¹/₂ cup blanched almonds							
1 teaspoon cornstarch							
¹/₂ teaspoon sugar							
2 tablespoons soy sauce							
2 tablespoons dry sherry							
1 medium onion, cut into thin wedges							
¹/₂ cup water chestnuts, thinly sliced							
¹/₂ cup bamboo shoots							
Total Exchanges:							
Exchanges per Serving:							
TAG per Serving:							

Adherence Tool 6-12   Weighing and Measuring (Informational Device)

STANDARD:	Weight	Carbo-hydrate	Protein	Fat
Apple, raw, 1 medium, with skin (without core)	138 grams	21.1	0.3	0.5

ACTUAL:
Your apple weighs 200 grams
(without core).

$$\frac{\text{Weight of Standards}}{\text{Carbohydrate (g) of Standard}} = \frac{\text{Weight of Actual}}{\text{Carbohydrate (g) in Actual}}$$

$$\frac{138}{21.1} = \frac{200}{X}$$

$$138X = 200 \times 21.1$$

$$X = \frac{200 \times 21.1}{138}$$

$$X = 30.6 \text{ g of Carbohydrate in your actual serving}$$

Adherence Tool 6-13   Total Available Glucose (TAG) for Mixed Food

---

1. Philly Sandwich	Carbo-hydrate	Protein	Fat
	45 grams	28 grams	24 grams

---

2. How much of the 28 grams of protein is vegetable protein? How many bread exchanges are in 45 grams of carbohydrate? 45/15 grams carbohydrate in each exchange = 3 bread exchanges. Protein = 3 grams in 1 bread exchange.

    $3 \times 3 = 9$ grams vegetable protein.

3. Subtract grams of vegetable protein from grams of total protein to get grams of animal protein:

    $28 - 9 = 19$ grams of animal protein

4. Use TAG formula:

$$\begin{aligned} \text{TAG} &= \text{Carbohydrate grams} + (\text{Animal Protein} \times 0.58) \\ \text{TAG} &= 45 + (19 \times 0.58 \text{ grams}) \\ \text{TAG} &= 45 + 11.02 \\ \text{TAG} &= 56.02 \text{ grams} \end{aligned}$$

Adherence Tool 6–14   Calculating Total Available Glucose (TAG)

1. Look for food value in Pennington.*

Standard Value:	3.5 oz Meat
	25.2 g Protein

2. Determine (by weighing) your meat portion.

    $$\frac{\text{2 oz Meat}}{X}$$

3. Calculate the ratio and proportion.

    $$\frac{\text{3 oz}}{\text{25.2 grams Protein}} = \frac{\text{2 oz}}{X}$$

    $$3X = 2 \times 25.2$$
    $$3X = 50.4$$
    $$X = 16.8 \text{ grams Protein}$$

4. Calculate TAG = grams Protein × 0.58

    $$\text{TAG} = 16.8 \times 0.58$$
    $$\text{TAG} = 9.74 \text{ grams}$$

5. Add this TAG to total Carbohydrate in rest of meal.

*Pennington JAT, Douglass JS. *Bowes and Church's Food Values of Portions Commonly Used*, Eighteenth Edition. Philadelphia: Lippincott Williams & Wilkins, 2005.

Adherence Tool 6-15 Your Favorite Meals: Are They Meeting Your Goals?

<table>
<tr><td align="center">**Breakfast**</td><td align="center">**Lunch**</td></tr>
<tr><td>CHO or TAG gms ____ = GOAL</td><td>CHO or TAG gms ____ = GOAL</td></tr>
<tr><td></td><td></td></tr>
<tr><td align="center">Total CHO gms ____</td><td align="center">Total CHO gms ____</td></tr>
<tr><td align="center">**Dinner**</td><td align="center">**Snack**</td></tr>
<tr><td>CHO or TAG gms ____ = GOAL</td><td>CHO or TAG gms ____ = GOAL</td></tr>
<tr><td></td><td></td></tr>
<tr><td align="center">Total CHO gms ____</td><td align="center">Total CHO gms ____</td></tr>
</table>

Adherence Tool 6-16   Worksheet for Food Labeling (Informational Device)

1. Select a label and obtain the following information:

    Product name _____

    Serving size   _____

    Number of servings per container   _____

    Calories _____

    Protein (g) _____

    Carbohydrates (g) _____

    Fat (g) _____

    Ingredients _____

    _____

    _____

    _____

2. From the information listed above, calculate the exchanges and TAG contained in this product.

3. Use this product with other foods to create a balanced meal (breakfast, lunch, or dinner), using your meal pattern.

CHAPTER 7

NUTRITION COUNSELING IN TREATMENT OF RENAL DISEASE

Chapter Objectives

1. Identify factors that lead to inappropriate eating behaviors associated with protein-modified regimens.

2. Identify specific nutrients using step 1, assessment, in the nutrition care process that should be emphasized in assessing a baseline eating pattern before providing dietary instruction in step 3, intervention.

3. As a part of step 3, identify strategies to treat inappropriate eating behaviors associated with low-protein patterns.

4. As a part of step 3, negotiate strategies to facilitate problem solving for clients who are following a protein-modified eating pattern.

5. Recommend dietary adherence tools for clients on protein-modified eating patterns.

This chapter guides the nutrition counselor who is working on potential prevention of dialysis or predialysis therapy for the person diagnosed with chronic renal insufficiency. Current facts and theories are discussed as researched by some of the foremost nephrologists in the world. The focus of this chapter is on the out-patient in a predialysis state.

Theories and Facts about Nutrition and Chronic Renal Failure

Many nephrologists recommend low-protein diets as a means of halting deterioration of renal function. Protein restriction and control of blood pressure delay the progression of renal disease in laboratory animals.[1-3] Most studies in humans[4-10] suggest that a restriction of dietary protein is beneficial, especially in patients with advanced renal disease,[4,10] but some of these studies were inconclusive because of deficiencies in their design or because changes in renal function were assessed only by measurements of serum creatinine, which may be affected by diet.

In 1978, Ibels and colleagues theorized that hyperphosphatemia was responsible for renal function deterioration,[11] and in 1982 Brenner and colleagues developed the glomerular hyperfiltration theory.[12] The Brenner hypothesis suggests that a low-protein diet halts the progression of chronic renal insufficiency in two ways: (1) by preventing the increase in glomerular plasma flow and (2) by preventing high capillary pressures. Accompanying proteinuria and structural alterations of epithelial cells seem to be less severe when persons are placed on low-protein diets predialysis. In the absence of a low-protein diet, glomerular hyperfiltration continues.[13,14] As the function of sclerosing glomeruli is lost, less severely affected glomeruli undergo further compensatory hyperfiltration with subsequent injury. This process favors progression of kidney damage and eventual total loss of glomerular and renal function.

To provide data beyond the above studies, the National Institutes of Health funded the Modification of Diet in Renal Disease (MDRD) Study that included two randomized, multicenter trials involving a total of 840 patients ages 18 to 70 with various chronic renal diseases. It tested two hypotheses: (1) that two interventions— a reduction in dietary protein and phosphorus intake and the maintenance of blood pressure at a level below that usually recommended[15]—retard the progression of renal disease; and (2) that these interventions are safe and acceptable to patients for long-term use.[16-18]

In the MDRD Study, clients with moderate renal insufficiency experienced a slower decline in renal function four months after the introduction of the low-protein diet when compared with clients on a moderate-protein diet. This suggests a small benefit of low-protein diet in slowing the progression of renal disease in patients with moderate renal insufficiency. Among clients with more severe renal insufficiency, a very-low-protein diet, as compared with a low-protein diet, did not significantly slow the progression of renal disease.[19]

Following the MDRD study, a moderately reduced protein intake has been recommended for clients with diabetes and pre-end stage disease. The Institute of Medicine, Food and Nutrition Board, in 2000 using a consensus of a panel of experts provided recommendations for persons with two types of glomerular filtration rates (GFR).[20]

In 1994, a panel of nephrologists following the MDRD Study reached a consensus on management recommendations for chronic renal disease. For persons with a GFR of 25–55 mL/min/1.73 m², a standard protein intake of >0.8 grams of protein per kilogram body weight per day is recommended. If there are signs of uremia or progression of renal insufficiency, an intake of 0.8 g/kg/day is recommended as appropriate. In persons who have a GFR of 13–25 mL/min/1.73 m², an intake of 0.6 g/kg/day is deemed appropriate.[21]

The American Diabetes Association recommends that clients with diabetic nephropathy restrict intake to ~0.8 g/kg/day.[22] For clients with pre-end stage renal disease, the Renal Dietitians Dietetic Practice Group of the American Dietetic Association prescribes 0.6 to 0.8 g/kg/day.[23]

The principle of reducing dietary protein and maximizing the biological quality of protein intake in predialysis clients has been generally accepted for decades. These measures increase the efficiency with which nitrogen is used for synthesis and reduce the ingested quantities of total nitrogen, nonprotein nitrogen, potassium, phosphorus, and sulfur. This results in a reduction of the requirements for excretion of urea, uric acid, potassium, phosphate, sulfate, and organic acid and decreases the tendency of such persons to develop azotemia, acidosis, hyperkalemia, and hyperphosphatemia with their consequences.

The levels of dietary protein recommended for persons suffering from chronic renal failure to maintain nitrogen balance are controversial. Unlike persons with normal renal function, a person with renal insufficiency requires more protein because of the altered metabolism associated with uremia, which may promote protein catabolism.[24] The most obvious effects of renal insufficiency are proteinuria and occult gastrointestinal bleeding. These problems increase protein requirements not only because blood proteins may not be completely reabsorbed, but also because they cannot be resynthesized with complete efficiency. Hormonal disturbances such as hyperglucagonemia and carbohydrate intolerance along with other biochemical abnormalities in uremic persons may increase protein requirements.[25-28]

Positive nitrogen balance depends directly on caloric intake. Energy requirements depend on the level of physical activity, and an intake of 35–40 kcal/kg of body weight/day is recommended for adults not involved in heavy physical activity.[28]

Use of protein in uremia also depends, in part, on the biological value of protein. The literature indicates a range for intake of protein of high biological value from 70–75%.[29]

The role of serum phosphate in the progression of renal disease is also controversial.[11,30] Walser has found excellent clinical results with dietary phosphorus restrictions in persons with modest protein restrictions (40 grams).[31] Phosphorus was reduced by restricting intake of milk, milk products, cheese, cola beverages, and instant powdered beverages to bring the level of phosphorus down to approximately 600 milligrams, approximately one-half the usual daily intake. The MDRD Study also describes a phosphorus restriction as a part of the dietary prescription.[19]

Early in the course of renal failure, intestinal calcium absorption is reduced before serum vitamin D levels fall.[32] Later, vitamin D deficiency further aggravates this problem. Both azotemia and acidosis independently increase renal excretion of calcium.[33] Calcium balance is usually negative in uremic persons unless calcium supplementation is prescribed.[32]

Nutritionists should be aware of sodium, potassium, and acid–base balance. Persons with renal insufficiency suffer from uremic acidosis, a condition caused by accumulation of phosphate, sulfate, and organic acids, impaired ammonia excretion, and renal bicarbonate wastage. The degree of renal bicarbonate wastage is variable; therefore, the requirement for sodium bicarbonate also varies—from 0 to 14 milliequivalents per kilogram (mEq/kg) of body weight.

Decreasing dietary protein results in some improvement in acidosis because the major source of acid in acid-ash diets is dietary protein (particularly its sulfur content). Treating acidosis is important for several reasons:

- prevention of dissolution of bone salt
- reduction in symptoms associated with decreased pH (which usually are not apparent until serum bicarbonate is 16 mmol or lower)

- prevention of the protein catabolic effect of acidosis; an alka-line-ash diet, comprised mostly of fruits and vegetables, may help, but it is rather monotonous

Persons with chronic uremia differ markedly from normal persons in their ability to vary renal excretion of sodium. They excrete a large, relatively fixed fraction of filtered sodium.

Various techniques have been developed to determine an optimal level of dietary sodium in a given client. Generally, the sodium bicarbonate requirement should be assessed first, because it affects the level of sodium chloride to be given. Ideally, 24-hour sodium output should be determined first. Providing an amount of sodium chloride equal to this quantity (in milliequivalents) minus the sodium bicarbonate intake will then maintain sodium balance.

Diuretics are indicated in most cases of moderate or severe renal failure.[34] When the diuretic is administered chronically, the same extracellular fluid volume may be maintained with higher salt intake, making the diet less difficult to follow.

Potassium balance in the chronic uremic client is less of a problem than sodium balance. However, hyperkalemia is quite common in more advanced stages of renal disease. Modest reductions in high-potassium foods such as tomatoes, bananas, potatoes, and oranges can be effective. A small number of persons with renal failure may exhibit a tendency toward hypokalemia. Increasing foods high in potassium and/or potassium supplements is recommended for these individuals.

A few clients may develop hyponatremia, especially those whose intake of sodium is severely restricted or those with congestive heart failure. Water intake must be restricted to correct and prevent hyponatremia.

Vitamin and mineral levels must be assessed in the chronically uremic client. Supplements of B vitamins and vitamin C are indicated. Serum levels of vitamin A and of retinol-binding protein are commonly elevated.[35] Because these substances are normally cleared by the kidney, vitamin A should not be given. Uremic persons have low concentrations of zinc in their plasma leukocytes and hair, so supplementation is recommended.[36]

In summary, the client with chronic renal failure requires careful, consistent nutrition monitoring through blood and urine values.

Research on Adherence to Eating Patterns in Treatment of Renal Disease

Treatment for patients with renal disease involves major adjustments and stress for clients. Although compliance with renal diets can be easily monitored with laboratory tests, many physiological factors can modify the results of these tests. For persons who are losing weight because calorie intake on low-protein diets tends to be low, loss of muscle mass may contribute to urinary nitrogen, which is used as a marker for dietary compliance. There is much to learn about urinary nitrogen and the possible effect of chronic renal disease on that biological marker. In many cases, very compliant persons whose intake by self-report may look excellent are classified as noncompliant on analysis of urinary nitrogen. Researchers have found that food diaries underestimate dietary intake for a variety of reasons. In one study, subjects believed they were consuming a diet containing 0.6 grams of protein per kilogram of standard body weight based on their food record calculations, but estimated protein intake indicated they consumed approximately 0.8 grams of protein per kilogram of standard body weight.[37] Subject errors in calculating the protein content of food and/or discrepancies between protein values on the patient education materials and computerized database accounted for part of this discrepancy. Researchers in this study noted that educating subjects on how to classify foods for protein content and calculate protein intake might have narrowed the difference between self-report records and the biological marker (urinary nitrogen). Nutritionists and physicians should be aware that discrepancies between urinary nitrogen excretion and reported protein intake may reflect factors other than willful noncompliance.

When patients with renal disease were asked which parts of a diet intervention program were most helpful, they indicated self-monitoring and dietitian support.[38] Clients who were satisfied with a low-protein eating pattern at the final visit in the MDRD Study had mean protein intakes closer to their assigned protein goals.[39]

The MDRD Study focused on behavioral dietary interventions and analyzed the factors that contributed to dietary adherence.[40] The dietary program emphasized appropriate food choices that promoted healthful long-term eating patterns rather than food restrictions. Adherers indicated more favorable attitudes about their eating patterns and perceived themselves as more successful than nonadherers. More frequent telephone contacts were made with nonadherers. Dietitians made telephone calls to solve problems, reinforce strategies discussed during the visit, and provide contact between monthly visits. Results of this study indicate that adherence to low-protein eating patterns requires social support and assistance to replace energy lost by decrease in protein intake. Adherence did not seem to require ongoing provision of guidelines for reducing protein intake. Adherent patients reported that the eating pattern did not interfere with their ability to socialize. Providing patients with protein-modified products and recipes and samples of products was beneficial in promoting adherence. The frequency of self-monitoring increased with those who were adherent. As many as 51% of adherent clients self-monitored on an average of six to seven days per week throughout the two-year period of this study.[40]

Inappropriate Eating Behaviors

The person with chronic renal insufficiency who is seen as an outpatient requires a great deal of assistance in dietary adherence. The MDRD Study showed that visits during months 1 through 4 lasted for a mean of 2 to 3 hours.[41] The regimen for a predialysis client is extremely complicated and requires extra time and assistance from the dietitian. The exchange lists alone can be overwhelming for many clients who have followed other diets in the past. The MDRD Study used protein counting as a means of streamlining the renal diet.[40] A low-calorie diet in principle contrasts directly with the renal diet, so a person who has followed low-calorie diets in the past may find it difficult to readjust to the new principles of the renal diet. For example, on a low-calorie diet, fat and pure carbohydrate foods are discouraged, but on a low-protein diet they are encouraged. With reduction in protein, an increase in calories through fat and carbohydrate is essential. Weight maintenance is crucial.

A family member who is diabetic may influence a renal client to avoid foods high in simple sugars. The renal client may have difficulty accepting the idea that simple sugars are necessary on a low-protein diet to maintain adequate caloric intake.

Like clients on other restricted eating patterns, clients who have difficulties adhering to low-protein diets must struggle with social pressures that are multiplied by the large number of restrictions. Clients may drop out of social affairs to avoid the embarrassment of having to explain their health problems. "Everything in my life has changed!" is a common remark. Old eating habits are replaced by a constant preoccupation with restriction. The tradition of enjoying all food is replaced by a feeling that meals are never spontaneous but always associated with don'ts. For clients with a protein restriction, eating can become only a means of existence instead of a means of recreation.

On a protein- and phosphorus-restricted diet, usual foods may be replaced by low-protein and low-phosphorus foods that are less moist, have an aftertaste, and are lower in fiber (due to the phosphorus restriction). The result is less enjoyment in taste and texture sensations, and frequently an initial side effect is constipation because of the reduction in fiber. These negative associations with the protein-restricted diet can lead to inappropriate eating behaviors.

Assessment of Eating Behaviors

Early assessment of the client with chronic renal insufficiency is crucial to dietary success. Identification of potential problems is important. Because many of these clients suffer from uremic symptoms, signs of depression may be more frequent than in the normal population. Prior to instruction on an involved eating pattern, some clients may require psychological counseling. It is important to look for predictors of adherence, especially in clients for whom the dietary and medication regimens are very complicated. Along with the diet, there are many medications that must be taken daily (for example, multivitamins, calcium, iron, blood pressure regulators).

Identifying the support of others is crucial. Support from a spouse or significant other may signal excellent future adherence. Lack of support may signal poor adherence.

The assessment of the person with renal insufficiency also requires close attention to personal indicators. For example, before instituting a low-protein eating regimen, counselors should identify past dietary behaviors. Has the patient tried without success to follow a low-sodium diet? Good past performance is an indicator of future success with a new eating pattern. Initial assessment might include eliciting a list of reasons that the client sees as positives for following the new eating pattern and taking medications. Later, when commitment wanes, a review of the reasons and circumstances in the client's life that have altered commitment can improve adherence.

The nutrition counselor should provide an opportunity for the client to try out behaviors before actually starting a regimen. For example, holding a special event for clients centered around a holiday buffet can give them an opportunity to try some foods they might like to serve during the holiday season. Vegetable fettuccine made with low-protein pasta and nondairy creamer along with black forest cake prepared with low-protein flour and without eggs are examples of festive, low-protein dishes clients may wish to serve.

Careful, detailed assessments of dietary intake should include the protein content of the diet along with other baseline information on dietary phosphorus, potassium, sodium, calcium, and magnesium. Intake assessment might include several diet records (three a month for three months) and diet recalls (once a month for three months). In addition, a food frequency or diet history may be valuable. The questionnaire in Adherence Tool 7-1 can provide valuable information on past eating habits. Once the client is placed on the new eating pattern, Adherence Tool 7-2 might be used to monitor intake.

An assessment of medication-taking habits is also important. Many renal clients have taken blood pressure medications. Potential problems with taking medications at certain times of day may be apparent from a description of past habits.

Before providing information about a new eating pattern, the counselor should assess the client's knowledge of diets. What information does the client presently have concerning dietary exchange patterns? What impact will these patterns have on learning a new dietary exchange list? What basic principles taught in relation to past diets may no longer be true? For example, a client who has followed low-calorie diets in the past may have difficulty switching to a totally new exchange list in which foods are categorized based on protein content rather than calories. The idea of limiting high-carbohydrate, high-fat foods is no longer valid. It is extremely difficult to assure a client that on a low-protein diet, it is not only good but *mandatory* to eat high-carbohydrate, high-fat foods on a daily basis for adequate caloric intake.

Assessment of adherence to a low-protein regimen may involve medication counting, review of urine urea nitrogens, a corresponding estimated protein intake,* and a review of laboratory serum and urine values. Adherence Tool 7-3 includes a worksheet to help calculate percent adherence to medications. Adherence Tool 7-4 is an accompanying list of adherence rates at each visit that serves as a monitoring device for clients and clinicians. Graphs can also be used to track diet adherence (Adherence Tool 7-5). It is extremely important to track serum and urine laboratory values for clients on low-protein eating regimens. The laboratory data can help determine how well the client is adhering to diet and medication. Adherence Tool 7-6 includes space for recording laboratory values and corresponding normal ranges for each chemistry value. This data should be reviewed with the client, observing trends and changes in intake and describing why those changes occurred. The counselor is a facilitator asking open-ended questions, such as, "What does this graph of your intake tell you? What was happening in your life at these times?"

Treatment Strategies

Problems with low-protein eating patterns fall into the three categories mentioned for other diets: lack of knowledge, lack of planning, and lack of commitment. As with all dietary regimens, lack of planning can be easily remedied. Cueing devices can provide help when planning is a problem. Lack of commitment is the most difficult problem to solve.

---

*Equation: 6.25 × [Urine Urea Nitrogen + (0.31 × Standard Body Weight) + Urine Protein] = Estimated Protein Intake (grams per kilogram).

If urine protein is greater than 5, add it into this equation. If it is less than 5, set urine protein equal to 0. Standard body weight is rounded to the nearest 10.

Strategies Dealing with Lack of Knowledge

Before dealing with problems involving lack of knowledge (Nutrition Education; see Part II, Exhibit 2), counselors have at their disposal large quantities of information to present to the client in a variety of ways. The most potent strategy to solve lack of knowledge is tailoring. The ideal situation for tailoring allows for an individual dietary pattern and an individualized exchange list for each person. The pattern shows exchanges with amounts tailored to each client's preferred eating style, such as X ounces or grams of meat, X servings of vegetables, X servings of fruits, X servings of milk, and so on. The tailored exchange list includes only foods the client eats; all others are eliminated from the list. The tailored list is preferred over one general list for the following reasons:

- A tailored list can be very short and thus less cumbersome. Fewer items mean less work for the person learning the list.
- It allows for much greater detail. With fewer items, more information can be included for each item, such as protein, phosphorus, and calories, automatically giving the person using the list more information about the eating pattern.
- It stimulates learning because it can create a feeling of ownership.

Along with individualizing exchanges, individualized menu planning with active client participation can be an aid to later adherence. The MDRD Study used protein counting as a method of facilitating dietary adherence. When other nutrients or calories required monitoring, the nutrition counselor specified changes in certain foods which were favorites for the client.

Once counselors have presented individualized crucial information to each client, they must stage changes in eating habits to coincide with the recommended dietary components. Counselors should avoid creating the impression that they are the "experts" and in sole control. Too often, counselors present forms, lists, and other documents in a way that leaves clients feeling totally removed from the process of change. Clients begin to regard themselves as unwilling objects to be moved, shaped, and molded by the counselors. The goal during the sessions should be to shape the eating patterns with clients as they continue to follow the dietary prescription.

Researchers in the MDRD Study found that the need to provide knowledge decreased over time,[38] and the behavioral skills discussed below increased.

Staging or setting priorities for the components of a diet with several restrictions, all of which clients must follow as a package, can be difficult. Staging allows clients to solve one problem at a time while continuing to follow all restrictions to the best of their ability. Once again, clients must be very actively involved in the developmental process. In choosing which problems to work on first, counselors should consider several factors:

- Which problem, if solved, will allow the most success? Initial success can be very important to continued improvement in dietary adherence.
- Which problem is the most difficult and inhibiting from the standpoint of dietary adherence? The counselor and client may need to deal first with a very large problem that precludes following the diet. A client who refuses to comply with any recommendations may need to be seen by a psychologist or psychiatrist before any instruction on a dietary regimen.
- Which problems will be moderately difficult to solve? Once the client feels he or she is in an action stage ready for change (Nutrition Intervention Terminology: Nutrition Counseling; Theoretical Basis/Approach: Transtheoretical Model; Strategy: Motivational Interviewing; see Part II, Exhibit 2), the nutrition counselor should focus on the easiest problems to solve, then rank the more difficult problems and discuss each separately. The ultimate choice should be a product of client-counselor teamwork.

In dealing with a client on a low-protein eating pattern, staging learning can be very important. Counselors should begin by focusing on selecting appropriate amounts of food from an exchange group high in protein, choosing a group less preferred by the client so that cutting back is not impossible. The counselor should try to ensure success. The area listed as most difficult should be the last. Staging makes it possible to use attribution to facilitate adherence to a more difficult problem. For example, the counselor might say, "You have done so well in eating the required amounts of food in the milk category (Attribution). You should eventually do well in cutting back on meat." Staging may also take the form of menu planning initially to provide direct guidance in dietary adherence.

As time passes, the client will become comfortable assuming personal responsibility for menu planning.

Lack of knowledge can often be the major problem in a variety of issues. One of clients' most commonly voiced concerns is social eating, which includes eating at friends' homes and in restaurants. Tracking adherence to diets and medications shows major decreases in group adherence rates during holidays such as Hanukkah and Christmas and during vacation periods. These times involve accelerated social eating. Initial assistance in this area can be informational. Counselors can involve clients by asking them to plan a menu (Adherence Tool 7-7). Adherence Tools 7-8 and 7-9 provide practice in learning exchanges and modifying recipes, and listing favorite low-protein foods. During the holidays, counselors can help clients adhere to the eating pattern by giving information as shown in Adherence Tool 7-10. This tool was designed to allow a client who has used up all exchanges for breakfast, lunch, and dinner to select foods spontaneously at a late-night party. It shows many "free" items in terms of protein content, allows a few lower-protein foods, and says "stop" to many high-protein foods. Adherence Tool 7-11 is a birthday card that includes a recipe for a low-protein birthday cake. When signed by all clinical staff, the card becomes an important reminder and aid in following the new eating pattern at a difficult time.

Restaurant eating can be very difficult for clients following a low-protein eating pattern. It is important to provide adequate information so clients can follow the diet when eating out. A file of menus for the client's favorite restaurant is extremely valuable. Counselors can ask clients to plan a day's menu that includes eating out. It is helpful to call the restaurant before; use a menu and elicit as much information as possible on serving sizes. By giving clients enough information, counselors can make restaurant eating much less difficult.

Eating at home when following restricted-protein eating patterns can be easier if the client has access to low-protein products that provide added calories. Adherence Tool 7-12 provides space to identify low-protein products along with company names. These products make it possible to include a greater amount of some high-protein foods. For example, by eating rice, which has minimal protein content, more protein can come from meat products rather than regular bread products.

Lack of knowledge may be evidenced by the lack of ability to identify circumstances preceding and following a behavior (Nutrition Intervention Terminology: Nutrition Counseling; Theoretical Basis/Approach: Cognitive/Behavioral Theory; Strategy: Problem Solving and Stimulus Control; Part II, Exhibit 2). For example, if snacking in the evening seems to be a behavior that pushes protein intake over the recommended amount, examining events leading to that behavior may help determine how to modify it. The chain of events might be as follows: Eat dinner, wash dishes, watch TV (antecedents), eat snack of cheese and crackers (behavior), tell myself how bad I've been, feel depressed, eat a peanut butter sandwich (consequences).

Identifying the ABCs of behavior (antecedents, behavior, and consequences) makes a variety of solutions available. First, the counselor can determine how important regular, as opposed to low-protein, crackers are. It is very easy to suggest low-protein crackers and jelly as an alternative to regular crackers and cheese. If this change is too drastic, a compromise might be a mixture of mayonnaise and very small amounts of cheese (0.2 ounces), mixed and microwaved, on low-protein crackers. The positive self-reinforcement that replaces the negative reinforcement indicated in the above chain will probably make the additional peanut butter sandwich less tempting. By saying, "This is great! I can eat this snack without increasing my protein intake significantly," the client can eliminate the feelings of depression and subsequent eating.

The more self-management through self-reinforcement a counselor can help the client achieve, the greater the likelihood of dietary success.

Strategies Dealing with Lack of Planning

Cueing devices can be very helpful in avoiding lack of planning. A note on the refrigerator saying, "Eat rice with margarine today" may help keep protein low and calories high. Placing hard candy in jars throughout the house can cue the client to eat adequate calories without added protein.

Forgetting along with planning is often a problem in dealing with medication taking. Pill boxes with sections for each day's doses (morning, noon, evening, and before bed) are useful. If placed in visible areas, such as the kitchen table or counter, they can serve as prompts to taking medication (see Adherence Tool 7-13).

During vacation times, a postcard (Adherence Tool 7-14) with cues to remind the client to take medications during the trip can help avoid poor adherence. Calendars (Adherence Tool 7-15) can help document times when clients forget to take medication. Recording the amount of medication taken at each time of day can help clients see when they miss medications, and the recording may be a cue to improve adherence.

Strategies Dealing with Lack of Commitment

On a low-protein regimen with many restrictions, almost every client inevitably faces periods when commitment wanes. The degree is directly related to the number of adherence predictors identified during the initial assessment. Counselors should watch persons prone to depression for periods of decreased commitment to diet and adherence to medication. Lack of support or constant negative reinforcement by a spouse or significant other may set the stage for more frequent and longer periods of decreased commitment. Clients who have tried in vain to follow an eating pattern in the past will probably experience periods of poor adherence to the low-protein eating pattern.

The first indication of reduced commitment may be a comment such as, "I'm tired of taking medications and following this strict diet." Assuming the counselor has provided enough information about the diet and the medication regimen and has offered cueing devices that the client is using, this comment indicates the following:

- More dietary information will probably only aggravate the situation. The client is not looking for more information at this point.
- Failing to remember to take the medication and follow the diet is not the major problem. Offering more cueing devices will only make the client angry because, as a counselor, you are not listening to what the client is saying.

At this point, the skills of communication discussed in Chapter 2 become very important. The counselor may either alienate the client by giving short, un-insightful answers such as "You just need to eliminate meat products," or, more positively, retrieve a potential non-adherer and improve adherence at the same time. The dialogue that follows illustrates one way to approach the person who lacks commitment:

Client: "I'm really tired of following this diet and taking all those medications." (Theory: Transtheoretical Model; Strategy: Motivational Interviewing; Part II, Exhibit 2)

Nutrition Counselor: "When you say you are 'tired,' what specifically do you mean?"

Client: "I have lost the desire to fight. I look at my pill dispenser and notice that I should take a noon dose of blood pressure medication, but I don't have the desire to do it. So I don't. I have started eating a second serving of meat at night."

Nutrition Counselor: "You were so committed when we started. I remember you listed several reasons for wanting to do well. I have the list here: (1) "I don't want my disease to get worse." (2) "I want to feel better." (3) "I want to succeed." (Attribution)

Client: "Yes, I remember, but many things have changed since then. I lost my job. My husband was laid off. It is hard to succeed or even see a reason to succeed if your future looks so bleak. We have so many financial problems that the diet and taking my medications have taken a back seat."

In many cases, lack of commitment may mean that other stressful life events have taken priority over adhering to an eating pattern or medication regimen. One of the most positive aspects in maintaining adherence to the low-protein regimen is that in the pre-dialysis client, it can result in uremic symptoms that are less severe. During life events when the stress factor is temporary, a short time of reducing dietary and medication monitoring requirements until life events stabilize may be necessary. For example, if a client is going through a divorce, the counselor can help the client identify the most difficult time period and arrange a way of decreasing monitoring during that time, or set up a contract (Adherence Tool 7-16) (Strategy: Contingency Management; Part II, Exhibit 2). The client can agree to monitor medication and dietary intake for one meal with a calendar every other week and try to do well without monitoring during the other weeks.

In some cases a client may adhere poorly to diet for a few days when eating at home is impossible. Once again, a contract (Adherence Tool 7-17) can avoid monumental indiscretions and create controlled ones (Strategy: Contingency Management; Part II, Exhibit 2). Instead of following a pattern of 0.8 grams per kilogram of protein, for a time the diet might be 0.9 grams per kilogram of protein. This process of relaxing the rules can help in times of crisis and serve as a way of staging back to the original prescription—from 0.9 grams per kilogram of protein to 0.85 grams per kilogram and finally back to 0.8 grams per kilogram. The contract written during this period should clearly indicate the times during which the rules will be relaxed and state exactly what relaxing the rules involves. The contract should make it very clear that the rules will be relaxed only while the client is recovering from an experience that precludes following the diet. The counselor should stress that the ultimate goal is to follow the diet 100% of the time.

At certain points, constructive confrontation may be necessary:

Nutrition Counselor: "I've enjoyed working with you over the past few weeks and I really thought you were making progress. (Personal and Relationship Statements) Let's look at a graph of your urine urea nitrogen levels. What do they tell you?"

Client: "It is evident that I have not been following my low-protein eating pattern. My diet records also show that I have an increase in my daily protein intake. I really want to do well, but particularly during breaks at work I just can't resist." (Description of Behavior by the Client)

Nutrition Counselor: "Keep in mind as you look at this how far you have come. You began eating 90 grams of protein and now you are down to 45 grams. Would it be OK to look at some of the negatives of continuing to follow your diet?"

Client: "OK. One of the negatives is that it is so hard to say 'no' to my friends."

Nutrition Counselor: "Anything else?"

Client: "Sometimes I just want to forget that I am ill. I want to be like everyone else."

Nutrition Counselor: "What are some positives related to changing your eating habits?"

Client: "I feel better and have more fun with my family. That is a super positive!"

Nutrition Counselor: "Great. You want to follow the diet, but the urgings of friends during breaks push you into eating more protein than you would like. You want to be like everyone else. But you know that you feel better when you follow your diet and you have more fun with your family. (Reflective Listening) After having looked at both sides of the issue what are your thoughts?" (This is constructive feedback for this person who has slipped into a contemplation stage. Note that no advice is given.)

Client: "It is overwhelmingly the positive side of being able to have fun with my family." (Theory: Transtheoretical Model; Strategy: Motivational Interviewing; Part II, Exhibit 2)

For the client with little support from a spouse or significant other and who is in the action phase (wanting to change), several alternatives are valuable. One is to identify another support person—a friend, daughter, sister, brother, cousin, or someone on a similar diet—who is doing well. A second alternative is to train the spouse to give positive reinforcement. For example, the counselor can provide many examples of positive reinforcement during a counseling session when a husband and wife are present. A third alternative is to help clients with self-reinforcement. Counselors can ask clients to record thoughts about eating and help the client turn negative to positive thoughts during the next counseling session. (Theory: Transtheoretical Model; Strategy: Motivational Interviewing; Part II, Exhibit 2)

For example, a client might say, "I ate the cottage cheese, and I know it is increasing my protein intake beyond what is recommended. I might as well give up." A more positive way to approach the situation is to say, "I ate more protein at this meal than I should have, but tonight at supper I can keep the amount of protein down by eating a small lettuce salad, toasted low-protein bread and margarine, 7-Up, low-protein Jell-O, and two low-protein cookies. I don't have to go over my protein allowance just because I have a problem with one meal." Adherence Tool 7-18 is a form on which to record both positive and negative monologues. (Theory: Cognitive-Behavioral Theory; Strategy: Cognitive Restructuring; Part II, Exhibit 2)

In summary, major problems with adherence to new eating patterns and supplementary medications involve information regarding the protein content of foods and means of applying this knowledge to specific situations. Planning techniques and cueing devices can be helpful in altering events to take medications and follow low-protein eating patterns. The most difficult problem involving lack of commitment might be approached with strategies such as motivational interviewing, self-monitoring, contracting, reinforcement, and positive thinking (cognitive restructuring).

Review of Chapter 7

1. List four factors associated with inappropriate eating behaviors when following a protein-modified eating pattern:

   a.

   b.

   c.

   d.

2. Identify five possible nutrients that should be identified as to baseline intake:

   a.

   b.

   c.

   d.

   e.

3. List four strategies to treat inappropriate eating behaviors associated with protein-modified patterns:

   a.

   b.

   c.

   d.

4. The following is an exercise to help in applying the ideas just discussed:

   John is a 31-year-old minister who eats all of his meals at home except for a few social gatherings. His major problem is his wife's reluctance to help him modify his diet because she feels there are too many restrictions. Explain what you would do, and why, to change the wife's feelings about the diet. (Don't presume the significant other's behavior will change.)

References

1. Klahr S, Buerkert J, Purkerson ML. Role of dietary factors in the progression of chronic renal disease. *Kidney Int* 1983;24(5):579–587.
2. Brenner BM. Hemodynamically mediated glomerular injury and the progressive nature of kidney disease. *Kidney Int* 1983;23(4):647–655.
3. Keane WF, Anderson S, Aurell M, de Zeeuw D, Narins RG, Povar G. Angiotensin converting enzyme inhibitors and progressive renal insufficiency. Current experience and future directions. *Ann Intern Med* 1989;111(6):503–516.
4. Mitch WE, Walser M, Steinman TI, Hill S, Zeger S, Tungsanga K. The effect of a keto acid-amino acid supplement to a restricted diet on the progression of chronic renal failure. *N Engl J Med* 1984;311(10):623–629.
5. Rosman JB, ter Wee PM, Meijer S, Piers-Becht TP, Sluiter WJ, Donker AJ. Prospective randomised trial of early dietary protein restriction in chronic renal failure. *Lancet* 1984;2(8415):1291–1296.
6. Hunsicker LG. Studies of therapy of progressive renal failure in humans. *Semin Nephrol* 1989;9(4):380–394.
7. Ihle BU, Becker GJ, Whitworth JA, Charlwood RA, Kincaid-Smith PS. The effect of protein restriction on the progression of renal insufficiency. *N Engl J Med* 1989;321(26):1773–1777.
8. Levey AS, Gassman JJ, Hall PM, Walker WG. Assessing the progression of renal disease in clinical studies: effects of duration of follow-up and regression to the mean. Modification of Diet in Renal Disease (MDRD) Study Group. *J Am Soc Nephrol* 1991;1(9):1087–1094.
9. Fouque D, Laville M, Boissel JP, Chifflet R, Labeeuw M, Zech PY. Controlled low protein diets in chronic renal insufficiency: meta-analysis. *BMJ* 1992;304(6821):216–220.
10. Walser M, Hill SB, Ward L, Magder L. A crossover comparison of progression of chronic renal failure: ketoacids versus amino acids. *Kidney Int* 1993;43(4):933–939.
11. Ibels LS, Alfrey AC, Haut L, Huffer WE. Preservation of function in experimental renal disease by dietary restriction of phosphate. *N Engl J Med* 1978;298(3):122–126.
12. Brenner BM, Meyer TW, Hostetter TH. Dietary protein intake and the progressive nature of kidney disease: the role of hemodynamically mediated glomerular injury in the pathogenesis of progressive glomerular sclerosis in aging, renal ablation, and intrinsic renal disease. *N Engl J Med* 1982;307(11):652–659.
13. Hostetter TH, Olson JL, Rennke HG, Venkatachalam MA, Brenner BM. Hyperfiltration in remnant nephrons: a potentially adverse response to renal ablation. *Am J Physiol* 1981;241(1):F85–F93.
14. Olson JL, Hostetter TH, Rennke HG, Brenner BM, Venkatachalam MA. Altered glomerular permselectivity and progressive sclerosis following extreme ablation of renal mass. *Kidney Int* 1982;22(2):112–126.
15. The fifth report of the Joint National Committee on Detection, Evalua-

tion, and Treatment of High Blood Pressure (JNC V). *Arch Intern Med* 1993;153(2):154–183.

16. Klahr S. The modification of diet in renal disease study. *N Engl J Med* 1989;320(13):864–866.

17. Beck GJ, Berg RL, Coggins CH, et al. Design and statistical issues of the Modification of Diet in Renal Disease Trial. The Modification of Diet in Renal Disease Study Group. *Control Clin Trials* 1991;12(5):566–586.

18. The Modification of Diet in Renal Disease Study: design, methods, and results from the feasibility study. *Am J Kidney Dis* 1992;20(1):18–33.

19. Klahr S, Levey AS, Beck GJ, et al. The effects of dietary protein restriction and blood-pressure control on the progression of chronic renal disease. Modification of Diet in Renal Disease Study Group. *N Engl J Med* 1994;330(13):877–884.

20. The Institute of Medicine, Food and Nutrition Board. *The Role of Nutrition in Maintaining Health in the Nation's Elderly.* Washington, DC: National Academy Press, 2000.

21. Striker GE. Report on a workshop to develop management recommendations for the prevention of progression in chronic renal disease Bethesda (MA) April 1994. *Nephrol Dial Transplant* 1995;10(2):290–292.

22. Standards of medical care in diabetes—2006. *Diabetes Care* 2006;29(Suppl 1):S4–S42.

23. Renal Dietitians Dietetic Practice Group of the American Dietetic Association. *National Renal Diet: Professional Guide.* Chicago, IL: The American Dietetic Association, 1993.

24. Bergstrom J, Lindholm B. Nutrition and adequacy of dialysis. How do hemodialysis and CAPD compare? *Kidney Int* 1993;40(Suppl.):S39–S50.

25. Bilbrey GL, Faloona GR, White MG, Knochel JP. Hyperglucagonemia of renal failure. *J Clin Invest* 1974;53(3):841–847.

26. DeFronzo RA, Alvestrand A. Glucose intolerance in uremia: site and mechanism. *Am J Clin Nutr* 1980;33(7):1438–1445.

27. Young VR. Nutritional requirements of normal adults. In: Mitch WE, Klahr S, eds. *Nutrition and the Kidney.* Boston: Little, 1993:1–34.

28. Slomowitz LA, Monteon FJ, Grosvenor M, Laidlaw SA, Kopple JD. Effect of energy intake on nutritional status in maintenance hemodialysis patients. *Kidney Int* 1989;35(2):704–711.

29. Acchiardo SR, Moore LW, Cockrell S. Does low protein diet halt the progression of renal insufficiency? *Clin Nephrol* 1986;25(6):289–294.

30. Tomford RC, Karlinsky ML, Buddington B, Alfrey AC. Effect of thyroparathyroidectomy and parathyroidectomy on renal function and the nephrotic syndrome in rat nephrotoxic serum nephritis. *J Clin Invest* 1981;68(3):655–664.

31. Walser M. Nutrition in renal failure. *Annu Rev Nutr* 1983;3:125–154.

32. Coburn JW, Hartenbower DL, Brickman AS, Massry SR, Kopple JG. Intestinal absorption of calcium, magnesium and phosphorus in chronic renal insufficiency. In: David DS, ed. *Calcium Metabolism in Renal Failure and Nephrolithiasis.* New York: John Wiley & Sons, 1977:77–109.

33. Marone CC, Wong NL, Sutton RA, Dirks JH. Acidosis and renal calcium excretion in experimental chronic renal failure. *Nephron* 1981;28(6):294–296.
34. Wollam GL, Tarazi RC, Bravo EL, Dustan HP. Diuretic potency of combined hydrochlorothiazide and furosemide therapy in patients with azotemia. *Am J Med* 1982;72(6):929–938.
35. Smith FR, Goodman DS. The effects of diseases of the liver, thyroid, and kidneys on the transport of vitamin A in human plasma. *J Clin Invest* 1971;50(11):2426–2436.
36. Mahajan SK, Abraham J, Hessburg T, et al. Zinc metabolism and taste acuity in renal transplant recipients. *Kidney Int* 1983;16(Suppl.):S310–S314.
37. Snetselaar LG, Chenard CA, Hunsicker LG, Stumbo PJ. Protein calculation from food diaries of adult humans underestimates values determined using a biological marker. *J Nutr* 1995;125(9):2333–2340.
38. Gillis BP, Caggiula AW, Chiavacci AT, et al. Nutrition intervention program of the Modification of Diet in Renal Disease Study: a self-management approach. *J Am Diet Assoc* 1995;95(11):1288–1294.
39. Coyne T, Olson M, Bradham K, Garcon M, Gregory P, Scherch L. Dietary satisfaction correlated with adherence in the Modification of Diet in Renal Disease Study. *J Am Diet Assoc* 1995;95(11):1301–1306.
40. Milas NC, Nowalk MP, Akpele L, et al. Factors associated with adherence to the dietary protein intervention in the Modification of Diet in Renal Disease Study. *J Am Diet Assoc* 1995;95(11):1295–1300.
41. Dolecek TA, Olson MB, Caggiula AW, et al. Registered dietitian time requirements in the Modification of Diet in Renal Disease Study. *J Am Diet Assoc* 1995;95(11):1307–1312.

Adherence Tool 7–1   Client Questionnaire for Protein-Restricted Eating Patterns (Monitoring Device)

Name:_____

Address: _____

Sex: M _____ F _____

Birthdate: _____

Home Phone: _____

Office Phone: _____

Doctor's name:_____

Anthropometry:

   Elbow Breadth _____

   Frame Size _____

   Standard Body Weight _____   (Use Metropolitan Life Insurance Tables)

WEIGHT HISTORY

1. Your present weight _____ height _____

2. Describe your present weight (check one).

   _____ Very overweight

   _____ Slightly overweight

   _____ About average

   _____ Average

   _____ Slightly underweight

3. Are you dissatisfied with the way you look at this weight? (check one)

   _____ Completely satisfied

   _____ Satisfied

   _____ Neutral

   _____ Dissatisfied

   _____ Very dissatisfied

4. What do you do for physical exercise and how often do you do it?

ACTIVITY	FREQUENCY
(for example, swimming, jogging, and dancing)	(daily, weekly, monthly)

_____

_____

_____

_____

continued

Adherence Tool 7–1 *continued*

PAST DIETS

(If you have never followed a special diet, skip to question 12.)

5. Have you followed a low-protein diet in the past? _____ If "yes,"
   what was the number of grams of protein eaten per day? _____
   When did you start this diet? _____ Are you still following it? _____

6. How would you describe your ability to follow the diet? (check one)

   _____ Excellent

   _____ Good

   _____ Fair

   _____ Poor

7. What were or are the attitudes of the following people about your
   attempts to follow the low-protein diet? (Place an *X* in the appropriate box.)

	Negative (They disapprove or are resentful.)	*Indifferent* (They don't care or don't help.)	*Positive* (They encourage me and are understanding.)
Husband			
Wife			
Children			
Parents			
Employer			
Friends			

8. Did or do these attitudes affect your ability to follow the low-protein
   diet? _____. If "yes," please describe: _____

   _____

   _____

   _____

   _____

9. What other diets have you followed in the past or are you currently
   following? (Check as many as apply.)

   _____ High-calorie   _____ Diabetic

   _____ Low-cholesterol, low-fat   _____ Low-potassium

   _____ Low-calorie   _____ High-potassium

   _____ Low-salt   _____ Low-phosphorus

   _____ Other

continued

Adherence Tool 7–1 *continued*

10. What special products did you use or are you currently using?

 _____ Low-protein products

 _____ Low-salt products

 _____ Sugar-free products

 _____ Other _____

11. Have you had a major mood change while or after following a special diet? Indicate any mood changes on the following checklist.

Mood	No Change	A Little Change	Moderate Change	A Lot of Change	Extreme Change
A. Depressed, sad, feeling down, unhappy, the blues					
B. Anxious, nervous, restless, or uptight all the time					
C. Physically weak					
D. Elated or happy					
E. Easily irritated, annoyed, or angry					
F. Fatigued, worn out, tired all the time					
G. A lack of self-confidence					

MEDICAL HISTORY

12. What was the date of your last physical exam? _____

13. Other than your kidney disease, do you currently have other medical problems? _____

14. What medications or drugs do you take regularly?_____

_____

_____

_____

_____

15. List any medications, drugs, or food to which you are allergic:

_____

_____

_____

continued

Adherence Tool 7–1   *continued*

16. List any hospitalizations or operations. Indicate how old you were at each hospital admission.

    Age   Reason for hospitalization

    _____

    _____

    _____

    _____

17. List any serious illnesses you have had that have not required hospitalization. Indicate how old you were during each illness.

    Age   Illness

    _____

    _____

    _____

    _____

    _____

18. How much alcohol do you usually drink per week? _____ounces

19. List any psychiatric contact, individual counseling, or marital counseling that you have had or are now having.

    Age   Reason for contact and type of therapy

    _____

    _____

    _____

    _____

    _____

20. List any recurring symptoms you are currently experiencing, vomiting, diarrhea, constipation, weak feeling, etc.

    _____

    _____

    _____

    _____

SOCIAL HISTORY

21. Circle the last year of school attended:

    1 2 3 4 5 6 7 8   9 10 11 12   1 2 3 4   MA/MS   PhD/MD
       Grade School   High School   College

continued

Adherence Tool 7–1 *continued*

22. Describe your present occupation:

_____

_____

(If self-employed, skip to question 24.)

23. How long have you worked for your present employer? _____

24. Present marital status (check one):

_____ Single _____ Widowed

_____ Engaged _____ Separated

_____ Married _____ Divorced

25. Describe spouse's occupation: _____

_____

_____

_____

26. Who lives at home with you? _____

_____

_____

_____

_____

FAMILY HISTORY

27. Is your father living? Yes _____ No _____

Father's age now, or age at and cause of death: _____

_____

_____

28. Is your mother living? Yes _____ No _____

Mother's age now, or age at and cause of death:_____

_____

_____

29. Please add any additional information you feel may be relevant to your dietary success. This includes interactions with your family and friends that might sabotage your ability to follow a low-protein diet and additional family or social history that you feel might help us understand problems you will encounter with eating low-protein meals.

_____

_____

_____

Adherence Tool 7–2   Daily Record of Foods Containing Protein
(Monitoring Device)

Time	Protein-Containing Food	Amount	Source

Adherence Tool 7–3   Calculating Adherence (Monitoring Device)

Last visit date _____

Last visit number _____

Start counting for next visit adherence on   (date)

                                                      _____
                                                      (AM, PM, or bedtime dose)

Number of days since last visit

Number of prescribed pills per day

a. Number of pills issued since last visit   _____

b. Returned by client this visit   _____

c. Left at home or accidentally destroyed _____

d. Not taken ($b + c$) _____

e. Subject has taken since last visit ($a - d$)   _____

f. Should have taken   _____

g. Percent adherence to nearest whole number_____
   ($a/f \times 100$)

h. Number of days missed ($f - e$)/number of pills _____

Since your last visit, have you stopped taking your medicine for any reason? _____
_____

Since your last visit, have you changed the dose of medicine for any reason? _____
_____

Adherence Tool 7–4   Record of Adherence Percentages (Monitoring Device)

Medication: _____

Dosage: _____

Date	Percent Adherence

Adherence Tool 7–5   Graph of Protein Intake (Monitoring Device)

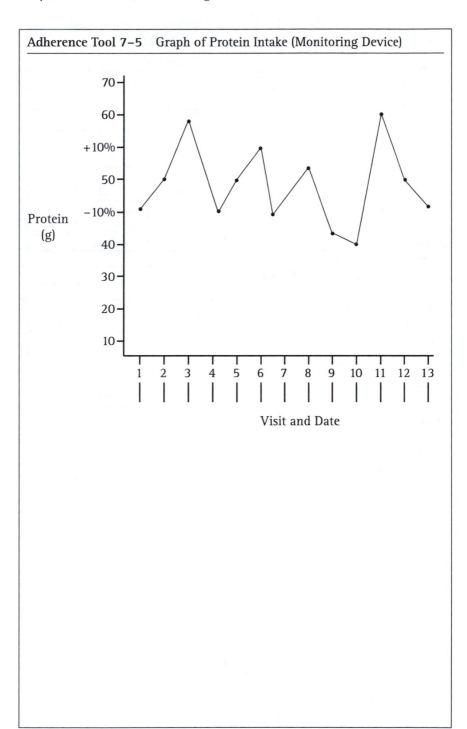

Adherence Tool 7–6   Laboratory Data (Monitoring Device)

Name: _____

Hospital Number: _____

Diagnosis: _____

	Normal Values					
Visit: ____ Date: ____						
Serum Values						
Total Protein						
Albumin						
Transferrin						
Urea nitrogen appearance (UNA)						
Creatinine						
Sodium						
Potassium						
Chloride						
Bicarbonate						
Calcium						
Phosphorus						
Magnesium						
Iron						
Glucose						
White Blood Cells						
Hemoglobin						
Hematocrit						
Urine Values						
Protein						
Creatinine						
Phosphorus						
pH						
Glucose						

Adherence Tool 7–7 Client Diet Basics and One-Day Menu
(Informational Device)

My diet should contain ____ grams of protein per day.

Examples of foods containing all essential amino acids:

Meats	Fish	Milk
Poultry	Eggs	Cheese

Examples of foods lacking one or more essential amino acids:

Breads	Fruits	Cereals
Vegetables	Gelatin	

Essential amino acids are:

Histidine	Threonine
Isoleucine	Tryptophan
Leucine	Valine
Lysine	

Plan one day's menu using protein-containing foods:

Breakfast	Lunch	Dinner	Snacks

Adherence Tool 7–8 Exchange Practice for Your Low-Protein Eating Pattern (Informational Device)

Please write in the amount of protein coming from the food in the list and its exchange amount.

Food	Amount of Protein	Amount of Phosphorus	Exchange*
$1/4$ cup corn			
$1/2$ cup ice cream			
8 ounces grape juice			
1 ounce hard candy			
4 saltine crackers			
$1/8$ of or 7" of apple pie			
$3/4$ cup applesauce			
$1/4$ cup mashed potatoes			
28 grams lean roast beef			
28 grams lean ham			
56 grams frankfurters			
28 grams cheddar cheese			
$1/4$ cup yogurt			

*Only the amount of protein may be important if exchanges are unnecessary.

Adherence Tool 7–9   Recipe Modifications for Your Low-Protein Diet (Informational Device)

Title of Recipe: _____

Ingredients	Amount	Grams of Protein	Milligrams of Phosphorus	Calories

Total Protein _____ grams

Animal Protein _____ grams

Total Phosphorus _____ milligrams

Calories _____

Exchanges _____

_____

_____

Adherence Tool 7–10	Holiday Eating (Informational Device)	
Christmas Goodies That Are "Go"	*Use Caution with These*	*Stop!*
Candy Canes	Raw Vegetables:	Sour Cream Dips
Lollipops	Carrot sticks (not more than	Chocolate Candies
Cut Rock (Prim Rose brand)	4[3"] sticks)	Fudge
Mint Filled Straws	Celery sticks (not more than	Meat and Cheese
(Prim Rose brand)	3[3"] sticks)	Appetizers and Snacks
Holiday Mints (Brachs)	Broccoli (not more than 1	Nuts
Yule Mints (Brachs)	floret)	Peanut Brittle
Christmas Jellies (Brachs)	Cherry Tomato (not more	Cheese Spreads
Cinnamon Santas (Brachs)	than 1 small)	Ice Cream
Starlight Mints (Brachs)	Radishes (not more than	Munchies: Pretzels,
Jelly Wreaths and Trees	5 small)	Crackers, Popcorn, Melba
(Brachs)	Mushrooms (not more than	Toast, Bread Sticks,
Ribbon Candy (Brachs)	2 tablespoons)	Potato Chips (over
Pastel Mints	Fruits:	$1/4$ cup), Cheese Curls,
(Richardson)	Kumquat, raw (not more	Corn Chips
Gumdrops (Brachs)	than 1 average)	
Lifesavers	Apple, raw (not more than	
Hard Candy	$1/2$ large)	
Spice Drop Candy (Sweets	Cranberry-Orange Relish	
and Treats Candy Shop)	(not more than $1/4$ cup)	
Christmas Gummy Bear	Pear, raw with skin (not	
(Sweets and Treats)	more than $1/2$ medium)	
Mini Fruit Balls (Sweets	Pineapple, raw, cubed (not	
and Treats)	more than $1/4$ cup)	
Rock Candy (Sweets and	Potato Chips (not more than	
Treats)	$1/4$ cup)	
Fruit Flavored Ices (Baskin	Mayonnaise Dips (not more	
Robbins)	than 1 tablespoon)	
Orange Ice (Sealtest)	Salad Dressing Dips (i.e.,	
Carbonated Beverages	Miracle Whip) (not more	
Apple Juice, Apple Cider	than 2 tablespoons)	
Cranberry Juice		
Wine		
Whiskey (mixed with water)		
Candied Apricots, Cherries,		
Citron, Lemons, Oranges		

Courtesy of Lisa Brooks and Dru Mueller.

Adherence Tool 7–11   Birthday Card (Informational Device)

[Insert Recipe Here]	Happy Birthday Linda *Barry* *Max* John Larry Joe Amy

Chocolate Cake

Number of Servings 12   Recipe makes 1 12-inch by 8-inch cake

1 cup margarine	$^1/_4$ teaspoon salt
$^1/_2$ cup cocoa	2 teaspoons vanilla extract
2 cups granulated sugar	$^3/_4$ cup chopped walnuts
4 teaspoons egg replacer mixed	1 cup miniature marshmallows
with 8 tablespoons water	
$1^1/_2$ cups low-protein baking mix	

1. Microwave margarine and cocoa in $2^1/_2$-quart glass casserole dish at high for 2 minutes.
2. Stir in sugar.
3. Add eggs and beat well.
4. Blend in flour, salt, vanilla, and nuts.
5. Pour batter into a 12-inch by 8-inch glass baking dish.
6. Microwave at high 10 to 11 minutes; rotate dish $^1/_2$ turn after 5 minutes.
7. Leave cake in pan, spread miniature marshmallows over warm cake.
8. Top with fudge frosting.

Fudge Frosting

$^1/_2$ cup margarine	1 pound box powdered sugar
$^1/_3$ cup Rich's liquid coffee creamer	dash of salt
2 tablespoons cocoa	1 teaspoon vanilla extract

1. Microwave margarine, Rich's liquid coffee creamer, and cocoa in a 2-quart glass casserole dish at high for 2 minutes.

continued

Adherence Tool 7–11   *continued*

2. Stir in sugar, salt, and vanilla.
3. Spread on warm cake.
Note: Do not freeze.

Protein	3.4 grams	Serving Size: $1/12$ cake
HBV* Protein	0.3 gram	Serving Weight: 130 grams
LBV** Protein	3.1 grams	
Calories	625	
Phosphorus	104 milligrams	

 *HBV = High biological value
**LBV = Low biological value

Adherence Tool 7–12   Low-Protein Foods for Your Diet (Informational Device)

Item Description	Company

Adherence Tool 7–13   Pill Box (Cueing Device)

	M	T	W	T	F	S	S
Morning							
Noon							
Evening							
Bed							

Adherence Tool 7–14		Vacation Postcard (Cueing Device)

Your travel checklist. Have you done the following?

Yes	No	
☐	☐	Temporarily canceled the newspaper
☐	☐	Put a stop on mail delivery
☐	☐	Locked all doors and windows
☐	☐	Counted your medication pills and added ones in case you stay longer than planned
☐	☐	Obtained a medication letter for customs clearance if traveling abroad
☐	☐	Checked and fueled your car, if driving
☐	☐	Left your destination phone number with a friend
☐	☐	Confirmed all reservations

Adherence Tool 7–15   Calendars (Cueing Device)

ONE-MONTH CALENDAR

Sun.	Mon.	Tues.	Wed.	Thur.	Fri.	Sat.

Month of _____ 20_____. If you have any questions, please call: _____

ONE-WEEK CALENDAR

NAME: _____

ATTN: _____   THANK YOU!

Adherence Tool 7–16   Reinstituting Commitment, Contract I (Behavioral Device)

During the week of January 2 (January 2–9) I agree to limit my monitoring of medication to every other day. For all other weeks in the month of January, I will monitor daily. I will record the exact amount of medication I take at breakfast, lunch, and dinner on the calendar provided. Each evening, I will allow myself to watch TV, call my friend, or read a book if I have been successful in recording for that week. If I fail to achieve this goal on designated weeks (all of those other than the week of January 2), I will not allow myself to engage in any of these behaviors. I will not reinforce during the week of January 2.

I understand that this break in my monitoring will be only temporary. Once life is back to normal (following the week of January 2), I will return to my old routine on January 10.

Client _____

Spouse/Parent/Friend _____

Nutrition Counselor _____

Physician _____

Adherence Tool 7–17   Reinstituting Commitment, Contract II
(Behavioral Device)

During the week of February 3 (February 3–9) I agree to limit my dietary intake to the new and temporary exchange list (0.9 grams per kilogram of protein per day) provided by my dietitian. Each day that I successfully follow this exchange pattern, I will reward myself by reading a book, going shopping, or visiting my cousin. If I do not follow the diet on a day, I will not allow myself to engage in any of these behaviors.

I recognize that this change in diet is temporary. On February 10, I will return to an intermediate dietary exchange pattern (0.85 grams per kilogram of protein per day). On February 17, I will return to my old exchange pattern (0.8 grams per kilogram of protein per day).

Client _____

Spouse/Parent/Friend _____

Nutrition Counselor _____

Physician _____

Adherence Tool 7–18   Reinstituting Commitment, Record of Monologues (Monitoring Device)

Time	Food Eaten	Thoughts

CHAPTER 8

NUTRITION COUNSELING IN TREATMENT OF HYPERTENSION

Chapter Objectives

1. Identify factors that lead to inappropriate eating behaviors associated with sodium-modified regimens.

2. Identify important steps in the assessment of a baseline diet for clients following a sodium-modified eating pattern.

3. In step 3, intervention, identify theories to use in counseling for inappropriate eating behaviors associated with sodium-modified patterns.

4. In step 3, intervention, generate strategies to use in facilitating behavior change for clients who are following sodium-modified patterns.

5. As a part of step 3 when the client is ready to make changes recommend dietary adherence tools for clients on sodium-modified eating patterns.

Theories and Facts about Nutrition and Hypertension

The Sixth Report of the Joint National Committee on Detection, Evaluation, and Treatment of High Blood Pressure states that the goal of treating patients with hypertension is to prevent morbidity and mortality associated with high blood pressure and to control blood pressure through lifestyle modification with or without medication by the least intrusive means possible.[1,2] The committee recommends lifestyle modifications including weight reduction, regular aerobic physical activity, reduced dietary sodium and alcohol intake, adequate dietary potassium, and maintaining a dietary pattern with reduced saturated and total fat that is high in fruits, vegetables, and low-fat dairy products (Exhibit 8–1).[2] These lifestyle factors form the basis for intervention strategies that have shown promise in the prevention of high blood pressure.[3–8]

The Dietary Approaches to Stop Hypertension (DASH) dietary plan (Table 8–1) demonstrated that lifestyle modifications offer multiple benefits at little cost and with minimal risk. Lifestyle modifications have been shown to prevent or delay hypertension and may reduce the number and doses of antihypertensive medications.[9,10] Researchers have found that lifestyle modifications are helpful in the majority of hypertensive patients who have additional risk factors for premature cardiovascular disease, especially dyslipidemias or diabetes.[8]

The Joint National Committee states that clinicians should vigorously encourage their patients to adopt these lifestyle modifications. The Joint National Committee also recommends the classification scheme and corresponding treatment in Table 8–2 for blood pressure levels. Optimal blood pressure is classified as a systolic of < 120 and diastolic of < 80 mm Hg. Normal is a systolic of < 130 and diastolic of < 85 mm Hg. These levels, along with

---

Exhibit 8–1   Lifestyle Modifications to Manage Hypertension

Weight reduction
Limit alcohol intake
Increase aerobic physical activity
Maintain dietary potassium intake
Maintain adequate intake of dietary calcium and magnesium
Stop smoking and reduce intake of dietary saturated and total fat

---

Table 8–1   The DASH Feeding Study

Food Group	Daily Servings
Grains	7–8
Vegetables	4–5
Fruits	4–5
Low-fat or non-fat dairy foods	2–3
Meats, poultry, and fish	≤ 2 Nuts, seeds, and legumes 4–5/wk

Table 8–2 Hypertension Risk and Treatments

Blood Pressure Stage (mm Hg)	Risk Group A (No risk factors; No target organ disease/ clinical CVD)	Risk Group B (At least 1 risk factor, not including diabetes; No target organ disease or clinical CVD)	Risk Group C [Target organ disease/ clinical CVD and/or diabetes, with or without other risk factors)
High Normal (130–139 systolic/ 85–89 diastolic)	Lifestyle modification	Lifestyle modification	Drug therapy for those with heart failure, renal insufficiency, or diabetes
Stage 1 (140–159/90–99)	Lifestyle modification (up to 12 months)	Lifestyle modification (up to 6 months)	Drug therapy
Stages 2 and 3 (≥ 160 / ≥ 100)	Drug therapy	Drug therapy	Drug therapy

Source: From *How to Stay on a Low-Calorie, Low-Sodium Diet.* Reprinted with permission of the American Spice Trade Association, © 1980.

those described in Table 8–2, are based on the average of two or more readings including a screening visit followed by two separate visits. Treatment recommendations include the assessment of major risk factors (smoking, dyslipidemia, diabetes mellitus, age older than 60, gender, specifically, men and postmenopausal women, and family history of cardiovascular disease for women under 65 or men under 55 years old) and the targeted organ damage/clinical cardiovascular disease (heart disease, stroke or transient ischemic attack, nephropathy, peripheral arterial disease, and retinopathy).[1]

Research on Weight Control and Hypertension

In overweight persons with hypertension, a weight loss of even 10 pounds can reduce blood pressure levels.[7,11,12] Additional evidence indicates that abdominal fat deposition is associated with risk of hypertension. This excess fat in the upper body region correlates with hypertension, dyslipidemia, diabetes, and increased coronary heart disease mortality.[13] This means that in persons whose waist circumference exceeds 34 inches in women and 39 inches in men treatment with blood pressure medication and/or lifestyle change should be considered.

Research correlating changes in blood pressure in hypertensive persons with changes in weight began in the 1920s. Rose found that weight reduction resulted in lower pressures,[14] and later many researchers reported reduced blood pressure with weight loss.[15–22] In the Chicago Coronary Prevention Evaluation Program, a considerable decrease in body weight was associated with decreases in blood pressure, heart rate, and serum cholesterol.[21] A later Israeli study indicated that most obese hypertensive persons achieved normal blood pressure when they lost only half of their excess weight, even though they remained very obese.[22] Achieving ideal body weight was not crucial to reducing blood pressure, and the pressure fall persisted as long as the decreased body weight was maintained. Researchers in the Dusseldorf Obesity study found that, for hypertensive persons not receiving antihypertensive medication over four and one-half years, the blood pressure decrease was greatest in those who lost 12 kilograms.[23] In another study, the decrease in blood pressure in subjects who lost weight was associated with contraction of plasma volume and a decline in cardiac output, which in turn was related to slower heart rate and decreases in plasma cholesterol, uric acid, and blood glucose.[24]

Weight reduction reduces blood pressure in a large proportion of hypertensive individuals who are more than 10% above
ideal weight.[25] A reduction in blood pressure usually occurs early
during a weight-loss program, often with weight loss as small as 10
pounds.[26]

Basic conclusions from these studies follow:

- Elevated blood pressure correlates with increased body mass.
- Decreases in blood pressure result when weight is reduced.
- With weight loss, cardiovascular morbidity and mortality will
  decrease even if pressure does not. For persons on antihypertensive drugs, the number and/or dosage of these agents may
  be reduced with decreases in blood pressure following weight
  loss.

The Joint National Committee on Detection, Evaluation, and Treatment of High Blood Pressure issued a recommendation about
weight control and hypertension. All hypertensive patients who are
above their desirable weight should initially be placed on an individualized, monitored weight-reduction program with reduced
calories and an increase in regular physical activity to 30–46 minutes most days of the week.[1]

Research on Dietary Sodium Restriction and Hypertension

A second nonpharmacological method for controlling high blood
pressure is restricting dietary sodium. Epidemiologic observations
and clinical trials support an association between dietary sodium
intake and blood pressure.[27]

An analysis of 17 randomized controlled trials that include
sodium restricted eating patterns in individuals 45 years and older
revealed an average urinary sodium reduction of 95 millimoles per
day (mmol/d) with an average blood pressure decrease of 6.3/2.2
mm Hg.[28] Additionally both controlled and observational studies
with moderately reduced sodium eating patterns have been associated with reduced need for antihypertensive medication and
reduced calcium excretion.[9,10,29-34] Based on linear regression
analysis within populations, a 100 mmol/d lower average sodium
intake was associated with a 2.2 mm Hg lower systolic blood pressure (SBP) in 10,000 people,[35] and a 5 to 10 mm Hg lower SBP in
multiple other studies involving 47,000 participants.[36] Furthermore, a 100 mmol/d lower sodium intake was associated with a 9

mm Hg reduction in the rise of SBP in persons between the ages of 25 and 55 years.[37]

Multiple therapeutic trials document a reduction of blood pressure in response to reduced sodium intake. In short-term trials, moderate sodium restriction in hypertensive individuals on average reduces SBP by 4.9 mm Hg and diastolic blood pressure (DBP) by 2.6 mm Hg.[38] In trials involving people aged 50 to 59 and lasting five weeks or longer, a 50 mmol/d reduction of sodium intake was associated with an average of 7 mm Hg reduction in SBP in hypertensive persons and a 5 mm Hg reduction in normotensive people.[39]

Individuals vary in their blood pressure response to changes in dietary sodium.[40] Sensitivity to changes in sodium intakes with resulting drops in blood pressure occur most frequently in African Americans, the elderly, and patients with hypertension or diabetes.[41-43]

The Joint National Committee on Detection, Evaluation and Treatment of High Blood Pressure issued the following recommendation about sodium restriction and hypertension. The committee indicated that because the average American consumes more than 100 mmol of sodium per day, moderate dietary sodium reduction to a level of less than 100 mmol/d (less than 6 grams of table salt or less than 2.4 grams of sodium per day) is recommended.[1]

Research on Alcohol and Hypertension

A third important nonpharmacological method of helping to lower blood pressure is reduction in alcohol consumption. Epidemiological surveys have shown that consuming more than 60 to 80 grams (1^1/$_2$ to 2 ounces) of alcohol per day is associated with a significantly higher prevalence of hypertension.[44-47] In one study, 51.5% of clients who consumed more than 80 grams of alcohol per day had hypertension (blood pressure greater than 140/90 mm Hg) on admission to a hospital.[48] Following elimination of alcohol, systolic and diastolic pressures decreased; only 9% remained hypertensive. Those who abstained from alcohol over time remained normotensive; most of those who reverted back to drinking also reverted to previous elevated levels of blood pressure. Although these studies point to the importance of abstinence from the standpoint of hypertension, almost all epidemiological evidence has shown lower morbidity and mortality from coronary heart disease in people who consume one to two ounces of ethanol per day compared with those who do not drink.[49,50]

The Joint National Committee on Detection, Evaluation and Treatment of High Blood Pressure provides the following recommendation about alcohol and hypertension. Persons with hypertension who drink alcohol-containing beverages should be counseled to limit their daily intake to 1 ounce of ethanol (2 ounces of 100-proof whiskey, 10 ounces of wine, or 24 ounces of beer).[51]

Women and lighter-weight people absorb more ethanol than men and heavier people. The Committee recommends that these groups limit their alcohol intake to no more than 0.5 ounces of ethanol per day.[51,52] Significant hypertension may develop during withdrawal from heavy alcohol consumption, but the pressor effect of alcohol withdrawal reverses a few days after alcohol consumption is reduced.[1, 53]

Research on Potassium and Hypertension

An adequate intake of dietary potassium (approximately 90 mmol/d) may protect against developing hypertension and cause positive changes in blood pressure for those diagnosed with hypertension, and potassium deficiency may increase blood pressure.[54]

The Joint National Committee on Detection, Evaluation, and Treatment of High Blood Pressure recommends the following:

- Normal plasma concentrations of potassium should be maintained, preferably from food sources such as fresh fruits and vegetables.
- If hypokalemia occurs during diuretic therapy, additional potassium may be needed either from potassium-containing salt substitutes, potassium supplements, or use of a potassium-sparing diuretic. Potassium chloride supplements and potassium-sparing diuretics must be used with caution in patients susceptible to hyperkalemia.[1]

Research on Calcium and Hypertension

In most epidemiologic studies, there is an inverse association between dietary calcium and blood pressure.[55] Calcium deficiency is associated with an increased prevalence of hypertension, and a low calcium intake may amplify the effects of a high sodium intake on blood pressure.[56] An increased calcium intake may lower blood pressure in some patients with hypertension. However, the overall effect is minimal, and there is no way to predict which patients will benefit.[57] Based on this evidence, there is currently no rationale for recommending calcium intakes in excess of the recommended daily allowance of 20 to 30 mmol (800 to 1200 mg) in an attempt to lower blood pressure.[1]

Research on Magnesium and Hypertension

Evidence suggesting an association between lower dietary magnesium intake and higher blood pressures exists. However, the Joint National Committee on Detection, Evaluation, and Treatment of High Blood Pressure states that, given no convincing data, they do not recommend an increased magnesium intake in an effort to lower blood pressure.[4]

Summary of Research Findings

In conclusion, three methods of dietary treatment, weight control, sodium restriction, and alcohol restriction, are recommended for management of hypertension (Table 8-2).

The research behind recommendations for low-calorie, low-sodium diets adds strength to the overall objective of reducing high blood pressure. The following sections provide research on adherence to changes in eating patterns: examples of inappropriate eating behaviors; methods of assessing those behaviors; and strategies to address lack of knowledge, lack of planning, and lack of commitment to low-sodium methods of altering high blood pressure. Indeed, persons who are hypertensive at ideal body weight may require only the low-sodium diet to normalize blood pressure. Suggestions for weight-loss strategies are covered in Chapter 4.

Adherence to Eating Patterns in Treatment of Hypertension

Many past research studies that included a dietary intervention component have targeted reduced blood pressure as an outcome. Steckel and Swain found contingency contracting effective in reducing weight in a hypertensive client population.[58] Further, a feasibility test for the Dietary Intervention Study of Hypertension showed that interventions for weight reduction and sodium-potassium modification among hypertensive persons can be relatively independent,[59] implying that a hypertension education program could be divided into these components or that these interventions could be used separately.

Monitoring of and feedback on urinary sodium levels resulted in successful sodium reductions in studies by Kaplan et al.[60] and Nugent et al.[61] The simplification of urine sodium estimation procedures through use of overnight instead of 24-hour urine samples and immediate feedback by analysis using chloride titrator strips are important advances in the practicality of these monitoring techniques.

Hovell and colleagues stressed the importance of regular monitoring of both behavioral (pill counts) and physiological outcome (blood pressure) data to avoid accidentally blaming clients for inadequate therapeutic response.[62] Indeed, a client may be an excellent adherer but show little physiological response if treatment is inappropriate or inadequate. Evers and associates suggested that the primary cause of dietary noncompliance may be inadequate dietary counseling.[63] Nurses trained by the medical director, a physician, counseled 489 subjects, who received information on the causes and results of hypertension and the elimination of salt at the table and in cooking, and discussed lists of high-sodium foods and substitutes. The 12 subjects in the control group were treated by family physicians in their usual manner, which generally included advice to restrict salt usage but no intensive dietary counseling or extra assistance. The failure to note differences in the two groups in this study was attributed to a lack of nutrition counseling as described by Tillotson, Winston, and Hall and others.[64–66] Evers also stated that the counseling sessions involved only the client; yet family support has been found to be important in successful adherence to dietary regimens.[63]

A study in Finland showed favorable results when cooperation between physician and client improved.[67] Physicians began providing oral and written information on hypertension that emphasized the importance of adherence to treatment. Clients also received a blood pressure follow-up card on which the blood pressure reading and the precise time of the next appointment were recorded. Clients who missed their appointments were sent a new invitation.

Miller, Weinberger, and Cohen stressed the importance of clients' belief that the benefits of hypertensive treatment outweigh the adverse effects.[68] Many clients believe that taking medicine should make them feel better. Since hypertension is an asymptomatic illness, the client does not obtain symptom relief from the medication or diet, thus making consistent adherence to each form of treatment difficult.

Kerr found that in chronic health care situations such as hypertension, a belief in shared control or cooperation between clients and health care providers lays the groundwork for optimum treatment outcomes.[69] This finding suggests that other, internal and powerful characteristics may interact in the best interest of the client. Shared responsibility in control of hypertension may be critical to increasing adherence in the client with uncontrolled hypertension.

Schlundt et al.[70] and Cohen[71] described components of a structured behavior modification program: (1) self-monitoring of sodium and/or calorie intake; (2) nutrient and behavior goal setting; (3) structured problem solving; and (4) skill training. Prevention of relapse should be addressed in the context of emotional, social, and environmental forces that impinge upon the individual's behavior. Elements in the relapse prevention program include (1) introducing the client to the concept of high-risk situations and assessing previous coping strategies; (2) including skill training and behavior rehearsal to increase the client's coping skills in response to negative emotions, interpersonal conflict, and social pressure; (3) enhancing motivation through an emphasis on the long-term consequences of engaging in prohibited behaviors; (4) teaching clients how to cope cognitively and behaviorally with slips; (5) tailoring the rules of a low-sodium, weight-loss eating pattern to the individual's unique situation; (6) teaching strategies for minimizing high-risk situations; and (7) teaching clients to seek and enhance the social support available for following an antihypertensive eating pattern. Schlundt and others also emphasized the importance of follow-up contact after completion of the initial program and recommended individual counseling, group meetings, telephone contact, and regular mail contact for at least the first three to six months—the time the majority of relapses occur.[70,72]

Inappropriate Eating Behaviors

Diets modified in sodium content may be extremely difficult for most clients with whom nutrition counselors must deal. Salt is used as a flavoring agent in nearly every food. Altering such dietary habits means drastic changes for most clients.

Nutrition counselors frequently hear the complaint, "I really miss familiar flavors," or "Everything I eat tastes like sawdust." For unconscious salters (those who salt without tasting), the true flavors of foods may never have been experienced. Clients can gradually discover the natural flavors in foods through strategies suggested in this chapter.

The new eating pattern limits clients' food options because most commercial products are very high in sodium. With the trend toward prepackaged commercial meals and other products, clients on a low-sodium regimen are left with fewer choices. This limitation has led to many alterations in old eating habits. Clients not only must change what they usually eat but also must become accustomed to a new and foreign range of food flavors.

The food industry, in an effort to assist these persons, has developed a variety of low-salt products. However, these generate comments such as, "Do you expect me to eat this low-sodium soup? It's terrible." Another complaint is that some salt substitutes leave a bitter aftertaste. Objections to commercial low-sodium products constitute a recurring problem for nutrition counselors.

Assessment of Eating Behaviors

For clients who must follow a low-sodium diet, a baseline assessment is crucial. Such regimens require changes in many foods that individuals routinely and even unconsciously consume. Identifying when, where, with whom, and how much sodium is consumed can be of great benefit in helping to reduce salt intake patterns. The format in Exhibit 8-2 can be used to collect baseline data.

In collecting this information, the clients self-monitor their sodium intake. Before using the form, clients might be asked simply to observe their general behaviors involving sodium consumption (for example, salting before tasting). They might be given ideas on which basic foods are high in sodium.

Exhibit 8–2   Sodium Intake Information

| Food | Amount | | Time | Place | Who Present |
	In Cooking	At Table			

During the baseline data collection, clients begin counting sodium intake occurrences, along with collecting related information indicated on the form. The following guidelines can be of help:

- The form must be portable and readily available for recording.
- Clients must be familiar enough with high-sodium foods to record all occurrences of the target behavior (sodium intake).
- Clients should record the data as the behaviors occur.

During this period, some changes in behavior may occur automatically and make the nutrition counselors' job that much easier. Unfortunately, not all clients respond with behavioral changes during this time, and some need guidance in the treatment phase. Counselors should emphasize to clients that treatment interventions should begin after, not before, the baseline data collection.

During data collection, clients will experience increasing awareness of and attention to sodium intake. For example, during a meal they may become conscious of salting food before tasting.

Clients might elicit help from friends and family. There are many ways family members can delicately and supportively point out excessive use of sodium.

Clients may eventually see recordkeeping as a punishment. Counselors might find ways to reinforce this function positively.

Clients should be aware of the importance of baseline data in identifying types of foods, amounts, and related factors—information that will improve their adherence to the dietary pattern. At this point, they might ask, "How long should I keep baseline data?" The reply depends on the following factors:

- The data collection should continue for at least one week, since the intake of sodium occurs daily.
- It is best to gather data for two weeks if an initial review reveals large variations in sodium intake from one day to the next.
- Data should be recorded for a long enough time to provide an accurate estimate of times in a day when the largest amounts of sodium are consumed.
- Data gathering can end when clients and counselors are satisfied that the records show the actual patterns and frequencies of sodium intake.

Clients may wonder when they have reached a stable baseline. Watson and Tharp provide the following guidelines:

- It is rare to get a stable baseline in less than one week. Data collection generally should run at least one "normal" week and should go beyond three or four weeks only rarely.
- The greater the variation from day to day, the longer it will take to get a stable baseline.
- Clients should be asked to be sure the period during which the data were gathered is representative of their usual lifestyle.[73]

In helping clients fill out the recording form, counselors might ask the following questions:

- Are the categories to be recorded defined specifically?
- Are sodium intakes and related factors recorded?
- Will the form always be present during times of food consumption?
- Is the format simple and not punishing or intimidating?
- Is it possible to reinforce the recordkeeping positively?

The sodium intake form in Exhibit 8-2 can identify a wealth of information related to eventual treatment. Assessment based on this form can lead to identification of causes of hypertension and of strategies to control blood pressure.

Treatment Theories and Strategies

The treatment theories and strategies that follow are organized around three topics—lack of knowledge, lack of planning, and lack of commitment. A variety of theories can be used in changing eating habits to bring blood pressure into normal ranges. Behavior modification where the counselor looks at the chain of events leading up to the inappropriate eating behavior may be helpful. By using the transtheoretical model, the counselor can assess the client's readiness to make dietary changes. Tailoring the intervention to specific stages of change is important. The cognitive behavioral theory may be of value in changing negative monologues to positive, thus increasing the likelihood of changing eating habits to decrease blood pressure.

Strategies to Address Lack of Knowledge

Initially, providing adequate information for the client who wishes to follow a low-sodium diet is crucial. Before recommending treatment strategies, counselors might identify a general problem to solve. Along with the statement of that problem, inappropriate regular eating patterns could be identified. Clients might be asked to help discover possible solutions, and the counselors then provide expertise by drawing from the strategies described below.

Tailoring and staging strategies help focus the dietary pattern on the clients' special needs. Behavior change is necessary for social occasions and for the routine alterations in eating style that the regimen requires.

Most nutrition counselors provide lists of standard dos and don'ts for low-sodium eating patterns. These do not allow for individualizing eating patterns to meet each client's needs. By carefully assessing dietary eating patterns and behaviors related to eating habits, the counselor can change dietary behaviors in a tailored fashion. The counseling session then is taken to a level beyond mere information giving. The counselor should tailor the eating pattern to the client, first by carefully studying the baseline information. Attention must be paid not only to consumption of sodium but also to other factors associated with its intake. If the client has a favorite high-sodium food, the counselor can discuss how it might be incorporated to meet a 2,000-milligram sodium limit, cautioning that other foods containing sodium may have to be eliminated or reduced. Compromises as to the amount of the favorite foods allowed might be discussed as well. In tailoring, the counselor should point out which foods on the diet record qualify for the sodium-restricted eating pattern. Foods the client routinely eats and likes should be discussed, and the counselor should explain the reasons for full acceptance, curtailment, or elimination. Any and all positive aspects of the low-sodium eating pattern should be emphasized.

Staging the diet can be crucial in maintaining adherence over time. It is very tempting for counselors to hand clients a list of foods high in sodium and send them on their way as the client complains that he or she will never will be able to follow the diet. In staging information there are two simple rules: (1) the beginning step can never begin too low and (2) the steps upward can never be too small. As the interviews progress, these rules should be individualized for each client. If the sessions move too slowly, the counselors can move up a step or discuss fewer steps. This type of staging helps clients feel that changes are easy and, therefore, that their chances for success are increased. Staging also can help in analysis of the component parts of these situations.

An alternative to this approach is to stage the dietary restrictions for sodium, with the client slowly adjusting to sets of restrictions. One way is to start with the group of foods easiest to begin using in low-sodium form, which enables the client to succeed with the initial food group. The baseline data can be used to prepare lists in consultation with the client.

Another strategy is to provide good substitutions for salt—other flavoring agents such as spices, herbs, fruit juices, etc.—as proposed in Table 8–3. Adherence Tool 8-1 provides a brief guide to low-sodium meal planning and space to practice applying the ideas. The average sodium content of all spices is less than 1 milligram per teaspoon. The spice highest in sodium is parsley flakes, which contain not quite 6 milligrams per teaspoon. In comparison, one gram of salt contains 2,300 milligrams of sodium.

Table 8–3　Chart of Spices that can Substitute for Salt

Spice	Appetizer	Soup	Meat & Eggs	Fish & Poultry	Sauces	Vegetables	Salad & Dressing	Desserts
Allspice Tapioca	Cocktail Meatballs	Pot au Feu	Hamsteak	Oyster Stew	Barbecue	Eggplant Creole	Cottage Cheese Dressing	Apple Pudding
Basil	Cheese Stuffed Celery	Manhattan Clam Chowder	Ragout of Beef	Shrimp Creole	Spaghetti	Stewed Tomatoes	Russian Dressing	
Bay Leaf	Pickled Beets	Vegetable Soup	Lamb Stew	Simmered Chicken	Bordelaise	Boiled new Potatoes	Tomato Juice	
Caraway Seed	Mild Cheese Spreads		Sauerbraten		Beef á la Mode Sauce	Cabbage Wedges		
Cinnamon	Cranberry Juice	Fruit Soup	Pork Chops	Sweet and Sour Fish	Butter Sauce for Squash	Sweet Potato Croquettes	Stewed Fruit Salad	Chocolate Pudding
Cayenne	Deviled Eggs	Oyster Stew	Barbecued Beef	Poached Salmon Hollandaise	Bearnaise	Cooked Greens	Tuna Fish Salad	
Celery Salt and Seed	Ham Spread (Salt)	Cream of Celery (Seed)	Meat Loaf (Seed)	Chicken Croquettes (Salt)	Celery Sauce (Seed)	Cauliflower (Salt)	Cole Slaw (Seed)	
Chervil	Fish Dips	Cream Soup	Omelet	Chicken Sauté	Vegetable Sauce	Peas Francaise	Caesar Salad	
Chili Powder	Seafood Cocktail Sauce	Pepper Pot	Chile con Carne	Arroz con Pollo	Meat Gravy	Corn Mexicali	Chili French Dressing	
Cloves	Fruit Punch	Mulligatawney	Boiled Tongue	Baked Fish	Sauce Madeira	Candied Sweet Potatoes		Stewed Pears
Curry Powder	Curried Shrimp	Cream of Mushroom	Curry of Lamb	Chicken Hash	Orientale or Indienne	Creamed Vegetables	Curried Mayonnaise	

continued

Table 8–3 *continued*

Spice	Appetizer	Soup	Meat & Eggs	Fish & Poultry	Sauces	Vegetables	Salad & Dressing	Desserts
Dill Seed	Cottage Cheese	Split Pea	Grilled Lamb Steak	Drawn Butter for Shellfish	Dill Sauce for Fish or Chicken	Peas and Carrots	Sour Cream Dressing	
Garlic Salt or Powder	Clam Dip	Vegetable Soup	Roast Lamb	Bouillabaisse	Garlic Butter	Eggs and Tomato Casserole	Tomato and Cucumber Salad	
Ginger	Broiled Grapefruit	Bean Soup	Dust lightly over Steak	Roast Chicken	Cocktail	Buttered Beets	Cream Dressing for Ginger Pears	Stewed Dried Fruits
Mace	Quiche Lorraine	Petite Marmite	Veal Fricassee	Fish Stew	Creole	Succotash	Fruit Salad	Cottage Pudding
Marjoram	Fruit Punch Cup	Onion Soup	Roast Lamb	Salmon Loaf	Brown	Eggplant	Mixed Green Salad	
Mint	Fruit Cup	Sprinkle over Split Pea	Veal Roast	Cold Fish	Lamb	Green Peas	Cottage Cheese Salad	Ambrosia
Mustard Powdered Dry	Ham Spread	Lobster Bisque	Virginia Ham	Deviled Crab	Cream Sauce for Fish	Baked Beans	Egg Salad	Gingerbread Cookies
Nutmeg	Chopped Oysters	Cream Du Barry	Salisbury Steak	Southern Fried Chicken	Mushroom	Glazed Carrots	Sweet Salad Dressing	Sprinkle over Vanilla Ice Cream
Onion Powder, Salt, Flakes, and Instant Minced Onion	Avocado Spread (Powder)	Consommés (Flakes)	Meat Loaf (Instant Minced Onion)	Fried Shrimp (Salt)	Tomato (Powder)	Broiled Tomatoes (Salt)	Vinaigrette Dressing (Instant Minced Onion)	
Oregano	Sharp Cheese Spread	Beef Soup	Swiss Steak	Court Bouillon	Spaghetti	Boiled Onions	Seafood	

continued

Table 8–3 *continued*

Spice	Appetizer	Soup	Meat & Eggs	Fish & Poultry	Sauces	Vegetables	Salad & Dressing	Desserts
Paprika	Creamed Seafood	Creamed Soup	Hungarian Goulash	Oven Fried Chicken	Paprika Cream	Baked Potato	Cole Slaw	
Parsley Flakes	Cheese Balls	Cream of Asparagus	Irish Lamb Stew	Broiled Mackerel	Chasseur	French Fried Potatoes	Tossed Green Salad	
Rosemary	Deviled Eggs	Mock Turtle	Lamb Loaf	Chicken á la King	Cheese	Sautéed Mushrooms	Meat Salad	
Sage	Cheese Spreads	Consommés	Cold Roast Beef	Poultry Stuffing	Duck	Brussels Sprouts	Herbed French Dressing	
Savory	Liver Paste	Lentil Soup	Scrambled Eggs	Chicken Loaf	Fish	Beets	Red Kidney Bean Salad	
Tarragon	Mushrooms á la Greque	Snap Bean Soup	Marinated Lamb or Beef	Lobster	Green	Buttered Broccoli	Chicken Salad	
Thyme	Artichokes	Clam Chowder	Use sparingly in Fricassees	Poultry Stuffing	Bordelaise	Lightly on Sautéed Mushrooms	Tomato Aspic	

Source: From *How To Stay on a Low-Calorie, Low-Sodium Diet.* Reprinted with permission of the American Spice Trade Association, © 1980.

The importance of reading labels carefully should be stressed, because some spices are prepared in combination with salt. Anyone on a low-sodium diet should avoid the spice-salt combination products. Table 8-4 indicates the sodium content of spices prepared without salt. Adherence Tool 8-2 provides estimates of the natural sodium content of foods.

Strategies to Address Lack of Planning

Calendars may serve as reminders to take blood pressure medications. For clients who must take medication, forgetting to take medications can result in increased blood pressure. The calendar in Adherence Tool 7-16 provides a means of checking on days or on times of day when patients find it most difficult to take medications. The calendar can also function as a cueing device to remind the client to take medication.

Table 8–4   Sodium Content of Spices

Spice	Milligrams/ teaspoon	Spice	Milligrams/ teaspoon
Allspice	1.4	Nutmeg	0.2
Basil Leaves	0.4	Onion Powder	0.8
Bay Leaves	0.3	Oregano	0.3
Caraway Seed	0.4	Paprika	0.4
Cardamom Seed	0.2	Parsley Flakes	5.9
Celery Seed	4.1	Pepper, Black	0.2
Cinnamon	0.2	Pepper, Chili	0.2
Cloves	4.2	Pepper, Red	0.2
Coriander Seed	0.3	Pepper, White	0.2
Cumin Seed	2.6	Poppy Seed	0.2
Curry Powder	1.0	Rosemary Leaves	0.5
Dill Seed	0.2	Sage	0.1
Fennel Seed	1.9	Savory	0.3
Garlic Powder	0.1	Sesame Seed	0.6
Ginger	0.5	Tarragon	1.0
Mace	1.3	Thyme	1.2
Marjoram	1.3	Turmeric	0.2
Mustard Powder	0.1		

Source: Reprinted from *Low-Sodium Spice Tips* with permission of the American Spice Trade Association, © 1980.

Adherence Tool 8-3 is a monitoring device that can be used to record when a client eats a high-sodium meal. If lunch has been targeted as a difficult meal, marking an X on days when lunch was high in sodium lets the counselor and the client know on what days the client needs special assistance in changing habits. The calendar helps remind the client, "I must watch Monday lunches." By planning ahead, the client may avoid slipping into old high-sodium eating habits.

Strategies to Address Lack of Commitment

Frequently, model adherers to diet revert to old habits. They tire of always choosing low-sodium meals and decide to "live a little." In some cases, this lack of commitment is short-lived and may end after one or two days. Indeed, a client who can limit indiscretions to a two-day period should be commended. But others may have difficulty working back to appropriate eating habits and need assistance in renewing commitment.

A common experience in following a low-sodium eating pattern is the plateau. Week after week, clients make excellent progress; then, suddenly, they stop—they enter the contemplation phase of the strategy called "stages of change." Moving up through all the previous steps may have seemed so easy, but now a new step—the same size as all the rest—seems very difficult. The first step to facilitate the move from contemplation to action is to show the client progress. "Look at this graph of your sodium intake (Figure 8-1). See how far you have come?" If action seems possible, move to small steps of change and provide constant reinforcement. The easiest way to continue to progress is to subdivide the difficult step. If this does not help, the counselor should try increasing reinforcement.

Many clients confide to practitioners that they are guilty of cheating—taking the reinforcers even though they have not achieved a particular step. In such cases, the counselor must redesign the staged schedule so that clients can be reinforced at a level they find achievable.

Some clients complain that they are losing the willpower to follow the low-sodium diet. They may experience this in two ways: (1) if they cannot get started, counselors and clients may not have set the initial step low enough (this can be resolved by moving to a

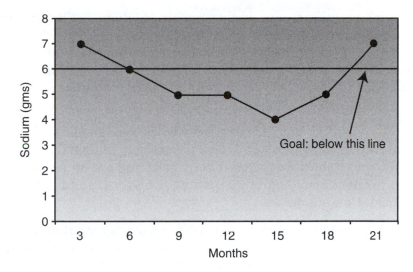

FIGURE 8–1 Tracking Sodium Intake

lower step); (2) if they have started but insist that they see no progress, smaller steps are necessary.

In changing eating behaviors, counselors must review with clients the antecedent-behavior-consequence sequence. The counselors begin to identify antecedents (events that precede a behavior) by asking the clients to think about the following questions as they relate to an eating occurrence:

- What were the physical circumstances? (i.e., was the client surrounded by large tables of food?)
- What was the social setting?
- What was the behavior of others?
- What did you think or say to yourself?[71]

The client should be asked to collect data on these antecedents.

One tactic in changing eating behaviors is to lengthen the chain of events before partaking of a desired item, such as high-sodium cheese. By pausing before eating, immediate gratification is delayed and the behavior eventually may not occur at all. It also may be possible to interrupt the chain by identifying an early link; a discontinuance or prolonged pause at that point may prevent the inappropriate behavior. The events also may be scrambled so that the eventual behavior is never reached.

Social occasions can present special problems. Clients can begin to learn to cope with such situations by collecting data on what types of reinforcers lead them to eat high-sodium foods during social events. The same reinforcer that maintains an undesired eating behavior can be used to strengthen appropriate conduct. For example:

Client (at a party): "Boy, do those salty chips look good. But I know that they aren't on my diet. Over here, though, are some fresh vegetables. They look just as good and are on my diet. I feel really good about myself after eating them and I haven't cheated on my diet."

A list of positive reinforcers may help clients maintain a low-sodium diet. Watson and Tharp provide a set of questions clients might be asked when making a list of positive reinforcers:

1. What kinds of low-sodium foods do you like to eat?
2. What are your major interests?
3. What are your hobbies?
4. What people do you like to be with?
5. What do you like to do with these people?
6. What do you do for fun, for enjoyment?
7. What do you do to relax?
8. What do you do to get away from it all?
9. What makes you feel good?
10. What would be a nice present to receive?
11. What kinds of things are important to you?
12. What would you buy if you had an extra five dollars? Ten dollars? Fifty dollars?
13. What behaviors do you perform every day?
14. Are there any behaviors that you usually perform instead of the target behavior?
15. What would you hate to lose?
16. Of the things you do every day, what would you hate to give up?[73]

Counselors can construct additional questions. Determining the best reinforcers will depend upon each individual client. Before choosing a reinforcer, counselors should consider how closely the consequence meets a client's needs and desires. The reinforcer must be manageable from the client's point of view and must be contingent on performance of the desired behavior—eating low-sodium foods. The reinforcer should be strong enough to help in changing behavior.

The next step in helping to alter behavior is to set up a contract (Exhibit 8-3) that should specify stages of the change in eating habits, kinds of reinforcers to be gained at each step, and self-agreement to make gaining those reinforcers contingent on changing eating behavior involving high-sodium foods.

Ideally, a contract should be written and signed and should specify each detail of dietary change. Each element of this intervention plan should be very specific. A plan—a written contract—will help clients in those inevitable moments of weakness.

Reinforcers should fall within the realm of possibility or be readily accessible. They also should be potent. For example, buying clothes is not a potent reinforcer if the client does not enjoy doing it. The clients might be told to use "intuition" or estimate potency. The counselors' own data, collected during intervention, can indicate whether the chosen reinforcer is sufficiently powerful. A desired eating behavior might be reinforced immediately after the

---

Exhibit 8–3   Contract for a Sodium-Modified Diet

I agree to carry out each of the following steps and supply each reinforcer listed as each step is achieved:

Steps	Reinforcer
1. Eliminate salting before tasting.	Read a new cookbook.
2. Slowly eat unsalted foods to allow detection of true flavors.	Buy a new scarf.
3. Add new spices to foods in place of salt.	Buy a new pair of shoes.

Signed: _____

Cosigned (nutrition counselor): _____

Date: _____

client has performed it. The longer reinforcement is delayed, the less effective it will be.

Cognitive restructuring is an important concept that has the ability to prevent a slip from turning into a total dietary set-back. Below is an example.

Client: "I don't know why I am doing this. It is too difficult. I totally blew my diet at lunch today."

Counselor: "One slip is not the end of all your efforts. Everyone has slips. (Normalization) Learning from slips is the key. Slips can actually be a major positive in dietary change." (Cognitive Behavioral Theory and Restructuring Cognitive Thinking; Part II, Exhibit 2)

As described in Chapter 3, the transtheoretical model is based on varied counseling strategies depending on how ready the client is to make dietary changes. For the client who really isn't ready to make a change, the following dialogue might occur:

Client: "It is hard to make huge changes in my diet. I loved salty foods and now having to avoid them is difficult." (Transtheoretical Model and Contemplation; Part II, Exhibit 2)

Counselor: "Tell me more about why you would like to go back to old eating habits."

Client: "I just love eating salty foods and feel deprived when I can't."

Counselor: "What are positives to maintaining your low-sodium diet?" (Open Question)

Client: "I know that I can avoid serious health problems if I avoid very salty foods."

Counselor: "Comparing the positive and negative aspects of your diet, what are your thoughts now?" (Open Question)

Client: "My health means a lot to me; it has to be the most important aspect and reason for continuing on my low-sodium diet."

In summary, treatment strategies for low-sodium eating patterns involve tailoring and staging with calendars as a means of dealing with forgetting. To address a lack of commitment, it is important to make a list of self-reinforcers, use contracting, and stage the steps toward a goal.

Review of Chapter 8

1. List four factors that lead to inappropriate eating behaviors associated with sodium-modified patterns.

   a. _____

   b. _____

   c. _____

   d. _____

2. Identify three important steps in the assessment of a baseline diet for clients following a low-sodium regimen.

   a. _____

   b. _____

   c. _____

3. List three theories and four strategies to use in treating problems associated with eating patterns low in sodium.

   a. _____

   _____

   b. _____

   _____

   c. _____

   _____

   d. _____

   _____

4. Mrs. B. is 40 years old and has just been placed on a low-sodium diet. She has collected baseline information. She says she has tried and failed to follow a low-sodium diet previously. She loves cheese and cold cuts. What other facts would be beneficial to know? Based on hypothetical answers to

those facts, what theories and strategies would you recommend to facilitate dietary behavior change with low-sodium eating patterns? Explain why you would use these theories and strategies.

References

1. The sixth report of the Joint National Committee on prevention, detection, evaluation, and treatment of high blood pressure. *Arch Intern Med* 1997;157(21):2413–2446.
2. Whelton PK, He J, Appel LJ, et al. Primary prevention of hypertension: clinical and public health advisory from The National High Blood Pressure Education Program. *JAMA* 2002;288(15):1882–1888.
3. Stamler R, Stamler J, Gosch FC, et al. Primary prevention of hypertension by nutritional-hygienic means. Final report of a randomized, controlled trial. *JAMA* 1989;262(13):1801–1807.
4. Stamler J, Caggiula AW, Grandits GA. Relation of body mass and alcohol, nutrient, fiber, and caffeine intakes to blood pressure in the special intervention and usual care groups in the Multiple Risk Factor Intervention Trial. *Am J Clin Nutr* 1997;65(1 Suppl):338S–365S.
5. The Hypertension Prevention Trial: three-year effects of dietary changes on blood pressure. Hypertension Prevention Trial Research Group. *Arch Intern Med* 1990;150(1):153–162.
6. The effects of nonpharmacologic interventions on blood pressure of persons with high normal levels. Results of the Trials of Hypertension Prevention, Phase I. *JAMA* 1992;267(9):1213–1220.
7. Effects of weight loss and sodium reduction intervention on blood pressure and hypertension incidence in overweight people with high-normal blood pressure. The Trials of Hypertension Prevention, phase II. The Trials of Hypertension Prevention Collaborative Research Group. *Arch Intern Med* 1997;157(6):657–667.
8. Appel LJ, Moore TJ, Obarzanek E, et al. A clinical trial of the effects of dietary patterns on blood pressure. DASH Collaborative Research Group. *N Engl J Med* 1997;336(16):1117–1124.
9. Neaton JD, Grimm RH, Jr., Prineas RJ, et al. Treatment of Mild Hypertension Study. Final results. Treatment of Mild Hypertension Study Research Group. *JAMA* 1993;270(6):713–724.
10. Singer DR, Markandu ND, Cappuccio FP, Miller MA, Sagnella GA, MacGregor GA. Reduction of salt intake during converting enzyme inhibitor treatment compared with addition of a thiazide. *Hypertension* 1995;25(5):1042–1044.
11. Whelton P, Applegate W, Ettinger W. Efficacy of weight loss and reduced sodium intake in the Trial of Nonpharmacologic Interventions in the Elderly (TONE). *Circulation* 1996;94(Suppl I):1–78.
12. U.S. Department of Health and Human Services. *Physical Activity and*

Health: A Report of the Surgeon General. Atlanta, GA: Centers for Disease Control and Prevention, National Center for Chronic Disease Prevention and Health Promotion, 1996.

13. Pouliot MC, Despres JP, Lemieux S, et al. Waist circumference and abdominal sagittal diameter: best simple anthropometric indexes of abdominal visceral adipose tissue accumulation and related cardiovascular risk in men and women. *Am J Cardiol* 1994;73(7):460–468.

14. Rose R. Weight reduction and its remarkable effect on high blood pressure. *NY Med J* 1922;115:752–759.

15. Hovell MF. The experimental evidence for weight-loss treatment of essential hypertension: a critical review. *Am J Public Health* 1982;72(4):359–368.

16. Reisin E, Abel R, Modan M, Silverberg DS, Eliahou HE, Modan B. Effect of weight loss without salt restriction on the reduction of blood pressure in overweight hypertensive patients. *N Engl J Med* 1978;298(1):1–6.

17. Fagerberg B, Andersson OK, Isaksson B, Bjorntorp P. Blood pressure control during weight reduction in obese hypertensive men: separate effects of sodium and energy restriction. *Br Med J (Clin Res Ed)* 1984;288(6410):11–14.

18. Maxwell MH, Kushiro T, Dornfeld LP, Tuck ML, Waks AU. BP changes in obese hypertensive subjects during rapid weight loss. Comparison of restricted v unchanged salt intake. *Arch Intern Med* 1984;144(8):1581–1584.

19. Tuck ML, Sowers JR, Dornfeld L, Whitfield L, Maxwell M. Reductions in plasma catecholamines and blood pressure during weight loss in obese subjects. *Acta Endocrinol* (Copenh) 1983;102(2):252–257.

20. Stokholm KH, Nielsen PE, Quaade F. Correlation between initial blood pressure and blood pressure decrease after weight loss: A study in patients with jejunoileal bypass versus medical treatment for morbid obesity. *Int J Obes* 1982;6(3):307–312.

21. Stamler J, Farinaro E, Mojonnier LM, Hall Y, Moss D, Stamler R. Prevention and control of hypertension by nutritional-hygienic means. Long-term experience of the Chicago Coronary Prevention Evaluation Program. *JAMA* 1980;243(18):1819–1823.

22. Eliahou HE, Iaina A, Gaon T, Shochat J, Modan M. Body weight reduction necessary to attain normotension in the overweight hypertensive patient. *Int J Obes* 1981;5(Suppl 1):157–163.

23. Jörgens V. Long-term effects of weight changes on cardiovascular risk factors over 4.7 years in 247 obese patients. Paper presented at: the 4th International Congress of Obesity, 1983, New York.

24. Reisin E, Frohlich ED, Messerli FH, et al. Cardiovascular changes after weight reduction in obesity hypertension. *Ann Intern Med* 1983;98(3):315–319.

25. Langford HG, Davis BR, Blaufox D, et al. Effect of drug and diet treatment of mild hypertension on diastolic blood pressure. The TAIM Research Group. *Hypertension* 1991;17(2):210–217.

26. Schotte DE, Stunkard AJ. The effects of weight reduction on blood pressure in 301 obese patients. *Arch Intern Med* 1990;150(8):1701–1704.

27. Elliott P, Stamler J, Nichols R, et al. Intersalt revisited: further analyses of 24 hour sodium excretion and blood pressure within and across populations. Intersalt Cooperative Research Group. *Br Med J* 1996;312(7041):1249–1253.

28. Midgley JP, Matthew AG, Greenwood CM, Logan AG. Effect of reduced dietary sodium on blood pressure: a meta-analysis of randomized controlled trials. *JAMA* 1996;275(20):1590–1597.

29. Devine A, Criddle RA, Dick IM, Kerr DA, Prince RL. A longitudinal study of the effect of sodium and calcium intakes on regional bone density in postmenopausal women. *Am J Clin Nutr* 1995;62(4):740–745.

30. Ram CV, Garrett BN, Kaplan NM. Moderate sodium restriction and various diuretics in the treatment of hypertension. *Arch Intern Med* 1981;141(8):1015–1019.

31. Antonios TF, MacGregor GA. Salt—more adverse effects. *Lancet* 1996;348(9022):250–251.

32. Cirillo M, Laurenzi M, Panarelli W, Stamler J. Urinary sodium to potassium ratio and urinary stone disease. The Gubbio Population Study Research Group. *Kidney Int* 1994;46(4):1133–1139.

33. Liebson PR, Grandits GA, Dianzumba S, et al. Comparison of five antihypertensive monotherapies and placebo for change in left ventricular mass in patients receiving nutritional-hygienic therapy in the Treatment of Mild Hypertension Study (TOMHS). *Circulation* 1995;91(3):698–706.

34. Messerli FH, Schmieder RE, Weir MR. Salt. A perpetrator of hypertensive target organ disease? *Arch Intern Med* 1997;157(21):2449–2452.

35. Intersalt: an international study of electrolyte excretion and blood pressure. Results for 24 hour urinary sodium and potassium excretion. Intersalt Cooperative Research Group. *Br Med J* 1988;297(6644):319–328.

36. Law MR, Frost CD, Wald NJ. By how much does dietary salt reduction lower blood pressure? I—Analysis of observational data among populations. *Br Med J* 1991;302(6780):811–815.

37. Sodium, potassium, body mass, alcohol and blood pressure: the INTERSALT Study. The INTERSALT Co-operative Research Group. *J Hypertens* 1988;6(4 Suppl):S584–S586.

38. Cutler JA, Follmann D, Elliott P, Suh I. An overview of randomized trials of sodium reduction and blood pressure. *Hypertension* 1991;17(1 Suppl):I27–33.

39. Law MR, Frost CD, Wald NJ. By how much does dietary salt reduction lower blood pressure? III—Analysis of data from trials of salt reduction. *Br Med J* 1991;302(6780):819–824.

40. Sullivan JM. Salt sensitivity. Definition, conception, methodology, and long-term issues. *Hypertension* 1991;17(1 Suppl):I61–68.

41. Flack JM, Ensrud KE, Mascioli S, et al. Racial and ethnic modifiers of the salt-blood pressure response. *Hypertension* 1991;17(1 Suppl):I115–121.

42. Grobbee DE. Methodology of sodium sensitivity assessment. The example of age and sex. *Hypertension* 1991;17(1 Suppl):I109–114.
43. Weinberger MH. Salt sensitivity of blood pressure in humans. *Hypertension* 1996;27(3 Pt 2):481–490.
44. Alcohol and hypertension—implications for management. A consensus statement by the World Hypertension League. *J Hum Hypertens* 1991;5(3):227–232.
45. Hennekens CH. Alcohol. In: Kaplan NN, Stamler J, eds. *Prevention of Coronary Heart Disease.* Philadelphia: W.B. Saunders, 1983:130–138.
46. MacMahon SW, Blacket RB, Macdonald GJ, Hall W. Obesity, alcohol consumption and blood pressure in Australian men and women. The National Heart Foundation of Australia Risk Factor Prevalence Study. *J Hypertens* 1984;2(1):85–91.
47. Friedman GD, Klatsky AL, Siegelaub AB. Alcohol, tobacco, and hypertension. *Hypertension* 1982;4(5 Pt 2):III143–150.
48. Saunders JB, Beevers DG, Paton A. Alcohol-induced hypertension. *Lancet* 1981;2(8248):653–656.
49. Marmot MG. Alcohol and coronary heart disease. *Int J Epidemiol* 1984;13(2):160–167.
50. Gordon T, Kannel WB. Drinking and mortality. The Framingham Study. *Am J Epidemiol* 1984;120(1):97–107.
51. Frezza M, di Padova C, Pozzato G, Terpin M, Baraona E, Lieber CS. High blood alcohol levels in women. The role of decreased gastric alcohol dehydrogenase activity and first-pass metabolism. *N Engl J Med* 1990;322(2):95–99.
52. U.S. Department of Agriculture, U.S. Department of Health and Human Services. *Nutrition and Your Health: Dietary Guidelines for Americans.* 4th ed. Washington, DC: USDA, 1995.
53. Maheswaran R, Gill JS, Davies P, Beevers DG. High blood pressure due to alcohol. A rapidly reversible effect. *Hypertension* 1991;17(6 Pt 1):787–792.
54. Whelton PK, He J, Cutler JA, et al. Effects of oral potassium on blood pressure. Meta-analysis of randomized controlled clinical trials. *JAMA* 1997;277(20):1624–1632.
55. Cappuccio FP, Elliott P, Allender PS, Pryer J, Follman DA, Cutler JA. Epidemiologic association between dietary calcium intake and blood pressure: a meta-analysis of published data. *Am J Epidemiol* 1995;142(9):935–945.
56. Hamet P, Mongeau E, Lambert J, et al. Interactions among calcium, sodium, and alcohol intake as determinants of blood pressure. *Hypertension* 1991;17(1 Suppl):I150–154.
57. Allender PS, Cutler JA, Follmann D, Cappuccio FP, Pryer J, Elliott P. Dietary calcium and blood pressure: a meta-analysis of randomized clinical trials. *Ann Intern Med* 1996;124(9):825–831.
58. Steckel SB, Swain MA. Contracting with patients to improve compliance. *Hospitals* 1977;51(23):81–82, 84.
59. Wing RR, Caggiula AW, Nowalk MP, Koeske R, Lee S, Langford H. Dietary approaches to the reduction of blood pressure: the independence

of weight and sodium/potassium interventions. *Prev Med* 1984;13(3):233–244.

60. Kaplan NM, Simmons M, McPhee C, Carnegie A, Stefanu C, Cade S. Two techniques to improve adherence to dietary sodium restriction in the treatment of hypertension. *Arch Intern Med* 1982;142(9):1638–1641.

61. Nugent CA, Carnahan JE, Sheehan ET, Myers C. Salt restriction in hypertensive patients. Comparison of advice, education, and group management. *Arch Intern Med* 1984;144(7):1415–1417.

62. Hovell MF, Geary DC, Black DR, Kamachi K, Kirk R, Elder J. Experimental analysis of adherence counseling: implications for hypertension management. *Prev Med* 1985;14(5):648–654.

63. Evers SE, Bass M, Donner A, McWhinney IR. Lack of impact of salt restriction advice on hypertensive patients. *Prev Med* 1987;16(2):213–220.

64. Tillotson JL, Winston MC, Hall Y. Critical behaviors in the dietary management of hypertension. *J Am Diet Assoc* 1984;84(3):290–293.

65. U.S. Department of Health and Human Services. *Report of the Working Group Critical Patient Behaviors in the Dietary Management of High Blood Pressure.* Bethesda: National Institutes of Health, NIH Publication 1981.

66. Glanz K. Compliance with dietary regimens: its magnitude, measurement, and determinants. *Prev Med* 1980;9(6):787–804.

67. Takala J, Leminen A, Telaranta T. Strategies for improving compliance in hypertensive patients. *Scand J Prim Health Care* 1985;3(4):233–238.

68. Miller JZ, Weinberger MH, Cohen SJ. Advances in non-pharmacologic treatment of hypertension: a new approach to the problem of effective dietary sodium restriction. 1. Sodium in the diet: patient compliance. *Indiana Med* 1985;78(10):893–895.

69. Kerr JA. Multidimensional health locus of control, adherence, and lowered diastolic blood pressure. *Heart Lung* 1986;15(1):87–93.

70. Schlundt DG, McDonel EC, Langford HG. Compliance in dietary management of hypertension. *Compr Ther* 1985;11(8):59–66.

71. Cohen SJ. Improving patients' compliance with antihypertensive regimens. *Compr Ther* 1985;11(10):18–21.

72. Perri MG, Shapiro RM, Ludwig WW, Twentyman CT, McAdoo WG. Maintenance strategies for the treatment of obesity: an evaluation of relapse prevention training and posttreatment contact by mail and telephone. *J Consult Clin Psychol* 1984;52(3):404–413.

73. Watson DL, Tharp RG. *Self-Directed Behavior: Self-Modification for Personal Adjustment.* Monterey, CA: Brooks/Cole Publishing; 1972.

Adherence Tool 8–1   Spices for Low-Sodium Diets (Informational Device)

Spices for Use with Meats:

Dill seed for fish or chicken sauces
Garlic powder for bouillabaisse
Ginger for roast chicken
Mace for fish stew
Marjoram for salmon loaf
Mint for veal or lamb roast
Mustard for cream sauce on fish

Nutmeg for Southern fried chicken
Oregano for Swiss steak
Rosemary for chicken á la king
Savory for chicken loaf
Tarragon for marinated beef
Thyme for clam chowder

Spices for Use with Vegetables:

Allspice for eggplant creole
Basil for stewed tomatoes
Bay leaf for boiled new potatoes
Caraway seed for cabbage wedges
Cinnamon for sweet potatoes
Celery seed for cauliflower
Chili powder for Mexican-style corn
Cloves for candied sweet potatoes
Curry for creamed vegetables
Dill seed for peas and carrots
Garlic for stewed tomatoes

Ginger for beets
Mace for succotash
Mint for green peas
Powdered dry mustard for baked
    beans
Nutmeg for glazed carrots
Rosemary for sauteed mushrooms
Sage for brussels sprouts
Savory for beets
Tarragon for broccoli
Thyme lightly on sauteed
    mushrooms

Plan menus for three meals. The menus should be low in sodium and should use the spices suggested above. Choose spices you think you and your family would enjoy.

Breakfast	Lunch	Dinner

Adherence Tool 8–2   Estimated Natural Sodium Content of Foods (Informational Device)

A rough guide follows for the natural sodium content of foods that are grown or produced and processed without the addition of sodium.

8 oz. milk	=	120 mg of sodium
1 oz. meat	=	25 mg of sodium
1 egg	=	70 mg of sodium
$1/2$ cup vegetable	=	9 mg of sodium
$1/2$ cup fruit	=	2 mg of sodium
1 slice of bread	=	5 mg of sodium
1 teaspoon of fat	=	0 mg of sodium

Source: Reprinted with permission from Mitchell H. S., et al., *Nutrition in Health and Disease*, p. 430, ©1976; Lippincott-Raven.

Adherence Tool 8–3   Daily Food Record with Emphasis on Sodium
Intake (Monitoring Device)

Time	Food Eaten	Amount	Low in Sodium*	Moderate in Sodium*	High in Sodium*

*Place an X in the column to indicate whether the food is high, moderate,
or low in sodium.

CHAPTER 9

NUTRITION COUNSELING FOR CANCER RISK PREVENTION

Chapter Objectives

1. Identify common inappropriate eating behaviors associated with following a fat-controlled eating pattern.

2. In step 1, assessment, identify how to assess problems associated with inappropriate eating patterns in following a fat-controlled regimen.

3. In step 3, intervention, list theories and strategies to overcome inappropriate eating behaviors associated with eating patterns controlled for fat.

Cancer and Nutrition

Cancer is the second most common cause of death in Western societies. Because cancer is largely a disease of old age, as the population ages, the number of cancer deaths increases. Most research in this area has been directed toward treatment and cure of cancers as they arise, a singularly unsuccessful public health policy. The prognosis of individuals with cancer of the lung, breast, large bowel, stomach, prostate, and pancreas is encouraging, with death rates for all cancer sites combined decreasing by 1.6% per year from 1993 to 2003 in males and by 0.8% per year in females from 1992 to 2003.[1] Successful approaches to diseases such as smallpox, rabies, plague, cholera, whooping cough, and diphtheria have focused on prevention rather than treatment.[2]

In the 1970s and 1980s, Doll and Peto,[3] as well as Wynder,[4] estimated that approximately 35% (with a range of 10%–70%) of human cancers might have dietary causes and might also be prevented by diet. Several review articles discuss the potential mechanisms behind diet-induced cancers and review the methodologic problems with dietary data collected through self-report.[5-9]

A variety of dietary factors have been associated with cancer. This chapter focuses on modifications in fat intake. Other approaches include an increase in fruits, vegetables, and grains to maximize fiber.

Theories and Facts about Nutrition and Cancer

Role of Dietary Fats in Cancer

Despite some inconsistencies in the data relating dietary fat to cancer causation, animal studies show an effect of dietary fat on carcinogenesis and suggest that dietary fat has a cancer-promoting role. International epidemiologic studies have suggested that differences in dietary fat intake may provide a meaningful key to prevention of cancer.

Animals fed a high-fat diet often have higher rates of carcinogen-induced cancers of the breast, colon, and pancreas than those fed low-fat diets.[10] Evidence of the positive connection between fat intake and cancer was shown in studies of experimental animals.[11] The combination of high fat and low dietary fiber is associated most highly with increased rates of cancers.[12]

The arguments and counterarguments based on human epidemiologic data are well summarized based on a 1990 symposium on the topic.[13-17] Studies of migrant populations have found that people who move to a country with a higher incidence of breast cancer than their native country tend to acquire the dietary habits of their new country of residence and may experience a cancer incidence that changes with the change in dietary fat.[18,19] Epidemiological studies show positive and negative associations for breast cancer and total fat consumption.[20-24] While methodological problems may have obscured a true risk association in the studies that have found negative associations,[24-26] these studies reinforce the need for cautious interpretation and additional study of diet and breast cancer risk.[27]

Substantial epidemiologic and animal evidence supports a relationship between dietary fat and the incidence of both breast cancer[28] and colon cancer.[29] Indeed, a comparison of populations indicates that death rates for cancers of the breast, colon, and prostate are directly proportional to estimated dietary fat intakes.[30,31] Other cancers that have been related to fat intake are those of the rectum,[32] ovaries,[33] and endometrium.[34] Considerable uncertainties remain to be resolved about these relationships. For example, the effects of different types of dietary fat (i.e., saturated versus unsaturated, animal versus plant origin) have not been separately analyzed in most human studies. In some human studies, diets low in both fat and polyunsaturated fatty acid (PUFA) (omega-6 acid) are associated with enhanced natural killer cytotoxicity for tumor cells in vitro, with especially pronounced effects; however, the results are not entirely clear. The low-fat diets in two studies (where fat was less than 25% or 30%, respectively, of calories) did have such an effect; alterations in polyunsaturated to saturated fat ratio (P/S ratio) did not.[35,36] Thus, at present, the role of PUFA is not clear; several reports suggest that the data are mixed.[37,38] Investigators have studied the role of the omega-3 fish oils in animal models and have concluded that many effects operate through prostaglandin metabolism. Because the omega-3 and omega-6 fatty acids are metabolized to prostaglandins of different types and different activities, their effects may be quite different. The omega-3 fatty acids give rise to prostaglandins that appear to have lower biological activity than those formed from the omega-6 fatty acids, affecting not only natural killer cell activity, but other mediators such as the lymphokines, leukotrienes, and thromboxanes.[39] Although the mechanisms are not yet clear, immunosurveillance is thought to be involved.[40] Studies in humans are now being completed.

Table 9-1 summarizes several past feasibility studies testing the hypothesis that low-fat diets are achievable among women living in various Western countries. The Women's Health Initiative (WHI) is a study funded by The National Institutes of Health and designed to address the issue in a clinical trial design.[41] Primary evidence from that study is presented in two research articles in the *Journal of the American Medical Association*. The results from these articles are summarized below.

The WHI began in 1992 with a randomized, controlled trial design including a dietary intervention and comparison group. The dietary intervention group consumed a diet consisting of 20% of

Table 9–1 Characteristics of Selected Feasibility Studies for Reducing Dietary Fat

Characteristic	NAS[1-4]	WHT[5-7]		Swedish Breast Cancer Study[8]		AHF Study[9]	
Study							
		Intervention Group	Control Group	Intervention Group	Control Group	Cancer	Cystic Disease
Group Size							
Treatment	17	220		121 randomized, 63 completed (52%)		19 breast cancer 16 fibrocystic disease	
Control	11			119 randomized, 106 completed (89%)			
Diet assessment methods	4 DDR at baseline, 3 mo.	Baseline, 6, 12, 24 mo. SQFF, 24-hr. recall to compare to 4 DDR, fat score used to measure adherence		Diet histories (all) Food records (treatment only)		4DDR	
Study Duration, Months	3	12		24		3	
Calories							
Baseline	1840 (419)	7258 KJ (122)	7148 KJ (168)	7.7 MJ	8.2 MJ	1504	1743
3-month follow-up	1365 (291)						
% decrease	25%						
12-month follow-up		5460 (112)	6619 (158)				
% decrease		−24%	−7%				
24-month follow-up		5691	6675	6.8	7.6	1347 (3 mo.)	1344
% decrease from baseline		−22%	−5%	−11.6%	−7.3%	−10.4%	22.8%
% decrease from 12 months		+2%	+2%				

continued

Table 9–1 *continued*

| | | | Study | |
Characteristic	NAS[1-4]	WHT[5-7]	Swedish Breast Cancer Study[8]	AHF Study[9]
Fat, % Calories				
Baseline	38% (4.3)	39%	36.9%	35.6%
6-months follow-up	23% (7.8)		37.2%	33.5%
% decrease	56%			
12-month follow-up	22%	22%	37% / 34.1	(3 mo.) 20.7
% decrease	-17%	-2%	-3.1%	-12.8%
24-month follow-up	23%	37%	24.0	21.4
% decrease	+1%	0%	-12.9%	-14.2%
Weight Loss, g/day				
Actual	31 g	40 g (3 mo.)	Not reported precisely, but intervention group decreased slightly (most in first year) then increased, but not to baseline; controls increased	22.6 g / 66.33 / 64.29 ; 15.5 g/day / 59.3 / 57.9
Predicted from calorie deficit reported	65 g	53 g (3 mo.)	Should have decreased in both groups almost equally if reporting were equally erroneous	20.4 g / 51.9 g

Notes: NAS = Nutrition Adjuvant Study   DDR = Dietary Diary Record   MJ = Millijoules
WHT = Women's Health Trial   SQFF = Semiquantified Food Frequency
AHF = American Health Foundation   KJ = Kilojoules

Table 9–1 *continued*

Data sources:

1. Chlebowski RT, et al. Breast Cancer Nutrition Adjuvant Study (NAS): Protocol design and initial patient adherence, *Breast Cancer Res Treatment* 1987;10:21.

2. Buzzard IM, et al., Diet intervention methods to reduce fat intake: nutrient and food group composition of self-selected low fat diets, *J Am Diet Assoc* 1990;90:42.

3. Chlebowski RT, et al. Adjuvant dietary fat intake reduction in postmenopausal breast cancer patient management, *Breast Cancer Res Treatment* 1991;20:73.

4. Chlebowski RT, et al. The Nutrition Adjuvant Study: Experience and commentary, *Contr Clin Trials* 1989;10:368.

5. Prentice RL, et al. Aspects of the rationale for the Women's Health Trial, *J Natl Cancer Inst* 1988;80:802.

6. Prentice RL, Sheppard L. Validity of international, time trend, and migrant studies of dietary factors and disease risk, *Prev Med* 1989;18:167.

7. Insull W, et al. Results of a randomized feasibility study of a low fat diet. *Arch Intern Med* 1990;150:421.

8. Nordevang E, et al. Dietary intervention in breast cancer patients: effects on dietary habits and nutrient intake, *Eur J Clin Nutr* 1990;44:681.

9. Boyar AP, et al. Recommendations for the prevention of chronic disease: the application for breast disease, *Am J Clin Nutr* 1988;48:896.

Source: Johanna Dwyer, Director, Frances Stern Nutrition Center, Box 783, New England Medical Center Hospital, 750 Washington Street, Boston, MA 02111.

calories from fat with a prescription for fruits and vegetables greater than 5 servings per day and for grains greater than 6 servings per day. The primary outcomes of the trial were breast and colon cancer in women who were postmenopausal and whose age was between 50 and 79 at screening for the study. Details related to the dietary intervention arm of this study have been published.[42] Dietary intervention included group sessions focused on reducing total dietary fat and increasing fruits, vegetables and grains.

Study results showed that adherence to diet was reduced over time with differences comparing the control to the intervention group at year one of 10.7% of calories from fat. Then at year six the comparison percent dropped to 8.1%. After an average of 8.1 years of follow-up, the number of women who developed invasive breast cancer was 655 (0.42%) in the intervention group and 1072 (0.45%) in the comparison group (hazard ratio [HR], 0.91; 95% confidence interval [CI], 0.83–1.01 for the comparison between the two groups). Following a secondary analysis, the data suggested a lower HR among women who adhered to the dietary prescription, had a higher fat diet at baseline, and had specific hormone receptor tumor characteristics. Over the 8.1 years of follow-up, the low-fat dietary pattern did not result in a statistically significant reduction in invasive breast cancer risk. However, a nonintervention follow-up may yield more definitive results.[43] This follow-up component beyond the 8.1 years with data collection is in the planning stages.

Additionally, the WHI looked at colorectal cancer comparing the dietary intervention group with the comparison group. There were 201 women with invasive colorectal cancer in the dietary intervention group (0.13% per year) and 279 (0.12% per year) in the comparison group (HR, 1.08; 95% CI, 0.90–1.29). Secondary analyses suggested potential interactions with the use of aspirin at baseline and estrogen-progestin use. No differences were noted when adjustments for adherence to the intervention were completed. Colorectal exam rates were equal when the comparison and intervention groups were analyzed.[44]

The Women's Intervention Nutrition Study (WINS) was a secondary breast cancer study designed to look at recurrence of breast cancer comparing a fat-modified diet to a control diet for an average mean follow-up of 60 months. The hazard ratio in the intervention group in comparison to the control group for disease-free survival was 0.76 (95% CI, 0.60–0.98, $P = 0.034$). This indicated a reduced risk of 24%. Secondary analyses suggested a substantially greater dietary effect on receptor negative cancers. The final conclusion was that reduced dietary fat-intake including modest weight loss may improve relapse free-survival in breast cancer patients who receive conventional management.[45]

In summary, the majority of the studies to date are strongly suggestive of the role for dietary fat in the etiology of some types of cancer. This chapter focuses on total fat intake as a possible means of modifying cancer incidence. It should be kept in mind that type of fat may play a large role in cancer occurrence. The three studies above in women focused on total fat as the primary target of dietary intervention.

Research on Adherence to Eating Patterns in Cancer Risk Prevention

No systematic studies of the role of nutrition education in reducing cancer risk have been completed, although the National Cancer Institute has sponsored field trials for high-risk persons as well as the public. The WHI was one of the long-term clinical trials designed to look at the preventive effect of dietary fat intake with increases in fruits, vegetables, and grains. The WINS was designed to study a reduced fat diet (15% of calories from fat) with a different ratio of types of fat consumed and an increase in wheat fiber and its effect on tumor recurrence either with or without chemotherapeutic or antiestrogen therapy. The Polyps Prevention Trial was also designed to determine if diets low in fat and high in fiber affect polyp occurrence. (The results of this study showed no statistically significant differences comparing the intervention and control groups.)

Planning nutrition education programs for reducing cancer risk involves many issues. Considerable controversy still exists about the extent to which dietary changes alone can reduce cancer morbidity. There is also much room for confusion about the specificity of cancers that are affected by certain nutrients in the diet. References to cancer in public health education may unnecessarily raise both the fears and the expectations of clients. Health professionals who are planning nutrition education on cancer risk must weigh the implications of the strategies and messages they plan to use.[46]

Patterson and colleagues have provided data from the WHI on low-fat diet practices of older women.[47] These practices can provide valuable information on planning nutrition programs. This research showed that 69% of 7,419 women, aged 50–75 years, who responded to a food questionnaire rarely or never ate skin on chicken, 76% rarely or never ate fat on meat, 36% usually drank nonfat milk, 52% usually ate low-fat or fat-free mayonnaise, 59% ate low-fat chips/snacks, and 42% ate nonfat cheese. African American and Hispanic women of lower socioeconomic status reported significantly fewer low-fat practices than white women and women of higher socioeconomic status.[47]

Glanz stressed the importance of support from the family and health care providers.[46] Carson reported on a team approach to nutrition for persons with cancer, in which nutritionists helped clients solve a variety of diet-related problems and provided information or referral to other team members as necessary. Nutritionists also provided credible information and answered questions about unorthodox dietary practices. Carson's article gave case examples to illustrate these activities.[48] Campbell et al. taught systematic relaxation techniques to 22 persons with cancer in their homes in an effort to promote weight gain in underweight persons. Only 55% of these persons practiced the relaxation techniques regularly, but nutritional status and cancer performance status improved among the compliers.[49] This preliminary study suggested that for motivated persons, relaxation techniques may help with diet, pain control, and anxiety reduction.

Nutrition education for persons with cancer must be part of the comprehensive treatment program and account for individual needs and preferences. It will probably gain more attention as survival rates for various cancers increase in the years ahead.[46]

The discussion below focuses on a diet recommended in the two National Cancer Institute Trials, the WHI and the WINS. An example of how to apply counseling skills to a specific low-fat diet for cancer prevention is provided in the following text.

Inappropriate Eating Behaviors

For the client who has difficulty with simple math, adding up total grams of fat consumed in a day can be very difficult. For some, just finding the time to make the computations may be a problem. The low-fat diet may be very different from the client's traditional high-fat diet. For example, a client might state, "I miss fried meats, fried potatoes, gravy, and vegetables smothered with butter. I don't know how to avoid those favorite dishes."

Assessment of Eating Behaviors

Assessing intake of fat might require using several three-day diet records and a quantified food frequency. Initially, the Client Eating Questionnaire for clients following cholesterol- and fat-controlled eating patterns might be of value (see Adherence Tool 4-1 in Chapter 4).

Treatment Theories and Strategies

Treatment strategies can be divided into three categories: those addressing lack of knowledge, lack of planning, and lack of commitment.

Strategies to Address Lack of Knowledge

Three-day diet diaries can be used to identify problem areas. Once the counselor and client have mutually identified a problem area, the counselor can determine exactly where knowledge may be lacking. The following are examples of problem areas:

- using mathematical skills
- knowing what to look for on a label
- cooking high-fat, ethnic dishes in a low-fat manner
- eating in restaurants

Using Mathematical Skills

For the person who has problems using math skills, the counselor can identify exactly where problems are occurring (for example, whether the math calculations for certain meals like breakfast are easier while calculations for other meals may be more difficult because of the variations in foods). The counselor should praise the use of math skills at one meal and build upon those for a more difficult meal.

Client: "I especially have trouble calculating grams of fat in meat at dinner."

Counselor: "You have done an excellent job with breakfast. I'm glad you brought up this problem with dinner so that we can try to solve it."

Client: "I'm no good at math. I can't handle this problem."

Counselor: "You have proven that you can use math skills in more routine situations at breakfast. Let's use some of those same skills for the dinner meal. You have said meat is a major problem; let's try to calculate it."

Reading Labels

A second problem involves lack of knowledge of what to look for on a label. Sometimes examples are unclear or covered too quickly in a nutrition counseling session for the client to gain adequate understanding of how to apply the knowledge to all situations. In subsequent sessions, it is up to the counselor to assess a problem in this area and allow for enough rehearsal to transfer general information adequately to specific individual situations.

Client: "I just don't know what to look for on food labels. It's so frustrating."

Counselor: "Can you give me an example of a label that has been difficult to figure out?"

Client: "Yes, this ingredient list says that there is no fat in this macaroni dish. But I have added margarine when I cook the food using the dry ingredients from the box, so I know fat is included."

Counselor: "The ingredient list will not include those items added to a product, only items in the box as you buy it. It is very important to count the fat added because it will contribute to your total fat for the day."

Cooking High-Fat, Ethnic Dishes in a Low-Fat Manner

Some clients have a problem combining the low-fat diet with their past high-fat, ethnic eating patterns.

Client: "I have a difficult time avoiding fried foods. They have become such an important part of my usual eating habits."

Counselor: "Martha, what foods in particular are you concerned about?"

Client: "I mostly miss fried potatoes."

Counselor: "Let's try using PAM spray and frying your potatoes with very little fat. Would you be willing to try that?"

Client: "I hadn't thought of that. It's a great idea."

Eating in Restaurants

Eating in restaurants forces the client to make many decisions. Initially choosing the restaurant can be a problem. Controlling the amount of food eaten, making changes at the table, and making low-fat requests are all important when eating out (see Adherence Tool 9-1).

Applying Other Strategies to Address Lack of Knowledge

Knowledge about how to deal with low-fat substitutions when eating can be valuable in beginning a low-fat diet (see Adherence Tools 9-2 to 9-5).

Knowledge is seldom enough to increase motivation or adherence, but misinformation can definitely undermine success. If a client is motivated but doesn't understand a correct procedure, simply providing the appropriate information can make a great difference. It is important to provide information on what to do, how to do it, and why it should be done. The tips below are ways to be sure clients understand information adequately:

- Knowing the rationale for the new eating pattern helps the client remember what information has been provided.

- Asking the client to repeat information can help in knowledge retention.
- Adding new information on the low-fat eating pattern to what the client already knows helps retention.
- Using language the client understands is important.
- Reemphasizing the benefits of the new low-fat eating pattern can help clear up the client's misunderstandings about the regimen and increase the client's involvement in active change.
- Providing information slowly over time helps eliminate overloading the client with too much information at one time.
- Practicing use of information in an actual or simulated situation helps the client retain information.
- Providing identical written information that supports verbally presented material can help the client retain information.

Strategies to Address Lack of Planning

Cues to help remind a client to plan to eat a low-fat diet can be very important. Some occasions that call for cueing are: vacations, parties, holiday meals, and birthdays.

Client: "I forgot to ask the waitress to give me salad dressing on the side, and I know I ate too much on the salad."
Counselor: "What might you have done to avoid this situation?"
Client: "Sometimes I just need help remembering."
Counselor: "Who might help remind you?"
Client: "My husband might remind me."
Counselor: "That's a great idea. Sometimes reminders from a spouse can turn into nagging. Has that ever happened to you?"
Client: "Yes, it has. How can I avoid that?"
Counselor: "One way is to provide your husband with a few specific things that are key in helping to remind you. The salad dressing on the side might be one of three or four specific reminders. This will eliminate constant general nagging."

Parties, holiday meals, and birthdays may be made easier by preplanning. For example, by calling the hostess ahead of time, clients can check out all items on the menu to determine fat content. By preplanning, the client can choose those items lowest in fat and lessen the temptation just to forget about the diet during the special event.

Aids for remembering can also point to the client's achievements and allow for positive reinforcement of healthy behaviors. One woman keeps a list of all of those tasks she must do in a day (see Adherence Tool 9-6). A check when each task is completed helps clients feel they have accomplished something.

A sign on the refrigerator with fat scores (tally of total fat eaten in a day) for each day of the week serves as a reminder to strive for a fat score goal.

Strategies to Address Lack of Commitment

Three factors contribute to lack of commitment to following a low-fat diet: a history of defeats, a negative attitude, and self-doubts. Theories that are important to achieving behavior change include behavior modification, cognitive behavioral therapy, and the transtheoretical model. Strategies within these theories are covered in the text below.

A History of Defeats

A client with a history of poor adherence to other diets may have problems following the low-fat eating pattern. Many clients begin a new eating pattern expecting to fail. To overcome the client's feelings of failure the counselor provides support and encouragement. Counselors should encourage the attitude that success is possible and emphasize taking a break from the old habit of going on and off a diet, stressing instead the idea of permanent lifestyle change. The client should know that lapses will occur and that these seemingly negative occurrences can be turned into positive learning experiences. Building new skills from past problems is important (Cognitive Behavioral Therapy, Cognitive Restructuring).

Negative Attitude

Some clients who have watched family members die of cancer may be very afraid of its consequences. They may feel that nothing can really help them. Following an eating pattern that may reduce risk is at least one way of easing a troubled mind. Counselors can discuss the goal of the new eating pattern with such clients and emphasize that the eating plan is a healthy one (Cognitive Restructuring).

Self-Doubts

For some clients, self-doubts can begin to creep into thoughts. Counselors can help clients focus on their successes.

Client: "Life isn't spontaneous anymore. I always have to think about what I'm eating. I'm not sure this new eating plan is worth the trouble."

Counselor: "Look at the successes you have already had. Have you ever done anything that you were proud of or successful at in the past? How did you feel at that time? Did it become easier as time went on? Let's try to build on those past efforts and be successful with this diet also" (Cognitive Restructuring).

This is an example of a client who has reverted to the precontemplation stage (Transtheoretical Model). The counselor doesn't give advice, but rather tries to involve the client in looking back over past successes.

Counselors should assist the client in tearing down blocks to adherence, for example, by helping clients develop short-term goals that they can easily achieve. This technique allows for positive self-rewards. By shaping behavior in this way, the counselor helps the client develop a more positive outlook. Counselors can also guide clients in practicing positive self-talk to help identify negative monologues and change them to positive (Cognitive Restructuring). Positive self-talk can lead to positive changes in eating patterns (see Appendixes F and G).

Some clients may benefit from assertiveness training. Feeling confident enough to ask the ingredients of a dish ordered in a restaurant can be a step toward successfully following the low-fat eating pattern.

What a client believes is true can help or hinder success. Following are some examples. Some clients have misconceptions about a low-fat eating pattern.

Client: "I've been reading that diets too low in fat can be bad for you."

Counselor: "What is your source of information?" [Explain misconceptions]

Some clients have unrealistic beliefs about the low-fat eating style:

Client: "I already eat a low-fat diet. This will be easy."

Counselor: "Your diet diaries show that your current eating pattern is low in visible fat but high in hidden fat. Let me show you what I mean."

Client: "Wow, my diet is high in fat. I'd better start cutting back."

Some clients may begin by being unnecessarily fearful.

Client: "Life will never be the same. I can never again eat just what I want."

Counselor: "If you feel like forgetting the new eating plan, give yourself a controlled 'day off.' By that, I mean increase your fat intake, but in a controlled fashion. For example, set aside one meal a week as a higher-fat meal."

Many clients find that the higher-fat foods are not so terrific and that, indeed, they have lost their taste for them.

Some behavioral strategies that help increase commitment are:

1. shaping of behaviors
2. self-monitoring
3. contracts
4. self-reward
5. group support networks.

Shaping behavior requires a gradual, stepwise process toward change that helps build success in stages, which promotes further success.

Client: "I know skim milk is lowest in fat, but I grew up on a farm where skim milk was given to livestock. I will never be able to give up whole milk."

Counselor: "Would you be willing to try a gradual movement to skim milk?"

Client: "I guess I can try."

Counselor: "First try using 2% milk. You can begin by mixing 2% and whole milk and then moving solely to 2%. You could then mix 2% and 1% milk and eventually move to only 1%. The same combination of 1% and skim would then end in eventual use of only skim milk."

Self-monitoring, another important strategy, encourages self-reliance, provides immediate feedback, shows behavior patterns that undermine or build success, and provides a means of planning for future problems so that they can be minimized. Examples of self-monitoring tools include Adherence Tool 9-7, which records grams of fat consumed in a day, and Adherence Tool 9-8, which allows weekly budgeting, or eating a little more fat one day and a little less the following day. Adherence Tool 9-9 provides a list of low-fat eating behaviors along with a check-off system to determine success. Adherence Tool 9-10 is a form for recording accomplishments in switching to low-fat foods over one week. Adherence Tool 9-11 is a meal-planning chart.

Client: "Most of my problem eating times seem to be when I am alone and my husband is out of town."

Counselor: "Are there others with whom you can eat when your husband is away to help eliminate boredom?"

Client: "Yes, I have a close friend who might go to the movies with me."

Contracts may work well when nothing seems to help the client achieve the adherence goal of a set number of grams of fat per day. In a contract, the client and counselor write down the goal in a very specific manner, along with some reward. Specific tips on developing contracts include the following:

- Be sure the contract includes automatic self-rewards such as reading a book, sewing, or anything already available so that extensive shopping or time is not required to obtain the reward.
- Be sure the client is involved in planning and has responsibility for the outcome.
- Be sure the client signs the contract to indicate formal commitment.
- Be sure that rewards are self-administered when goals are achieved.

The counselor provides the support and encouragement while the client plans and carries out the terms of the contract. The client must be involved in making major decisions and striving to fulfill the contract. Adherence Tool 9-11 allows the client to take an active role in meal planning. The contract might specify this as a task instead of eating.

Although nutrition counselors can provide a great deal of reinforcement, teaching the client to provide self-administered rewards can be helpful. An example is a verbal pat on the back: "You followed your exact grams of fat today without going over your prescription. That's great!" For some clients, verbal rewards may be less important than tangible rewards such as spending the weekend alone with a friend, buying clothes, having hair styled, going to a movie, or reading a book.

Positive thinking as a part of rehearsing what will happen can be beneficial (Cognitive Restructuring). For example, if following the new eating pattern during a party is the goal, a client can imagine standing before the buffet table making only low-fat choices. This behavior can then be followed by a reinforcing outcome, like feeling healthy or taking a pleasant two-mile walk.

Support from groups can help to increase commitment to following a new, low-fat eating pattern. Support can come from others who are following the diet, fellow workers, friends, or family. The group that can have three or four members or be a buddy system can offer empathy for similar problems, provide helpful ideas for solving problems, give positive reinforcement when a goal is met, serve as role models, and help to minimize stress.

When goals are not met, reestablishing goals that are easily attainable is important. While a long-term goal may be to lower total fat to 20% of total calories, that goal does not tell the client how to develop realistic steps toward that goal.

Client: "I love meat. Since it is my major problem, I should probably set my goal at cutting back drastically on it. I really worry about being able to follow this diet."

Counselor: "Just because you see meat as a major barrier to following your new eating plan doesn't mean that you have to tackle it first. What other foods do you eat that are high in fat?"

Client: "I still use whole milk, but I don't use a lot of it and it won't be that difficult to switch to skim."

Counselor: "Let's start with that area first. It sounds as though you are confident that changes in that area won't be too burdensome."

Waning commitment to an eating pattern can begin with lack of support from a spouse, family members, a housemate, or friends. An otherwise supportive spouse may become unsupportive when faced with a rival, the low-fat diet. A spouse may become jealous, threatened, or hurt by the demands of a new eating style.

Client: "My husband is not supportive. This is an example of how he feels about my new eating style: 'This diet is all yours. I'm not joining you in a feast of rabbit food!'"
Counselor: "Have you ever asked how he feels about the low-fat eating pattern?"
Client: "No, but I think he is hurt that I no longer pay attention to him but devote all my energy to the new eating pattern."
Counselor: "How have you coped with problems like this in the past?"
Client: "We have always talked through our problems."
Counselor: "What might you say now? Perhaps being honest about your feelings would help. For example, 'It makes me feel angry and hurt when you make fun of my eating habits. You don't have to eat my 'rabbit food,' but your support of my new habits would be appreciated.'"

Sometimes children in a family make it difficult to change eating patterns. Children can also have many different feelings: jealousy, neglect, and deprivation of their favorite foods.

Client: "My children are so negative sometimes. They say things like 'Why do we have to eat this awful, low-fat stuff? We are playing basketball and need some good food.'"
Counselor: "What do you think your children would accept as a compromise?"
Client: "They might appreciate a homemade snack that is lower in fat."
Counselor: "That's a great idea."

Some children may not take efforts to follow a low-fat diet seriously: "This is just another crazy diet." The family should know that the new, low-fat eating pattern may be effective in preventing a disease and that it is very important to be supportive. Clients should involve children in meal planning, calculating a fat score, and helping to avoid temptations.

Here are several ways to help increase the support of family members:

- It is important to discuss openly feelings about the new, low-fat eating pattern. If the client tells the family members the importance of avoiding high-fat snacks, they will be more likely to comply.
- It is best to be patient. A family needs time to go through changes.
- The client must try to provide reinforcement when support is offered, no matter how minor the support.

Holidays, stressful periods, and eating out are all potential challenges to adherence. Adherence Tool 9-12 provides a way to plan ahead for a special event. Never going off the new, low-fat eating pattern is a very unrealistic expectation and should be avoided as a written goal. Adherence Tool 9-13 lists a variety of strategies to minimize difficult eating situations during vacations and holidays. Here are several suggestions for participants who have trouble during these times:

- Do not be afraid to ask for help from friends or relatives prior to a special holiday. If the request is made early, the hostess will appreciate having low-fat dishes for the client's benefit.
- View following the diet as a series of corrections, not as an undeviating straight line.
- Expect and predict setbacks in a holiday season.
- Practice saying "no."

Stressful periods can cause changes in strict observance of a dietary pattern. Adherence Tool 9-14 provides a few strategies to help save time and thus reduce stress associated with meal preparation. During stressful periods, it is important to identify the cause of the change and the emotion associated with it.

Client: "When I am depressed, tired, or in general under a lot of pressure at work, I turn to my favorite high-fat foods for comfort."

Counselor: "When eating is a way of consoling yourself, you

> might make a list of those things that provide comfort or positive reinforcement. These should be things that do not involve eating. Can you think of some things now?"
>
> Client: "Sometimes just going to talk with a friend boosts my spirits."

When clients need comfort, other activities that give reinforcement might be taking a bubble bath, listening to music, or calling a friend.

Tension or anxiety may also cause a lapse in adherence. Exercise, like walking or swimming, may relieve stress. Making a list of things to do, and then delegating and prioritizing this list can help manage stress.

When boredom causes the problem, keeping busy may be the answer. Clients can write a list of tasks to be completed or volunteer for an organization, take a class, learn a craft, or participate in any number of other activities.

Eating out is frequently a problem when others make the majority of the decisions. For example, a German meal served family style may lead to eating more than intended. A special occasion on which food is ordered for the client may result in eating inappropriately large amounts of fat. Many occasions call for spontaneity, such as beer and pizza after a bowling game or an office party.

Many options are available to help with social occasions:

- The client can call the restaurant ahead of time to determine what is on the menu and eliminate surprises.
- The client can bring in menus from favorite restaurants for review, and role play with the counselor in selecting from a menu in a safe environment.
- By saving all of the fat for the day and using it only at the special restaurant meal, clients can eat without worrying whether they are adhering to the low-fat eating plan.
- Positive monologues can help clients work through an adherence-challenging situation.
- Sometimes making a compromise can help the client through a difficult situation. For example, "I will order the cheese cake, but only eat one-third of it."
- Eating slowly allows for eating less and prevents others from offering second servings.

Lapses in following the new, low-fat eating pattern should not lead to feelings of guilt or anger (Cognitive Restructuring). Deviation from the new eating pattern is a way to make corrections; past actions are something to forget. Clients can start anew with more appropriate eating behaviors, viewing the setback as temporary or short-lived ("a bad day") rather than a forecasting of "never" getting better.

When commitment to the study begins to wane, a specific plan of action to help cope with adherence-challenging situations helps clients achieve goals in spite of the barriers. The following are two examples of plans to help eliminate barriers to adherence:

Client: "I find that I go overboard when I attend parties with my husband."

Counselor: "What are some preliminary planning steps that might help you?"

Client: "I suppose I could do what I've done on other days and save my fat for the cocktail party. This means all of my other meals are virtually fat free."

Counselor: "Are there ways to minimize your feelings of hunger during the party?"

Client: "I could snack on low-fat snacks at home. This might prevent eating on a whim during the party."

Counselor: "Great! One suggestion I might give is to avoid alcohol at the party. It can make you careless and less aware of what you are eating."

A second example of overcoming barriers to success in the new eating pattern follows:

Client: "I frequently eat more when I'm under stress."

Counselor: "Can you describe in detail when stresses occur and what causes them?"

Client: "Usually a hectic day at work when someone is on vacation is stressful."

Counselor: "What can you do in advance to avoid these situations?"

Client: "I could plan ahead by bringing a sack lunch on days when I know the potential for stress is greatest."

Counselor: "Great idea!"

To be effective, a strategy should include the following:

- a description of strategy A to be taken, plus an alternative strategy B if A does not work
- rehearsals of specific strategies through role playing or reviewing mentally
- application of these strategies to specific, predictable stressful situations.

Stressful life events, including death or illness in the family, divorce, marriage, or retirement, can cause major changes in commitment. During these times, it is best to maintain changes and avoid making others. Even if a lapse in following an eating pattern occurs at this time, it should be viewed as temporary (one week) with the plan of renewing efforts the next week and maintaining good adherence.

Some clients may feel discouraged at times. The counselor can remind them of how much progress they have already made, focus on these positive changes (such as coming to appointments), and let clients know that others experience this same discouragement.

At times, clients whose commitment wavers can be encouraged by being asked to use their talents to show they are accomplished in areas other than eating. For example, a client can bring in a favorite recipe to share with others, or an artistic client might help design a handout with patient information.

Conclusion

Counseling on a low-fat eating pattern involves knowledge of the fat content of food and an ability to use that knowledge in designing individualized eating patterns. Knowledge can provide assistance in making social eating more pleasant. Reminders to avoid high-fat foods can be beneficial in maintaining good dietary adherence. When commitment wanes, the counselor's ability to deal with goal setting, positive self-talk (Cognitive Restructuring), assertiveness training, shaping, self-monitoring, contracts, self-rewards, and group support is extremely important.

Review of Chapter 9

1. List two problems associated with inappropriate eating behaviors when following a fat-controlled eating pattern.

a. _____

b. _____

2. List two dietary components to assess in modifying a diet for possible cancer risk prevention.

   a. _____

   b. _____

3. List three theories and strategies that might help the client follow a fat-controlled eating pattern.

   a. _____

   b. _____

   c. _____

4. The following describes a problem situation with a client who has been instructed on a fat-controlled eating pattern to reduce risk of breast cancer.

   Mrs. B is trying to follow a low-fat diet. During an assessment of her current eating habits, it was apparent that most difficulties occur with the evening meal, which is traditionally high fat (potatoes with gravy, high-fat meat, buttered vegetable, and high-fat dessert). Mrs. B's family loves these high-fat meals. (a) What additional information might you request regarding current eating habits? (b) What strategies would you use to help alleviate the problem? (c) Why did you choose these strategies?

   a. _____

   b. _____

   c. _____

References

1. Jemal A, Siegel R, Ward E, Murray T, Xu J, Thun MJ. Cancer statistics, 2007. *CA Cancer J Clin* 2007;57(1):43–66.
2. Hill MJ. Diet and human cancer: A new era for research. In: Joossens

JV, Hill MJ, Geboers J, eds. *Diet and Human Carcinogenesis.* New York: Elsevier Science Publishers; 1985:3–12.

3. Doll R, Peto R. The causes of cancer: quantitative estimates of avoidable risks of cancer in the United States today. *J Natl Cancer Inst* 1981;66(6):1191–1308.

4. Wynder EL, Gori GB. Contribution of the environment to cancer incidence: an epidemiologic exercise. *J Natl Cancer Inst* 1977;58(4):825–832.

5. Key TJ, Schatzkin A, Willett WC, Allen NE, Spencer EA, Travis RC. Diet, nutrition and the prevention of cancer. *Public Health Nutr* 2004;7(1A):187–200.

6. Gotay CC. Behavior and cancer prevention. *J Clin Oncol* 2005;23(2):301–310.

7. McCullough ML, Giovannucci EL. Diet and cancer prevention. *Oncogene* 2004;23(38):6349–6364.

8. Michels KB. The role of nutrition in cancer development and prevention. *Int J Cancer* 2005;114(2):163–165.

9. Willett WC. Diet and cancer: an evolving picture. *JAMA* 2005;293(2):233–234.

10. Dwyer JT. Dietary fat and breast cancer: testing interventions to reduce risks. *Adv Exp Med Biol* 1992;322:155–183.

11. Carroll KK, Khor HT. Dietary fat in relation to tumorigenesis. *Prog Biochem Pharmacol* 1975;10:308–353.

12. Weisburger JH, Wynder EL. Dietary fat intake and cancer. *Hematol Oncol Clin North Am* 1991;5(1):7–23.

13. Cohen LA, Kendall ME, Zang E, Meschter C, Rose DP. Modulation of N-nitrosomethylurea-induced mammary tumor promotion by dietary fiber and fat. *J Natl Cancer Inst* 1991;83(7):496–501.

14. Prentice RL, Sheppard L. Dietary fat and cancer: consistency of the epidemiologic data, and disease prevention that may follow from a practical reduction in fat consumption. *Cancer Causes Control* 1990;1(1):81–97; discussion 99–109.

15. Prentice RL, Sheppard L. Dietary fat and cancer: rejoinder and discussion of research strategies. *Cancer Causes Control* 1991;2(1):53–58.

16. Willett WC, Stampfer MJ. Dietary Fat and Cancer: Another View. *Cancer Causes Control* 1990;1(1):102–109.

17. Howe GR. Dietary Fat and Cancer. *Cancer Causes Control* 1990;1(1):99–100.

18. Hiller JE, McMichael AJ. Dietary fat and cancer: a comeback for etiological studies? *Cancer Causes Control* 1990;1(1):101–102.

19. Kolonel LN, Nomura AM, Hirohata T, Hankin JH, Hinds MW. Association of diet and place of birth with stomach cancer incidence in Hawaii Japanese and Caucasians. *Am J Clin Nutr* 1981;34(11):2478–2485.

20. Gori GB. Dietary and nutritional implications in the multifactorial etiology of certain prevalent human cancers. *Cancer* 1979;43(5 Suppl):2151–2161.

21. Miller AB, Kelly A, Choi NW, et al. A study of diet and breast cancer. *Am J Epidemiol* 1978;107(6):499–509.
22. Lubin F, Wax Y, Modan B. Role of fat, animal protein, and dietary fiber in breast cancer etiology: a case-control study. *J Natl Cancer Inst* 1986;77(3):605–612.
23. Graham S, Marshall J, Mettlin C, Rzepka T, Nemoto T, Byers T. Diet in the epidemiology of breast cancer. *Am J Epidemiol* 1982;116(1):68–75.
24. Willett WC. Implications of total energy intake for epidemiologic studies of breast and large-bowel cancer. *Am J Clin Nutr* 1987;45(1 Suppl):354–360.
25. Willett WC, Stampfer MJ, Colditz GA, Rosner BA, Hennekens CH, Speizer FE. Dietary fat and the risk of breast cancer. *N Engl J Med* 1987;316(1):22–28.
26. Hebert JR, Wynder EL. Letter to the Editor. *N Engl J Med* 1987;317:165–166.
27. Wynder EL, Cohen LA, Rose DP, Stellman SD. Dietary fat and breast cancer: where do we stand on the evidence? *J Clin Epidemiol* 1994;47(3):217–222; discussion 223–230.
28. Self S, Prentice R, Iverson D, et al. Statistical design of the Women's Health Trial. *Control Clin Trials* 1988;9(2):119–136.
29. Kakar F, Henderson M. Diet and breast cancer. *Clin Nutr* 1985;4:119–130.
30. Kolonel LN, Le Marchand L. The epidemiology of colon cancer and dietary fat. In: Ip C, Birt DF, Rogers AE, Mettlin C, eds. *Dietary Fat and Cancer.* New York: Liss, 1986:69–91.
31. Wynder EL, McCoy GD, Reddy BS, et al. Nutrition and metabolic epidemiology of cancers of the oral cavity, esophagus, colon, breast, prostate and stomach. In: Newell GR, Ellison NM, eds. *Nutrition and Cancer: Etiology and Treatment.* New York: Raven Press, 1981:11–48.
32. Rose DP. The biochemical epidemiology of prostatic carcinoma. In: Ip C, Birt DF, Rogers AE, Mettlin C, eds. *Dietary Fat and Cancer.* New York: Liss; 1986:43–68.
33. Armstrong B, Doll R. Environmental factors and cancer incidence and mortality in different countries, with special reference to dietary practices. *Int J Cancer* 1975;15(4):617–631.
34. Rose DP, Boyar AP, Wynder EL. International comparisons of mortality rates for cancer of the breast, ovary, prostate, and colon, and per capita food consumption. *Cancer* 1986;58(11):2363–2371.
35. Mahboubi E, Eyler N, Wynder EL. Epidemiology of cancer of the endometrium. *Clin Obstet Gynecol* 1982;25(1):5–17.
36. Hebert JR, Barone J, Reddy MM, Backlund JY. Natural killer cell activity in a longitudinal dietary fat intervention trial. *Clin Immunol Immunopathol* 1990;54(1):103–116.
37. Barone J, Hebert JR, Reddy MM. Dietary fat and natural-killer-cell activity. *Am J Clin Nutr* 1989;50(4):861–867.
38. The diets of British schoolchildren. Sub-committee on Nutritional Surveillance. Committee on Medical Aspects of Food Policy. *Rep Health Soc Subj (Lond)* 1989;36:1–293.

39. Lee HP, Gourley L, Duffy SW, Esteve J, Lee J, Day NE. Dietary effects on breast-cancer risk in Singapore. *Lancet* 1991;337(8751):1197–1200.
40. Byham LD. Dietary Fat and Natural Killer Cell Function. *Nutr Today* 1991;31:31–36.
41. Women's Health Initiative. *Protocol for Clinical Trial and Observation Components.* Seattle, WA: WHI Clinical Coordinating Center, 1994.
42. Tinker L, Burrows E, Henry H, Patterson R, Rupp J, Van Horn L. The Women's Health Initiative: overview of the nutrition components. In: Krummel DA, Kris-Etherton PM, eds. *Nutrition in Women's Health.* Gaithersburg, MD: Aspen Publishers, 1996:510–549.
43. Prentice RL, Caan B, Chlebowski RT, et al. Low-fat dietary pattern and risk of invasive breast cancer: the Women's Health Initiative Randomized Controlled Dietary Modification Trial. *JAMA* 2006;295(6):629–642.
44. Beresford SA, Johnson KC, Ritenbaugh C, et al. Low-fat dietary pattern and risk of colorectal cancer: the Women's Health Initiative Randomized Controlled Dietary Modification Trial. *JAMA* 2006;295(6):643–654.
45. Chlebowski RT, Blackburn GL, Elashoff RE, et al. Dietary fat reduction in postmenopausal women with primary breast cancer: Phase III Women's Intervention Nutrition Study (WINS). *Proc Am Soc Clin Oncol* 2005;24:10.
46. Glanz K. Nutrition education for risk factor reduction and patient education: a review. *Prev Med* 1985;14(6):721–752.
47. Patterson RE, Kristal AR, Coates RJ, et al. Low-fat diet practices of older women: prevalence and implications for dietary assessment. *J Am Diet Assoc* 1996;96(7):670–679.
48. Carson JA. Nutrition in a team approach to rehabilitation of the patient with cancer. *J Am Diet Assoc* 1978;72(4):407–409.
49. Campbell DF, Dixon JK, Sanderford LD, Denicola MA. Relaxation: its effect on the nutritional status and performance status of clients with cancer. *J Am Diet Assoc* 1984;84(2):201–204.

Adherence Tool 9-1 Eating Out (Informational Device)

WHERE YOU EAT
- Choose restaurants with low-fat choices.
- Stay away from all-you-can-eat places.
- Avoid restaurants that serve only fried foods.

HOW MUCH YOU EAT
- Order small servings.
- Select from the appetizer list, not the main dish list.
- Share your meal.

WHAT CHANGES YOU CAN MAKE
- Trim fat from meat.
- Remove skin from chicken.
- Dip your fork into salad dressing and then eat your lettuce.

WHAT REQUESTS YOU CAN MAKE
- Request salad dressing on the side.
- Ask for broiled, poached, or steamed rather than fried foods.
- Ask to have the cheese removed.
- Ask for all foods to have the fat left off (e.g., vegetables and meats with high-fat sauces, burgers with mayonnaise).

Adherence Tool 9-2 Make Your Desserts Low in Fat (Informational Device)

- Add fresh fruits to all main dishes and desserts.
- Choose ice milk, sherbert, sorbets, fruit ices, nonfat yogurt, and fat-free puddings.
- Choose angel food cake, gingersnaps, fig bars, apple and strawberry bars, vanilla wafers, and animal crackers.
- Select hard candy, licorice, jelly beans, and gumdrops.

Adherence Tool 9-3   Make Your Dairy Food Choices Low in Fat
(Informational Device)

- Gradually change your milk from whole to skim.
- Chill your skim milk on ice.
- Use evaporated skim milk for cooking and baking.
- Try part-skim mozzarella and low- or fat-free cheese.
- Eat smaller servings of ice cream less often.
- Choose ice milk, sherbert, or the new fat-free frozen desserts.
- Use fat-free sour cream.
- Use fat-free cream cheese.
- Use low-fat or fat-free frozen whipped toppings.

Adherence Tool 9-4   Ways to Cut Down on Fat (Informational Device)

- Spread margarine thin.
- Use honey or jam, not margarine or butter.
- Do not set butter or margarine on the table.
- Use a tomato sauce for a gravy.
- Choose "light" mayonnaise.
- Stir-fry in broth, flavored vinegar, or wine.

Adherence Tool 9-5   Spicing Low-Fat Foods (Informational Device)

- Try barbeque, Tabasco, catsup, or Worcestershire sauce to season chicken, turkey, and lean meats.
- Try oriental sauces such as hoisin, oyster, or sweet-and-sour sauce on stir-fry vegetables.
- Use dijon mustard and other hot mustards to add flavor to marinades and sauces.
- Use seasoned rice vinegar as a dressing.
- Try flavored vinegars such as raspberry, balsamic, or herbed.
- Experiment with herbs and spices.

Adherence Tool 9-6   Stress Management Chart (Informational and Cueing Device)

When you feel overwhelmed, make a "to do" list of everything you need to get done.

Date   Item To Do

_____

_____

_____

When you have finished the list, ask yourself the following questions:
1. Can I delete anything from this list that might be classified as unnecessary?
2. What can I delegate to a relative or friend?
3. What can I pay someone else to do?
4. What is the most important task? Now begin by doing it first.

Courtesy of Laura Coleman, Joanne Csaplar, Johanna Dwyer, Carole Palmer, and Molly Holland.

Adherence Tool 9-7   Fat Grams for One Day (Monitoring Device)

Meal or Snack	*Grams of Fat*
Breakfast	Total _____
Snack	Total _____
Lunch	Total _____
Snack	Total _____
Dinner	Total _____
Snack	Total _____
	TOTAL _____

Adherence Tool 9-8   Budgeting for Fat in a Two-Day Period (Monitoring Device)

Day	Grams of Fat
1 _____	_____
_____	_____
_____	_____
_____	_____
_____	Total _____
2 _____	_____
_____	_____
_____	_____
_____	_____
_____	Total _____

Adherence Tool 9-9   Low-Fat Action List for a Day (Monitoring Device)

Make a list of specific types of eating behaviors involving low-fat eating that you wish to accomplish:

	Check off when accomplished
1.	( )
2.	( )
3.	( )
4.	( )
5.	( )

Examples: 1. Switch from high-fat wieners to lower-fat turkey franks.
2. Use skim milk instead of 1% milk.
3. Have fruit compote for dessert instead of a high-fat fruit cobbler.

Courtesy of Laura Coleman, Joanne Csaplar, Johanna Dwyer, Carole Palmer, and Molly Holland.

Adherence Tool 9-10 Low-Fat Eating Accomplishments (Monitoring and Cueing Device)

Sunday	Monday	Tuesday	Wednesday	Thursday	Friday	Saturday

Courtesy of Laura Coleman, Joanne Csaplar, Johanna Dwyer, Carole Palmer, and Molly Holland.

Adherence Tool 9-11   Client Planning Chart (Informational Device)

Meal planning can help you keep your total fat intake low. Before your next visit, plan three days of meals in which you avoid foods high in fat.

Meal	Day 1	Day 2	Day 3
Breakfast			
Snack			
Lunch			
Snack			
Dinner			
Snack			

Adherence Tool 9-12   Planning for a Special Event or Occasion (Informational Device)

- Where will I stay?
- What activities will I do?
- Who can help or hinder me in following my diet?
- How do I feel about this occasion, and how will these feelings affect what I eat?
- What foods will be available, and what specific foods do I want to eat?
- How long will I be in this situation, and what can I do to eat less fat before and after it?

Adherence Tool 9-13   Strategies to Minimize Difficult Eating Situations During Vacations and Holidays (Informational Device)

- Find new recipes or lower the fat in old favorites.
- Plan to eat less fat on days before and after the holidays.
- Plan fun activities that don't involve eating.
- Eat before you go, so that you are not so hungry.
- Prepare a low-fat or fat-free food to bring to the occasion.
- Fill most of your plate with low-fat foods or a salad.
- Plan to spend most of your time talking not eating.
- Eat only high-fat foods that are your favorites.

Adherence Tool 9-14   How to Save Time (Informational Device)

- Plan meals ahead of time.
- Have low-fat and fat-free foods in your pantry and refrigerator.
- Keep a low-fat shopping list.
- Use time-saving equipment to make your meals (pressure cooker, microwave, electric skillet, etc.).
- Use leftovers.
- Use a file of quick and easy recipes.
- Use time-saving ingredients (precut vegetables; boned, skinless chicken; cubed turkey; precut fruits, etc.).
- Use convenience foods (frozen, canned, instant, etc.).
- Make double quantities and freeze part for a later meal.
- Use quick-cooking methods (microwave, stir-fry, poach, broil, etc.).

PART III

ENDING COUNSELING SESSIONS

This section describes techniques for assessing each counseling session and gives suggestions for client follow-up.

CHAPTER 10

EVALUATION AND FOLLOW-UP

Chapter Objectives

1. Identify elements necessary for evaluating both client and counselor.

2. Identify strategies to ensure dietary adherence after ceasing reinforcement.

3. Generate the reinstitution of an intervention or treatment plan.

4. Identify elements of the termination process.

Evaluation of Counselor Progress

Evaluation of the counselor's individual progress forms an important part of the client's success. A counselor can be ineffective in facilitating client success for a variety of reasons. The questions below are a way to begin defining potential problems.

1. Did the counseling session address the client's major problem?
2. Was assessment prior to designing a modified eating pattern adequate to prepare a dietary regimen compatible with the client's lifestyle?
3. Did the client's goal appear to have been achieved?
4. Were the strategies for altering eating behaviors carried out efficiently?
5. Did the counselor use appropriate verbal and nonverbal communication skills? Where might changes have been made?
6. Did the counselor use appropriate counseling skills? Where might changes have been made?

7. What general changes might the counselor make in the next counseling interview with a similar client?

Each list of questions should be made more specific as the situation requires and can be adapted, depending on answers given during the interview.

Evaluation of Client Progress

Evaluating the client's progress is crucial to maintenance of a modified eating pattern. Booster sessions to assist in solving problems may be a direct result of careful evaluation.

Following each session, the counselor can appraise the client's success. Below is a list of questions the client might ask to determine whether behavior has changed successfully:

1. Are my dietary patterns different but still compatible with my lifestyle?
2. Have my misconceptions about foods and what they contain been replaced with factual information?
3. Are social occasions less of a problem now than when I first began my diet?
4. Is my family providing needed positive reinforcement?

These very general questions provide insight into potential problems with dietary adherence. Evaluation of client progress is an ongoing process that should be a part of all client counseling sessions. The client should feel a sense of control in changing inappropriate eating behaviors. Self-management of problem eating behaviors is crucial to eventual maintenance of dietary goals.

Strategies to Maintain Dietary Adherence

Follow-up interviewing sessions are extremely important to counseling on nutrition-related issues. The number of return visits depends on the success of efforts in following a diet. There is always a point at which the nutrition counselor and client must end a set of counseling sessions. This is the point at which the counselor must be sure that the client can follow the diet without continued help. At that time, the goal of the counseling session is tested: Can the client function adequately in the real world?

Counselors must be sure that their clients are given ample opportunity during the sessions to practice eating behaviors, and these new behaviors must be reinforced in the natural environment. This can be done by asking clients for records of foods consumed, times eating takes place, persons present during the meal or snack, and the type of situation (where and what type of function). These records should be discussed thoroughly with the clients, and problem areas and their solutions noted.

To help with reinforcement in the natural setting, clients are asked to list times and places where their eating behaviors can be supported. The counselors then help them plan for natural situations that reinforce the new eating pattern. If new behaviors are really adjustive, clients should find natural support and natural reinforcements.

In early stages of termination, counselors should help clients identify chains of events that bolster behavior. A woman who had succeeded in losing 10 pounds found that her colleagues at work responded very warmly to her. She was asked out more often and spent more time in discussions with colleagues. She eliminated her clothes-buying reinforcement and instead posted a sign on her refrigerator door: "Dieting keeps the telephone ringing!"

After an eating behavior has been solidified in relation to one antecedent condition, clients can make that behavior even more frequent by gradually increasing the range of situations in which reinforcement occurs. They should test for generalization by looking at how reinforcement can be a part of many situations. By keeping a list of all situations in which either appropriate or inappropriate eating behaviors occur, nutritionists can work on problem situations before counseling is terminated.

An important issue to address before termination is building in resistance to extinction. The best way to ensure that an appropriate eating behavior continues is to develop an intermittent reinforcement schedule. A treatment plan should never be stopped abruptly.

Once an acceptable upper level of behavior has been established, the ratio of its reinforcement can be reduced. Instead of clients' always buying presents for themselves (such as clothing) after eating an appropriate meal, sporadic buying can be used as a reinforcement (e.g., 75% of the time, then 50%, then 25%, and so on).

During this gradual reduction in positive reinforcement, both counselors and clients must continue to count the frequency of the appropriate behaviors. There is some danger that these will decline. Alternating between periods of 0% and 100% reinforcement can keep their frequency at an acceptably high level if the natural supporters are slow to evolve.

Counselors should ensure that adequate practice of the reinforcement has occurred during intervention or treatment. In general, acceptable behaviors are made more probable by providing a certain number of trials on a reinforcement schedule. Practice is important.

This need for practice implies, correctly, that nutrition counselors should not terminate the program as soon as the goal is reached. Instead, it would be wise to continue the plan for a week or two, or perhaps more, depending on the frequency of the opportunities to practice. The number of practices depends on many factors in the intervention plan. For example, a more complicated dietary regimen may require division of practice into small segments, each focusing on one exchange category or a single nutrient counting system.

However, a trial at reducing reinforcement is a good test of the degree to which an eating behavior can be maintained after termination. If the frequency of the targeted behavior drops alarmingly as soon as a reduction in reinforcement begins, it means more practice is necessary. In that case, the 100% reinforcement schedule should be resumed, along with more practice. For this reason, the frequency of an eating behavior should be recorded after termination of reinforcement until the rate has stabilized.

Reinstitution of Intervention or Treatment

Nutrition counselors may find that an intervention plan must be restarted if gradually decreasing reinforcement seems to be causing an appropriate eating behavior to decrease. At that point, practitioners must be closely attuned to client needs.

Because clients must deal with many life stresses, their attention to an intervention strategy of gradually decreasing reinforcement may be diverted, resulting in total lack of support. By working with clients' significant others, practitioners can suggest persons who are aware of the importance of reinforcing good eating behaviors in the absence of nutrition counseling sessions. Chapter 3 provides many ideas on how to move from contemplation to action and focuses on the importance of goal setting.

The Termination Process

The algorithm in Figure 10-1 indicates a step procedure to use in terminating nutrition counseling. Termination should always be approached gradually. The algorithm indicates four possible situations:

1. Some clients begin having negative thoughts. The algorithm suggests listing those thoughts and working on them.
2. Some clients may refuse to discuss their thoughts, in which

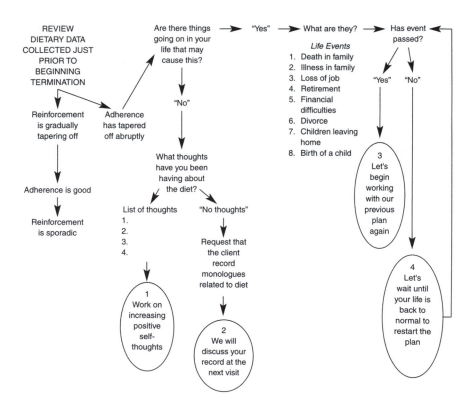

FIGURE 10–1   Algorithm for Nutrition Counseling Termination

case they should be asked to record both negative and positive monologues for discussion later.

3. Some other clients may admit to having a drastic change in their lifestyles. Those changes may be temporary. In that case, the intervention plan is reinstituted and reinforcements decreased gradually.

4. Clients in some cases may be in the midst of a change in lifestyle. If so, counselors should wait until clients seem ready to restart the intervention plan, meanwhile keeping in close contact so that the diet is not totally forgotten.

Termination is different for each client. Counselors should be prepared to restart a strategy to help ensure adherence to the diet over long periods. They might call or write to the client periodically to check on progress. Such attention to the client's needs after the counseling has ended will show a sense of caring and may help maintain the individual's motivation.

A gradual fading process of termination rather than an abrupt "goodbye" is essential. If clients are to be successful on their own, they must prove that success is possible. Nutrition counselors can help clients find this success on their own. A gradual termination can prevent regression to problem eating behaviors.

Review of Chapter 10

(Answers in Appendix H)

1. Identify questions you might ask to evaluate counselor progress.

   a.

   b.

   c.

   d.

   e.

   f.

   g.

    h.

    i.

2. Identify questions you might ask to evaluate client progress.

    a.

    b.

    c.

    d.

3. Identify five ways in which you as a counselor might facilitate the continuation of appropriate dietary behaviors in clients who no longer will be coming in for interviews and must live with the regimen in the real world.

    a.

    b.

    c.

    d.

    e.

4. Mr. Y. has been slipping in his adherence to the low-sodium regimen he was following so well when counseling sessions were frequent. What questions might you use to determine exactly what has happened to the reinforcement schedule?

_____

_____

_____

5. What intervention plan can you recommend to help clients maintain dietary adherence?

_____

_____

_____

CHECKLIST OF NUTRITION COUNSELOR SELF-IMAGE

Check the items that are most descriptive of you.

Competence Assessment

___ 1. Constructive negative feedback about myself doesn't make me feel incompetent or uncertain of myself.

___ 2. I tend to put myself down frequently.

___ 3. I feel fairly confident about myself as a helper.

___ 4. I often am preoccupied with thinking that I'm not going to be a competent nutrition counselor.

___ 5. When I am involved in a conflict, I don't go out of my way to ignore or avoid it.

___ 6. When I get positive feedback about myself, I often don't believe it's true.

___ 7. I set realistic goals for myself as a helper that are within reach.

___ 8. I believe that a confronting, hostile client could make me feel uneasy or incompetent.

___ 9. I often find myself apologizing for myself or my behavior.

___10. I'm fairly confident I can or will be a successful counselor.

___11. I find myself worrying a lot about "not making it" as a counselor.

___12. I'm likely to be a little scared by clients who would idealize me.

___13. A lot of times I will set standards or goals for myself that are too tough to attain.

___14. I tend to avoid negative feedback when I can.

___15. Doing well or being successful does not make me feel uneasy.

Power Assessment

____ 1. If I'm really honest, I think my counseling methods are a little superior to other people's.

____ 2. A lot of times I try to get people to do what I want. I might get pretty defensive or upset if the client disagreed with what I wanted to do or did not follow my direction in the interview.

____ 3. I believe there is (or will be) a balance in the interviews between my participation and the client's.

____ 4. I could feel angry when working with a resistant or stubborn client.

____ 5. I can see that I might be tempted to get some of my own ideology across to the client.

____ 6. As a counselor, "preaching" is not likely to be a problem for me.

____ 7. Sometimes I feel impatient with clients who have a different way of looking at the world than I do.

____ 8. I know there are times when I would be reluctant to refer my clients to someone else, especially if the other counselor's style differed from mine.

____ 9. Sometimes I feel rejecting or intolerant of clients whose values and lifestyles are very different from mine.

____10. It is hard for me to avoid getting in a power struggle with some clients.

Intimacy Assessment

____ 1. There are times when I act more gruff than I really feel.

____ 2. It's hard for me to express positive feelings to a client.

____ 3. There are some clients I would really like to be my friends more than my clients.

____ 4. It would upset me if a client didn't like me.

____ 5. If I sense a client has some negative feelings toward me, I try to talk about it rather than avoid it.

____ 6. Many times I go out of my way to avoid offending clients.

____ 7. I feel more comfortable maintaining a professional distance between myself and the client.

____ 8. Being close to people is something that does not make me feel uncomfortable.

___ 9. I am more comfortable when I am a little aloof.

___ 10. I am very sensitive to how clients feel about me, especially if it is negative.

___ 11. I can accept positive feedback from clients fairly easily.

___ 12. It is difficult for me to confront a client.

Learning Activity Reaction: Applications to Your Counseling

1. For each of the three assessment areas above, look over your responses and determine the areas that seem to be OK and the areas that may be a problem for you or something to watch out for. You may find more problems in one area than another.

2. Do your "trouble spots" seem to occur with mostly everyone, or just with certain types of people? In all situations or some situations?

3. Compare yourself now to where you might have been four years ago or where you may be four years from now.

4. Identify any areas you feel you could use some help with, from a colleague, a supervisor, or a counselor.

Source: From *Interviewing Strategies for Helpers: Fundamental Skills and Cognitive Behavioral Interventions* by W.H. Cormier and L.S. Cormier. Copyright © 1991, 1985, and 1975 Brooks/Cole Publishing Company, Pacific Grove, California 93950, a division of International Thomson Publishing Inc. By permission of the publisher.

CHECKLIST OF NUTRITION COUNSELOR'S NONVERBAL BEHAVIOR

Instructions: Determine whether the counselor did or did not demonstrate the desired nonverbal behaviors listed in the right column. Check "yes" or "no" in the left column to indicate your judgment.

Desired Behaviors	Demonstrated Behaviors	
	Yes	*No*
Eye contact–Maintained persistent eye contact without gazing or staring.	_____	_____
1. Eyes		
Facial expression–Punctuated interaction with occasional head nods.	_____	_____
2. Head nods		
Mouth–Punctuated interaction with occasional smiles.	_____	_____
3. Smiles		
Body orientation and posture–Faced the other person, slight lean forward (from waist up), body appeared relaxed.	_____	_____
4. Facing client		
5. Leaning forward	_____	_____
6. Relaxed body	_____	_____

Desired Behaviors	*Demonstrated Behaviors*	
	Yes	*No*
Paralinguistics–Completed sentences without "who" or hesitations in delivery, asked one question at a time, did not ramble.	_____	_____
7. Completed sentences		
	_____	_____
8. Smooth delivery–no speech errors		
Distance–Seats of counselor and client were between 3 feet, or 1 meter, and 5 feet or $1^1/_2$ meters apart.	_____	_____
9. Distance		

Source: From *Interviewing Strategies for Helpers: Fundamental Skills and Cognitive Behavioral Interventions* by W.H. Cormier and L.S. Cormier. Copyright © 1991, 1985, and 1975 Brooks/Cole Publishing Company, Pacific Grove, California 93950, a division of International Thomson Publishing Inc. By permission of the publisher.

APPENDIX C

MEASUREMENTS OF NUTRITIONAL STATUS

Anthropometry

Elbow breadth, upper arm circumference, and three skinfold thicknesses—triceps, biceps, and subscapular—are described below. The purpose of the elbow breadth measurement is to classify the subject's frame size according to the appropriate column of the standard weight tables. The skinfold and arm circumference measurements are used to determine body fatness and arm muscle area. The repeated measurements are used to assess change in body fat and muscle mass.

Preparation

The skinfold calipers must measure accurately at different thicknesses of skinfolds. Use the calibration block to check the caliper calibration before measuring each client. A constant error of 1 millimeter is acceptable and should be added to or subtracted from the actual reading. A greater error requires repair or replacement of the calipers.

Measurement

Elbow Breadth

The client extends the right arm forward, perpendicular to the body, with the arm bent so the angle at the elbow measure 90 degrees and with the fingers pointing up and the dorsal part of the wrist toward the measurer. Apply the sliding caliper across the greatest breadth of the elbow joint (at the medial and lateral condyles of the humerus) along the axis of the upper arm. Approximate the arms of the caliper with firm pressure and read the breadth in millimeters.

Have the client repeat the arm maneuver and remeasure. Repeat the reading aloud and record. If the two measurements are within 1 millimeter, use the second measurement as the elbow breadth for the weight table. If the second measurement differs by more than one millimeter from the first, repeat until two consecutive measurements are within one millimeter. Use the last of the measurements as the elbow breadth. Table C–1 gives frame size from height and elbow breadth.

Upper Arm Circumference

The client flexes the right arm to 90 degrees at the elbow. Use the steel tape to measure the distance from the acromion to the end of the humerus. Mark the lateral part of the arm at the midpoint with a pen or skin marker. With the arm hanging freely, place the lower edge of the tape at skin mark and measure the circumference. The tape should fit snugly to the arm without compressing tissue. State the reading in millimeters and record. Repeat the maneuver. Successive measurements should be within 5 millimeters. Record the last measurement as the midarm circumference.

Skinfolds

Pick up a fold of skin and subcutaneous tissue between the thumb and index finger of the left hand and lift it firmly away from the underlying muscle. Hold the fold between the fingers throughout the time the measurement is being taken. Apply the calipers to the fold 1 centimeter below the fingertip so that pressure on the fold at the point measured is exerted by the caliper faces only, and not by the fingers. The calipers are applied to the skinfold by removing the thumb of the right hand from the trigger lever of the caliper.

The value registered on the calipers sometimes decreases as one watches the pointer of the dial. This decrease can usually be stopped by taking a firmer pinch with the left hand; if it continues, the reading must be taken immediately after application of the spring pressure.

All measurements are read to the nearest 1 millimeter. Obtain two measurements at each site. If the two measurements are within 5%, record the last measurement as the skinfold thickness. If the difference between the measurements exceeds 5%, repeat the maneuver until two successive measurements are within 5%.

Table C–1   Frame Size from Height and Elbow Breadth[1]

Height* (centimeters)	Small Frame (millimeters)	Medium Frame (millimeters)	Large Frame (millimeters)
Men Elbow Breadth			
150–154	< 62	62–71	> 71
155–158	< 64	64–72	> 72
159–168	< 67	67–74	> 74
169–178	< 69	69–76	> 76
179–188	< 71	71–78	> 78
189–190	< 74	74–81	> 81
191–194	< 76	76–82	> 82
195–199	< 78	78–83	> 83
200–204	< 79	79–85	> 85
205–209	< 80	80–88	> 89
Women Elbow Breadth			
145–148	< 56	56–64	> 64
149–158	< 58	58–65	> 65
159–168	< 59	59–66	> 66
169–178	< 61	61–68	> 68
179–180	< 62	62–69	> 69
181–184	< 63	63–70	> 70
185–189	< 64	64–71	> 71
190–194	< 65	65–72	> 72
195–199	< 66	66–73	> 73

*Without shoes.
[1]The medium frame elbow breadths for men, < 155 cm or ≤ 191 cm, and women, ≤ 181 cm, were determined by extrapolation on a semilog graph. Courtesy of *Statistical Bulletin*, Metropolitan Life Insurance Company, 1983, New York, New York.

Most skinfolds are measured in the vertical plane except when the Lines of Linn (natural skinfold lines) result in torsion of the skinfold, in which case the skinfold is taken along these lines.

Triceps skinfold. The client should be standing with right arm relaxed and suspended along midaxillary line. The point of measurement is at the skin mark made for arm circumference measurement. Pinch the skin and subcutaneous tissue (do not include muscle) between the thumb and index finger of your left hand. The pinch should be 1 centimeter above the skin mark and parallel to the long axis of the arm. The jaws of the calipers are placed perpendicular to the fold at the marked level.

Biceps skinfold. The client should be standing with right arm relaxed and suspended along midaxillary line. Pick up the skinfold on the front of the right arm directly above the center of the cubital fossa at the same level as that at which the triceps skinfold is measured.

Subscapular skinfold. The client should be standing and relaxed. Grasp the skin and subcutaneous tissue just below the inferior angle of the right scapula between your left thumb and index finger. Lines of Linn will determine the angle of the skinfold.

Calculation of Body Percent

Percent body fat is determined from (1) a regression equation for the prediction of body density from the triceps, biceps, and subscapular skinfolds and (2) an equation using the known relationship between body density and the proportion of fat in the body.[1]

Body density (Y) is calculated as follows:

$$Y = C - M \text{ (log of the sum of the skinfolds)} \qquad \text{Eq. 1}$$

The coefficients C and M are obtained from Table C–2 for the appropriate age and sex group.

Percent body fat is calculated as follows:

$$\% \text{ Fat} = ([4.95 \div Y] - 4.5) \times 100 \qquad \text{Eq. 2}$$

Example: A 45-year-old female has a sum of the three skinfolds of 50 millimeters.

$$Y = 1.1303 - 0.0635 \text{ (log 50)}$$
$$= 1.0224$$

Table C–2   Linear Regression Coefficients for the Estimation of Body Density $\times\,10^3$ (kg/m^3) from the Logarithm of the Skinfold Thickness (Biceps + Triceps + Subscapular)

Age (Years)	Males		Females	
Age Categories	C	M	C	M
17–19	1.1643	0.0727	1.1509	0.0715
20–29	1.1593	0.0694	1.1605	0.0777
30–39	1.1213	0.0487	1.1385	0.0654
40–49	1.1530	0.0730	1.1303	0.0635
50+	1.1569	0.0780	1.1372	0.0710
Overall				
17–72	1.1689	0.0793	1.1543	0.0756

Source: Reprinted from Durnin JVGA, Wormersley J. Body fat assessment from total body density and its estimation from skinfold thickness: measurements on 481 men and women aged from 16 to 72 years. *Br J Nutr* 1974;32:77–97, with permission of Cambridge University Press, © 1974.

$$\% \text{ Fat} = ([4.95 \div 1.0224] - 4.5) \times 100$$
$$= 34.1$$

Arm Muscle Area

The arm muscle area (AMA) is determined by two measurements: (1) triceps skinfold (TSF) in millimeters and (2) midarm circumference (MAC) in millimeters.[2] The following formula is used to calculate arm muscle area:

$$AMA = \frac{(MAC - II \times TSF)^2}{4\,II}$$

A corrected AMA$_c$ ("available" arm muscle area) is then calculated separately for men and women as follows:

$$\text{Men AMA}_c = AMA - 19$$
$$\text{Women AMA}_c = AMA - 15.5$$

Evaluation

Continued decreases in arm muscle area may indicate early signs of malnutrition. Large decreases in weight to less than 75% of standard body weight (as indicated in height and weight Table C-3) should prompt the nutritionist to look at change in arm muscle area. In the weight-loss client, a decrease in body fat as opposed to muscle area is preferable.

References

1. Durnin JVGA, Wormersley J. Body fat assessment from total body density and its estimation from skinfold thickness: measurements on 481 men and women aged from 16 to 72 years. *Br J Nutr* 1974;32:77–97.
2. Heymsfield SB, et al. Anthropometric measurements of muscle mass: revised equations for calculating bone-free arm muscle area, *Am J Clin Nutr* 1982;36:680–690.

Table C–3　Height and Weight Tables[†]

	Men Weight in Kilograms				Women Weight in Kilograms		
Height[1] (cm)	Small Frame[2]	Medium Frame[2]	Large Frame[2]	Height[1] (cm)	Small Frame[2]	Medium Frame[2]	Large Frame[2]
153	59.0	61.2	64.7	145	48.5	52.4	56.8
154	59.3	61.5	65.2	146	48.8	52.8	57.2
155	59.7	61.9	65.6	147	49.0	53.1	57.7
156	60.0	62.2	66.0	148	49.3	53.6	58.1
157	60.4	62.6	66.5	149	49.6	54.1	58.6
158	60.7	62.9	66.9	150	50.0	54.5	59.0
159	61.1	63.3	67.4	151	50.4	55.0	59.6
160	61.4	63.7	67.8	152	50.9	55.4	60.2
161	61.8	64.1	68.4	153	51.3	55.9	60.7
162	62.2	64.6	68.9	154	51.7	56.4	61.2
163	62.5	65.0	69.4	155	52.3	57.0	61.9
164	62.9	65.5	70.0	156	52.8	57.5	62.5
165	63.2	66.0	70.6	157	53.3	58.1	63.1
166	63.7	66.6	71.2	158	53.8	58.6	63.7
167	64.1	67.1	71.8	159	54.4	59.1	64.3
168	64.6	67.6	72.4	160	54.9	59.6	64.9
169	65.0	68.1	73.0	161	55.5	60.2	65.5
170	65.5	68.7	73.7	162	56.0	60.7	66.1
171	65.9	69.2	74.3	163	56.6	61.3	66.8
172	66.3	69.7	74.9	164	57.1	61.9	67.5
173	66.8	70.3	75.5	165	57.6	62.4	68.1
174	67.3	70.8	76.2	166	58.2	62.9	68.7
175	67.7	71.3	76.8	167	58.7	63.4	69.3
176	68.1	71.9	77.4	168	59.2	63.9	69.9
177	68.6	72.4	78.1	169	59.7	64.5	70.5
178	69.1	73.0	78.7	170	60.3	65.0	71.2

continued

Table C–3 *continued*

Men — Weight in Kilograms

Height[1] (cm)	Small Frame[2]	Medium Frame[2]	Large Frame[2]
179	69.6	73.6	79.3
180	70.2	74.3	80.0
181	70.8	74.9	80.7
182	71.4	75.5	81.4
183	72.0	76.2	82.1
184	72.7	76.9	82.9
185	73.3	77.6	83.7
186	73.9	78.2	84.5
187	74.5	78.8	85.3
188	75.3	79.6	86.2
189	76.0	80.4	87.1
190	76.7	81.2	88.0
191	77.3	81.8	88.9
192	78.1	82.6	89.9
193	78.9	83.5	91.0
194	79.7	84.3	92.0
195	80.5	85.1	93.0
196	81.1	85.7	94.0
197	81.9	86.6	95.2
198	82.8	87.5	96.4
199	83.7	88.4	97.6

Women — Weight in Kilograms

Height[1] (cm)	Small Frame[2]	Medium Frame[2]	Large Frame[2]
171	60.8	65.5	71.7
172	61.3	66.0	72.2
173	61.9	66.6	72.6
174	62.5	67.2	73.3
175	63.0	67.7	73.8
176	63.5	68.3	74.4
177	64.0	68.9	74.9
178	64.6	69.3	75.5
179	65.1	69.8	76.0
180	65.6	70.3	76.5
181	66.1	70.8	77.0
182	66.6	71.3	77.5
183	67.1	71.8	78.0
184	67.6	72.3	78.5
185	68.1	72.8	79.0
186	68.6	73.3	79.5
187	69.1	73.9	80.0
188	69.6	74.4	80.5
189	70.1	75.0	81.0
190	70.6	75.5	81.5
200	84.6	89.3	98.8

†Weights for heights in men below 155 cm and over 190 cm and in women over 180 cm estimated by extrapolation.
[1]Height without shoes.
[2]Frame size from Table C-1.

Source: Reprinted with permission from Metropolitan Life Foundation, "Height and Weight Tables," *Statistical Bulletin* (January–June 1983).

BEHAVIORAL CHART

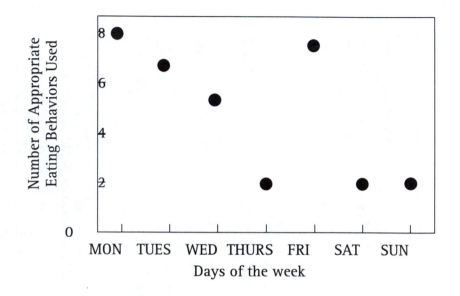

BEHAVIORAL LOG

Date	Time	Setting	Event	Actual Reaction	Desired Reaction

APPENDIX F

LOGS OF THOUGHTS RELATED TO FOOD

BASELINE LOG

Time	Thoughts
7:30	"I'd really like a doughnut, but I'm not going to blow my day."
8:15	"It's not fair, I'm really trying and I haven't lost anything."
9:10	"Wish I had a doughnut or something. I'm hungry."
10:00	"It's not fair, it's snack time and all I get is water."
11:30	"Nothing tastes as good when I know there's no dessert."
12:10	"Look at them. They stuff themselves with sweets and stay skinny."
1:15	"Maybe I could have just a couple of cookies after school. I've earned them."
2:30	"Look at them running off to their afternoon snacks. It's not fair."
3:15	"I don't care if I'm fat. I'll never lose anyway. It's not worth it."
4:30	"I might as well eat and enjoy it. I'll never lose anyway. It's not worth it."
5:45	"You pig. Now you feel stuffed and you've ruined your day."
7:30	"What a failure I am. I don't deserve to be thin."
9:00	"I'll never learn, will I? It's no use."
10:30	"I feel hopeless. I've tried everything and I always blow it."

Source: From Mahoney MJ, Mahoney K. *Permanent Weight Control: A Total Solution to the Dieter's Dilemma,* Copyright © 1976 by W.W. Norton & Company, Inc. Reprinted by permission of W.W. Norton & Company, Inc.

REPLACEMENT LOG

Problem Category	Negative Monologues	Appropriate Monologues
Pounds Lost	"I'm not losing fast enough." "I've starved myself and haven't lost a thing." "I've been more consistent than Mary and she is losing faster than I am. It's not fair."	"Pounds don't count. If I continue my eating habits, the pounds will be lost." "Have patience—those pounds took a long time to get there. As long as they stay off permanently, I'll settle for any progress." "It takes a while to break down fat and absorb the extra water produced. I'm not going to worry about it."
Capabilities	"I just don't have the willpower." "I'm just naturally fat." "Why should this work—nothing else has?" "I'll probably just regain it." "What the heck—I'd rather be fat than miserable. Besides, I'm not that heavy."	"There's no such thing as lack of willpower—just poor planning." "If I make a few improvements here and there and take things one day at a time, I can be very successful." "It's going to be nice to be permanently rid of all this extra baggage. I'm starting to feel better already."
Excuses	"If it weren't for my job and the kids, I could lose weight." "It's just impossible to eat right with a schedule like mine." "I'm just so nervous all the time—I have to eat to satisfy my psychological needs." "Maybe next time. . . "	"My schedule isn't any worse than anyone else's. What I need to do is be a bit more creative in how to improve my eating." "Eating doesn't satisfy psychological problems—it creates them." "Job, kids, or whatever, I'm the one in control."
Goals	"Well, there goes my diet. That coffee cake probably cost me two pounds, and	"What is this—the Olympics? I don't need perfect habits, just improved ones."

continued

Problem Category	Negative Monologues	Appropriate Monologues
	after I promised myself—no more sweets."	"Why should one sweet or an extra portion blow it for me? I'll cut back elsewhere."
	"I always blow it on the weekends."	"Those high standards are unrealistic."
	"Fine—I start the day off with a doughnut. I may as well enjoy myself today."	"Fantastic—I had a small piece of cake and it didn't blow the day."
Food Thoughts	"I can't stop thinking about sweets."	"Whenever I find myself thinking about food, I quickly change the topic to some other pleasant experience."
	"I had images of cakes and pies all afternoon—it must mean that I need sugar."	"If I see a magazine ad or commercial for food and I start thinking about it, I distract my attention by doing something else (phoning a friend, getting the mail, etc.)."
	"When we order food at a restaurant, I continue thinking about what I have ordered until it arrives."	

DAILY RECORD OF COGNITIVE RESTRUCTURING

Date: _____   Record of: _____

Description of Situation	Coping Thoughts Used	Positive Self-Statements Used	Date and Time

INDEX